Understanding

Hypermobile Ehlers-Danlos syndrome

and Hypermobility Spectrum Disorder

(previously known as Ehlers-Danlos syndrome hypermobility type & joint hypermobility syndrome, respectively).

by Claire Smith

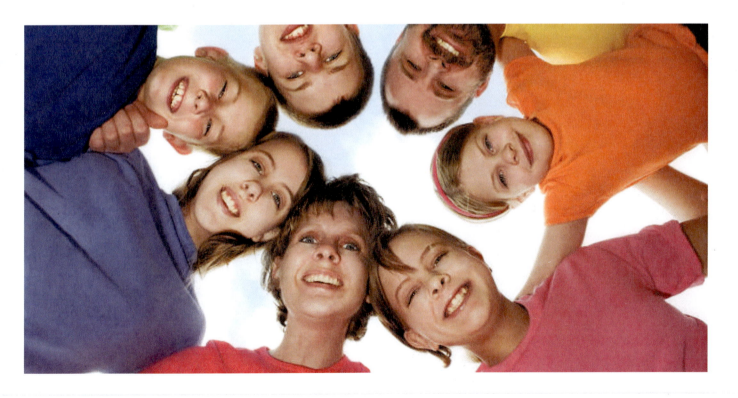

© Understanding hEDS and HSD by C. Smith

About the author

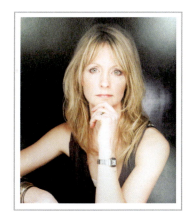

Claire Smith is Publications Editor & Partnership Director at the Hypermobility Syndromes Association (HMSA), a national charity supporting those with heritable disorders of connective tissue including Ehlers-Danlos syndrome, Marfan syndrome, Osteogenesis imperfecta and Stickler syndrome, and hypermobility spectrum disorders of all aetiologies.

On a daily basis, Claire works either in person, online or by telephone with individuals who have multi-systemic disorders. Many have struggled for years with lack of service provider knowledge, and find no clear treatment pathway available. Some describe medical treatment that has made them worse, not better, and most have received fragmented and single-body-system, rather than holistic, care; something which is not only detrimental to their physical and psychosocial wellbeing, but is also non-cost-effective for health care providers. They report feeling disbelieved and frustrated, and often lack confidence in the professionals they see. Inappropriate interventions and poor past experiences may have resulted in increased physical and mental stress and, in some cases, the understandable adoption of coping mechanisms that can sometimes become a barrier to further management. Claire works hard to provide reassurance and validation, advice and explanation. With this in mind, she has spent the past five years writing what she describes as *'the kind of book I would have liked to have been available when my own daughter was first diagnosed'*; clearly answering the questions to which people most want answers, and providing information on evidence based treatment and self-management. She hopes this book 'Understanding Hypermobile Ehlers-Danlos Syndrome and Hypermobility Spectrum Disorder' does just that.

Claire, who is herself affected by symptomatic hypermobility, is also a patient reviewer for the National Institute for Health Research, working to shape research and improve practice within the NHS and public health. Publications she has produced, on behalf of the HMSA, include 'Living Well With a Heritable Disorder of Connective Tissue', the biannual HMSA Journal, and the ever popular 'Educator's Guide to Hypermobile Students'. In her role as Partnership Director, Claire works collaboratively with charities such as Ehlers-Danlos Support UK and PoTS UK, establishing links and finding ways to share knowledge, skills and information, and has recently joined the expert patient panel as part of the EDS International Consortium. She works closely with the HMSA medical advisory board and trustees, and forms part of the team currently working alongside Dr Philip Bull, to set up a 'care web' model for patients with hypermobility related disorders; linking together a network of allied healthcare professionals keen to better support patients.

In her spare time (which she doesn't get a great deal of), Claire enjoys spending time with her family, laughing with friends, and taking her much loved Border Collie for long walks by the sea.

© Understanding hEDS and HSD by C. Smith

Preface

Both hypermobile Ehlers-Danlos syndrome (hEDS) and hypermobility spectrum disorder (HSD) can be very complex and daunting conditions.

Claire's approach to addressing this is methodical and thoughtful throughout, with great care given to the language used, and information provided. The result - a remarkably clear and concise text.

There is a wonderful balance to Claire's writing arising from her extensive experience as a writer and editor of patient information booklets and journals; her own health needs; being a carer herself; the exposure to, and the support of others with these conditions through her work with several charities, and the relationships she has developed world-wide with health and social care professionals in this field of Medicine.

Citing the literature and incorporating the reflections of patients and professional colleagues, Claire carefully guides us through the world of hEDS and HSD, dividing the book in to three chapters, each broken down into manageable sections, and flagging information through post-it notes along the way.

Claire takes us through the biology, classification, and diagnosis of hEDS and HSD, cutting through the medical language and bringing us right up to date with the latest knowledge of the associations between a variety of issues, their medical treatment, and ways to self-manage.

I commend this terrific book to anyone wishing to learn more about these conditions, the different concerns that can arise, the effects these can have on peoples' lives, and the modern methods of treatment.

This is very much a book for patients, carers, and health and social care colleagues alike.

By Alan Hakim MA PGCert-TM FRCP
Consultant in Rheumatology and Acute Medicine
Board member in Clinical Commissioning
Clinical Researcher & Author of Medical Texts
Chief Medical Advisor and Trustee to the Hypermobility Syndromes Association
Medical Advisor to Ehlers-Danlos Support UK
Member of the Medical and Scientific Board of the Ehlers-Danlos Society.

© Understanding hEDS and HSD by C. Smith

Acknowledgements

My grateful thanks to everyone who has helped me bring this book to fruition.

In particular, I would like to thank:

My husband and daughter for always believing in me and for putting up with me 'being absent' while I have been tucked away working on this book.

My wonderful family, for walking this road alongside us, and for your never ending love and support.

Dr Alan Hakim for his guidance and expertise in reviewing this entire book, and for his tireless work helping those affected by symptomatic hypermobility, including myself and my daughter.

Donna Wicks, CEO at the HMSA, for suggesting I write this book in the first place; for her friendship and unfailing support, and for her contributions to the self management section.

Dr Lesley Kavi for being the first to agree to review a section of my book, and for her much valued advice on autonomic dysfunction and postural orthostatic tachycardia syndrome.

Prof. Suranjith Seneviratne for his assistance in reviewing the section on mast cell activation syndrome and for boosting my confidence when I had moments of major self-doubt.

Dr Jessica Eccles for reviewing the section on anxiety

Dr Pradeep Chopra for reading and reviewing the sections on pain, complex regional pain syndrome and pain management.

Dr Phillip Bull for reviewing my chapter on diagnosis and management, and for his work in raising awareness of hypermobility related disorders amongst medical professionals.

Prof. Shea Palmer for reviewing the sections on physiotherapy, kinesiophobia, proprioception and 'why we are all affected so differently'.

The Hypermobility Syndromes Association (HMSA) for allowing me to quote text from their website, and for the support they have provided to our family - through them, I have learnt so much and made so many friends.

To Sarah Gurley-Green, for allowing me to use content from her letter to the Oxford Journals (2001). Reading that amazingly eloquent and accurate letter set me on my own journey to raise awareness.

To partner organisations and charities of the HMSA such as Ehlers-Danlos Support UK, Ehlers-Danlos Society, PoTSUK, EDS Wellness, Bindweefsel.be and many, many more worldwide, who work so hard to improve awareness and provide advice and support.

Benedikta Fones for her, much needed, proofreading skills.

Scott Ponton, Cathy Board, Emma Frith and Rebecca Karageorgopoulos for their valuable critique and assistance with proofreading.

Kendra Neilson Myles for her motivational guidance and invaluable advice on publishing.

To the colleagues, friends, and EDS community with whom I have shared my life. I cherish the close connections I share with the HMSA team, a group of wonderful volunteers who support those with hypermobility spectrum disorders, and heritable disorders of connective tissue.

Praise for this book

'You must publish this book Claire and as soon as possible. Do not let your self doubt stop you. I will be recommending your book to my patients - very well done.'
Prof Seneviratne, Director of the Centre for Mast Cell Disorders, and Consultant in Clinical Immunology and allergy, UCL

'Wow, this is incredibly helpful. I was diagnosed several years ago and I still didn't know about at least half of this. It explains SO much!'
Patient Reviewer

'Congratulations on writing a very comprehensive overview... I'm sure it will be a great success.'
Dr Lesley Kavi - Managing Trustee at PoTS UK

'Dear Claire, thank you for your noble initiative of writing this book!'
Dr Marco Castori - Clinical Genetics at the Division of Medical Genetics of the San Camillo-Forlanini Hospital in Rome

'Your wonderful book; it must and will be published.' Alan Hakim - Consultant in Rheumatology and Acute Medicine, and Chief Medical Advisor to the Hypermobility Syndromes Association

'This book is a 'must have' for anyone affected by HSD or hEDS (and the health care professionals caring for them). It clearly explains all the different aspects of these complex disorders, and also explains how each patient, and those supporting them, can best contribute towards treatment and management.'
Katie Allen, Patient Reviewer

'Happy to help in any way I can. I can see [the book] *has got the makings of a really useful publication.'*
Dr Philip Bull - Consultant Rheumatologist with a special interest in hypermobility spectrum disorder

'I am excited by the book concept - very much needed I think, good quality and accessible info.'
Emma Frith - Clinical Trial Manager, Oxford Brookes

'These sections [on physiotherapy and proprioception] *are really good and capture the main issues very well I think. This* [book] *seems like a fantastic venture and I am sure will be very helpful for patients and professionals alike. Best of luck with it and please let me know if you want any further help or advice.'*
Professor Shea Palmer, Professor of Musculoskeletal Rehabilitation, University of the West of England.

'Very well written, good job. I think it will help a lot of people. [I am] *delighted to help you on this wonderful project.'*
Dr Pradeep Chopra - Assistant Professor, Pain Medicine

© Understanding hEDS and HSD by C. Smith

© Understanding hEDS and HSD by C. Smith

Foreword

Our understanding of the complexities of hypermobile Ehlers-Danlos syndrome, and hypermobility spectrum disorder (previously known as Ehlers-Danlos syndrome hypermobile type, and joint hypermobility syndrome) has advanced significantly over the last 10 years, of that there is no doubt. Yet there is a lack of good quality publications covering the new information we have. Frequently, patients are expected to navigate a complex medical system and then manage more and more of their often complex care at home, so it is with great pleasure that I have read this book, which provides answers to the most frequently asked questions; describes signs, symptoms and co-morbidities, what to expect from clinical diagnosis, and management. If you are newly diagnosed; then this book tells you what you most need to know about the conditions. Professionals in health and social care will also benefit from reading this book; so as to gain a broader understanding of the complex issues surrounding what are multi-systemic conditions, and the impact on their patients on a day to day basis.

This book can be read cover to cover if the reader chooses. Alternatively, it could be effectively used as an encyclopaedic tool and relevant sections read when needed. Each bodily system is covered but, importantly, the book also focuses on how to live well with these conditions. Resources for readers have been added where possible, to allow further reading. I am pleased to note the section on anxiety based disorders, something which is often overlooked and yet must be managed successfully if a person is to progress to positive self-management.

One of the remarkable features of this book is the author's ability to provide insight and observations that help bridge the gap between the viewpoint of clinicians and that of their patients, helping them achieve effective communication and understanding. Communication barriers often go undetected in health care settings and can have serious effects on the health and safety of patients.

I would like to congratulate Claire – this book has been a 5 year project for her; it is extremely well written and great care has been taken to explain medical terms. Few people, regardless of experience, will read this book without having learned something. I recommend it without reservation to all of the hEDS/HSD community and those who support them.

Donna Wicks
CEO & Senior Medical Liaison Officer
Hypermobility Syndromes Association

Contents

Chapter 1 - Frequently asked questions   16

Introduction   17
Hypermobility   17
Heritable Disorders of Connective Tissue   18
Ehlers-Danlos syndrome   19
Hypermobile Ehlers-Danlos syndrome   20
Genetics and hypermobile Ehlers-Danlos syndrome   22
Joint hypermobility syndrome - where does it fit into the picture?   25
EDS Classification history   27
International Classification 2017   27
Introducing 'hypermobility spectrum disorder'   29
Concerns arising from the 2017 Classification   31
Why are people so differently affected?   33
Are hEDS or HSD progressive?   36

Chapter 2 - Symptoms & comorbidities   40

What are Symptoms, manifestations, syndromes and comorbidities   41

Part 1 - Widespread symptoms and comorbidities   44
   Joint hypermobility   45
   Recurrent musculoskeletal disorders   45
   Hyperextended alignment of joints   47
   Pain   48
   Complex regional pain syndrome   53
   Fatigue   55
   Proprioceptive dysfunction   57
   Muscle stiffness and tightness   59
   Habitual cracking of joints   60
   Frequent dislocations or subluxations   61
   Osteoarthritis   61
   Osteopenia   62
   Osteoporosis   62
   Skin involvement   63
   Local anaesthetic   65
   Anxiety   65
   Cardiovascular autonomic dysfunction   69
   Mast cell activation syndrome   77
   Raynaud's phenomenon and chilblains   81
   Fibromyalgia   82

Part 2 - Area specific symptoms and comorbidities   84
   Headaches   85
   Ocular features   85
   The nose and throat   86
   Asthma-like symptoms   86

Dental features	86
Chronic neck strain	87
The shoulders	88
The chest and ribs	89
The heart	90
The elbow	90
The wrist and hand	91
The spine	91
The bony pelvis	95
The hip	96
Gastrointestinal dysfunction	97
Rectal prolapse, and faecal incontinence	101
Contraception, pregnancy and childbirth	101
Urogynaecological symptoms	105
Male urinary tract dysfunction	110
Restless leg syndrome, and benign idiopathic nocturnal limb pains	111
Disorders of the knee	112
Disorders of the foot and ankle	113

Chapter 3 - Diagnosis and management of hEDS and HSD	116

Initial diagnosis by clinical assessment	118
A note to clinicians	118
Quick questions designed to assist GPs	119
Diagnostic criteria	120
2017 International Criteria for hypermobile Ehlers-Danlos syndrome	121
The Beighton Score to diagnose generalised joint hypermobility	122
Reaching a diagnosis	123
Summary of investigations and management of HSD and hEDS	126
The 2017 Classification Criteria for 8 of the 13 Ehlers-Danlos syndrome subtypes	127
What might a patient expect at a rheumatology clinical assessment	129
An overview of services who may be involved in patient care	132
Management strategy and multi-disciplinary referral	133
Why patients must be assessed on an individual basis	134
Physiotherapy	135
Occupational therapy	145
Joint protection	145
Splinting, bracing, taping, compression ware, and orthotics	146
Relief of severe pain, and using pain killers effectively	148
Self management	150
Cognitive behavioural therapy	156
Complementary and physical therapies	157
Making the most of your health care team	159
Dental management in hEDS and HSD	162
Surgical issues	165
Bibliography, and image attribution	166
Resources	184
EDS Types Chart	188

© Understanding hEDS and HSD by C. Smith

Chapter 1
Frequently asked questions

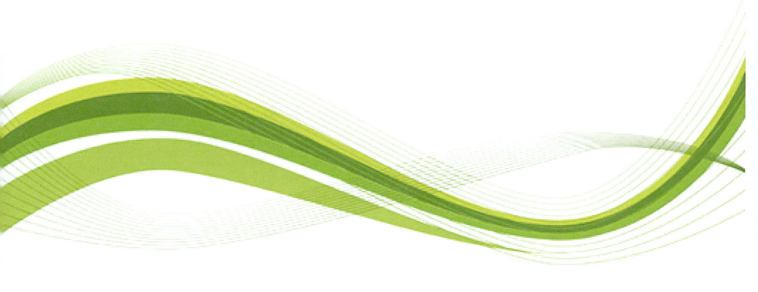

Introduction

If you have hypermobile Ehlers-Danlos syndrome, or hypermobility spectrum disorder, or you have an affected child or relative, please remember that, although it may sometimes feel like it, you are not alone; there are many people who are similarly affected and share the same concerns, and there are many strategies that can be put in place in order to help you to help yourself.

In 1597, Sir Francis Bacon wrote 'Knowledge is Power' and this phrase still holds true today.

The internet has unlocked almost unlimited medical information, providing an invaluable resource for researchers and healthcare professionals to learn from one another and from patients. Patient knowledge itself has flourished, with the internet providing a forum in which support groups can be built, stories swapped, treatments compared and information shared.

'Modern technology has allowed patients to find one another and be heard. A voice, previously unheard, gains strength in numbers...'
(Dr Heidi Collins MD 2011 at EDNF Educational Conference)

The concept of the 'expert patient' is, perhaps, nowhere better developed than in the hypermobile Ehlers-Danlos syndrome and hypermobility spectrum disorder community. However, trying to navigate the sheer volume of material available can lead to information overload, with some online sources lacking balance in their views, and many publications addressing the subject of Ehlers-Danlos syndrome as a whole rather than providing detailed information on each specific type.

Hypermobile Ehlers-Danlos syndrome (hEDS) and hypermobility spectrum disorder (HSD) are no longer seen as rare; hEDS is now considered the most prevalent type of heritable disorder of connective tissue in the world, thought to affect at least 1 in every 5000 people (Steinmann B. et al 2002), and the prevalence for association of generalised joint hypermobility and widespread pain is higher still (Mulvey M.R et al. 2013 / Hakim A.J. 2013e /Morris S.L. et al. 2016). This shift in understanding demands a different approach to information provision; one that is tailored specifically to those with hEDS and HSD, and provides a clear, concise and balanced overview - a book that allows you to 'see the woods from the trees'!

I hope that this book helps you to find answers to some of the questions and concerns you have, and that these answers leave you better informed and more able to navigate your way through the complexities of these conditions and their management. I have tried to communicate the content in a clear and concise manner, where possible avoiding the use of unnecessary, technical medical jargon that can be incomprehensible to many outside the medical profession. Questions relating to exercise, physiotherapy, surgery and the psychological effects of the disorder are discussed, as well as what to expect during clinical assessment, and much more. I am well aware, however, that not everything can be learnt from a book and that nothing can really replace the advice and help of an experienced and sympathetic doctor, physiotherapist, nurse or counsellor. Readers are urged to take appropriately qualified medical advice in all cases. The information in this book is intended to be useful to the general reader, but should not be used as a means of self-diagnosis, or for the prescription of medication.

Hypermobility

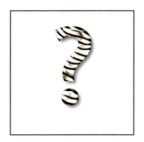

What is hypermobility?
Normally, the composition of connective tissue ensures ligaments are just tight enough, muscle tone just strong enough and the sockets just deep and well formed enough to ensure joints are stable and are restricted only to 'normal' ranges of motion. Such stability prevents joint injury. Variations in one or more of these structures, (e.g. connective tissue that is more easily stretched than usual, sockets that are shallow in formation, or muscle tone that is poor) can all result in a greater than average range of motion in the joint(s) being possible - this is described as 'joint hypermobility.' (Please see page 33 for more info on what causes people to be affected so differently).

Joint hypermobility is common in the general population. It is most common in childhood and adolescence, in females, and Asian and Afro-Caribbean races. For most people, it is just the way they are made; or has been developed through training for sports such as gymnastics or training for the performing arts. Indeed, where an athlete has as a certain degree of hypermobility, and is strong, active and fit, it may even be seen as an advantage (5/ HMSA 2014/ Tinkle B. et al 2017).

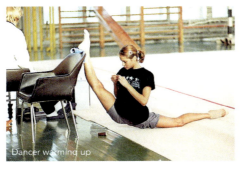
Dancer warming up

Hypermobility can occur in just a few joints or it may be widespread. For example, it is perfectly possible, and fairly common for people to only have hypermobile joints in the hands/feet (known as 'peripheral joint hypermobility'), or to inherit or acquire hypermobility in a single joint or body part (known as 'localised joint hypermobility'). Others may have body-wide joint hypermobility where most or all of their joints are affected. When hypermobility affects joints throughout the body, it is called 'generalised joint hypermobility.'

Regardless of how many joints are hypermobile, if the hypermobility gives rise to no symptoms it is described as 'asymptomatic' and is not considered a clinical disorder (Castori M. et al 2017).

Hypermobility itself is considered to be 'genetically influenced;' something which can be seen when studying family groups. However, this does not mean those who are hypermobile have an inherited disease. Instead, it is an inherited genetic trait(s) in the same way as an individual inherits the traits for eye colour, similar facial features or height. Some people with hypermobility are susceptible to injury and joint pain, others in the same family are not; it is not yet clear why this is the case.

For a small percentage of the population, symptomatic hypermobility can be a sign of more serious underlying disorders, although the levels of severity and the originating aetiology (causation) can differ significantly (HMSA 2014a)

Such disorders include:

- Heritable disorders of connective tissue
- Some chromosomal and neuro-developmental disorders
- Some skeletal dysplasias
- Some hereditary myopathies (diseases of the muscle) and congenital abnormalities
- Hypermobility spectrum disorders (see page 29)

(Voermans N.C. et al 2009, Donkervoort S. et al 2015, Bonafe L. et al 2015, Sugimoto J. et al 2000, Castori M. et al 2017).
(Photo attribution - irulandotnet 04.ShareAlike)

© Understanding hEDS and HSD by C. Smith

UNDERSTANDING

Over the following pages we will consider heritable disorders of the connective tissue in general and hypermobile Ehlers-Danlos syndrome in particular, the history of the disorder previously known as joint hypermobility syndrome, and hypermobility spectrum disorders in more detail.

Heritable disorders of connective tissue

What are heritable disorders of connective tissue?
Heritable disorders of connective tissue (HDCT) are conditions caused by changes to genes that build our connective tissues, which are passed down from parent to child.

There are more than 200 known HDCTs. Some affect how the tissues work within the body; others affect the joints, skin, bones, blood vessels, heart, lungs, ears and eyes. Many, but not all, HDCTs are rare.

What is the function of connective tissue?
Connective tissue performs many functions throughout our bodies. Fascia, which forms in sheets or bands beneath our skin, is made entirely of connective tissue; attaching, stabilising, enclosing, and separating muscles and other internal organs.

But connective tissue is responsible for a great deal more than that! It is also the major constituent of skin, bones, blood vessels, tendons and ligaments, and forms the extra-cellular matrix - that surrounds our cells, providing structural and biochemical support to the cells around it. In fact, the same proteins found in the extra cellular matrix are also found inside the cells of the body themselves; they give strength and form to each individual cell and allow them to function. Connective tissue is important to every aspect of life, so it is little wonder it can cause problems when it is defective!

What are the most common heritable disorders of connective tissue?
The most common heritable disorders of connective tissue that feature hypermobility include:

- Ehlers-Danlos syndrome
- Marfan syndrome
- Osteogenesis imperfecta

Continued...

- Stickler syndrome

Others include:
- Beals syndrome
- Loeys-Dietz syndrome
- Pseudoxanthoma Elasticum

What do these HDCTs have in common?
Alterations in the genetic make-up of those affected by an HDCT change the structure and development of many areas of the body made from the body's connective tissue proteins. At first glance the most common HDCTs appear to be very different diseases, with very different primary features i.e. marfanoid body-shape in Marfan syndrome; skin hyperextensibility and persistent pain in some forms of Ehlers-Danlos syndrome; and brittle bones and blue sclerae in osteogenesis imperfecta. However, they all share a broad commonality; the feature of 'hypermobility' - a range of movement in the joints that exceeds the norm, although the degree to which a person is hypermobile and how this affects them can vary enormously.

In fact, it is now recognised that these HDCTs can actually share more than 'just' hypermobility, and the so called 'cardinal features' are by no means uniquely linked to the disease with which they are most closely associated. Thus, stretchy skin (associated with some types of Ehlers-Danlos syndrome) also occurs in Marfan syndrome; the marfanoid body shape (associated with Marfan syndrome) is also seen in Ehlers-Danlos syndrome, as is osteoporosis (commonly associated with Osteogenesis imperfecta) (Grahame R. & Pyeritz R. 1995 / De Paepe A. 1996 / Dolan A. et al1998).

Ehlers-Danlos syndrome

What is Ehlers-Danlos syndrome?
Ehlers-Danlos syndrome (EDS) is a collection of heritable connective tissue disorders.

Either directly or indirectly, Ehlers-Danlos syndrome is thought to alter the biology of collagen in the body (the most abundant protein), which can lead to multi-systemic symptoms (1/Ehlers Danlos Society). EDS is described as genetically and clinically heterogeneous (Castori M. 2012 / Tinkle B. et al 2017). Heterogeneous means 'diverse or varied' referring to the fact that EDS can arise from one of a range of

mutations in one of a number of different genes associated with connective tissue. This means that, in the clinical setting, medical professionals see a widely varied pattern of signs and symptoms when they examine different patients with EDS.

Over the last 20 years, new variants of EDS have been identified and, as of 2017, thirteen different types have been formally recognised as follows:

- hypermobile Ehlers-Danlos syndrome (hEDS)
- Classical Ehlers-Danlos syndrome (cEDS)
- Classical-like Ehlers-Danlos syndrome (clEDS)
- Cardiac-valvular Ehlers-Danlos syndrome (cvEDS)
- Vascular Ehlers-Danlos syndrome (vEDS)
- Arthrochalasia Ehlers-Danlos syndrome (aEDS)
- Dermatosparaxis Ehlers-Danlos syndrome (dEDS)
- Kyphoscoliotic Ehlers-Danlos syndrome (kEDS)
- Brittle Cornea Ehlers-Danlos syndrome (BCS)
- Spondylodysplastic Ehlers-Danlos syndrome (spEDS)
- Musculocontractural Ehlers-Danlos syndrome (mcEDS)
- Myopathic Ehlers-Danlos syndrome (mEDS)
- Periodontal Ehlers-Danlos syndrome (pEDS)

Each of the types has certain physical traits, but there are also physical characteristics that are common to all types of Ehlers-Danlos syndrome, including hypermobile joints and differing levels of skin involvement (1/ Ehlers Danlos Society). It is highly improbable to have more than one type of Ehlers-Danlos syndrome, but as they have features and 'biology' in common, each type may appear to have variable features of other types (1/ Ehlers-Danlos Society). The 2017 international criteria for Ehlers-Danlos syndrome subtypes can be found in Chapter 3, p.127.

Which connective tissue protein is affected in those with Ehlers-Danlos syndrome?
Each heritable disorder of connective tissue is caused by a mutation, or multiple mutations, in the genes that encode the connective tissue proteins, such as collagen, elastin and fibrillin. For example, those with Marfan syndrome have a genetic mutation in the connective tissue protein, fibrillin.

Mutations in the various genes associated with EDS disrupt the production or processing of the connective tissue protein, collagen.

Geneticists have successfully identified the genes for many of the EDS sub types (see Chapter 3, page 126), but the underlying genetic causes for the biosynthesis of collagen in the most common form, hEDS, have yet to be definitively identified.

UNDERSTANDING

Hypermobile Ehlers-Danlos syndrome

Hypermobile Ehlers-Danlos syndrome (hEDS) is the newly defined term for the heritable disorder of connective tissue that has, until recently, been known synonymously as 'Ehlers-Danlos hypermobility type' and 'joint hypermobility syndrome'.

Important Note: For information relating to the history of joint hypermobility syndrome and its relevance to hEDS please see page 25, **Box 3.**

How is hypermobile Ehlers-Danlos syndrome defined?

Hypermobile Ehlers-Danlos syndrome (hEDS) is considered the most prevalent type of inherited genetic disorder of connective tissue in the world (Tinkle B. et al 2017) although the causational gene(s) has yet to be identified. It is defined by the association of generalised joint hypermobility, joint instability complications, widespread musculoskeletal pain, (minor) skin features and/or pelvic / rectal / uterine dysfunction, (Beighton P. 1998 / Castori M. 2012 / Castori M. et al 2017) and is now widely recognised as being associated with the potential to affect multiple systems of the body including the cardiovascular autonomic system (Hakim A et al 2017a), the gastrointestinal system (Fikree A. et al 2017) and mast cell activation (Seneviratne S. et al 2017). More in-depth information on associated conditions can be found in Chapter 2.

How do the effects of defective collagen manifest themselves as symptoms in hEDS?

The most commonly recognised symptom is hypermobility of the joints. In hEDS a person's joints are lax because they have inherited looser and stretchier connective tissues. Hypermobile people can easily injure soft tissues around joints because their joints can twist or over-extend easily. This reduced stability in the joints can lead to symptoms such as:

- Ligament sprains and pulled tendons
- Joint subluxations and dislocations; vertebral listhesis
- Tendon tears
- Disc prolapse and chronic pain
- Skin that may stretch, scar or bruise more easily

Of course, these injuries can happen to anyone, but they occur far more easily and more frequently in those who are hypermobile (1/ HMSA 2014).

What is the primary function of collagen proteins in the connective tissue?

Collagen is a major structural protein of the types of connective tissue found in the tough inner layer of the skin (the dermis), the tendons, the ligaments, the blood vessels, and in/around internal organs such as the bladder, bowel and pelvic organs. Collagen gives structure to the connective tissue, allowing it to resist deformation, give strength to the skin and have sufficient strength for tendons to attach muscles to bones. It allows ligaments to hold the many bones of a joint in position, and the internal organs to be protected and supported.

(Information on the manifestations (signs and symptoms) that result from the connective tissue variant seen in hEDS are discussed over the following pages and in Chapter 2).

> 'Connective tissue is something of an orphan child in medicine: although it is an integral part of the musculoskeletal system, connective tissue is basically absent from orthopaedic textbooks, which deal principally with bones, cartilage, and muscles. Orthopaedic interest is almost exclusively restricted to the "specialised" connective tissues such as tendons and ligaments, which connect bone to muscles and to other bones, respectively. Non-specialised connective tissues, which form what's known as the fasciae and envelop all muscles, nerves, bones, and blood vessels, are typically allotted a short paragraph in current textbooks, if mentioned at all.' (Langevin H.M. 2013)

What effect does this collagen defect, involved in EDS, have on the body's connective tissue?

Alteration in a collagen gene itself can result in the body producing connective tissue which is abnormal. A similar outcome can also be seen when there is an alteration in the genes that code for *the proteins* that are responsible for the collagen building blocks, or are responsible for assembling those building blocks into collagen fibres. Either way, the end result is collagen fibres, throughout the body, that lack the stiffness and strength required, that are too elastic, or that break too easily.

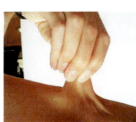

Mildly stretchy skin - individual with hEDS underlying connective tissue variant

© Understanding hEDS and HSD by C. Smith

Are there other signs and symptoms:

Aside from joint problems, the following are also commonly seen in those with hEDS, arising either as direct complications of hEDS or as associated disorders. (A person may have any combination of the conditions listed or, indeed, may never develop these problems):

- Persistent (chronic) fatigue.
- Acute (short-term) pain.
- Persistent pain (day in, day out), which is often widespread, and neuropathic pain can also arise.
- Poor proprioception (knowing where parts of one's body are in space) increase risk of injury.
- Reduced response to local anaesthetic (e.g., injections for dental work, minor surgery, or epidurals).
- Functional gastrointestinal disorders, which may include a sluggish bowel with bloating, pain and altered bowel habit.
- Bladder over-activity and pelvic floor weakness.
- Asthma-like symptoms.
- Cardiovascular autonomic dysfunction, which may include: heart palpitations and/or feeling faint.
- Anxiety, phobic states and depression.
- Reduced mobility.
- Earlier than 'normal' onset of osteoarthritis.
- Tethered cord and chiari malformation.
- Mast cell activation syndrome.

(Ref: 1/ HMSA 2014 & 2017 / Tinkle B. et al 2017 / Castori M. et al 2017 / Henderson Sr. F.C. et al 2017)

(Additional observations are shown in **Box 1.** More in-depth information on signs and symptoms can be found in Chapter 2).

The associated disorders (comorbidities) affect people in different ways, but in many cases are even more debilitating than the more commonly recognised musculoskeletal symptoms; they seriously affect quality of life and need to be properly managed as part of holistic treatment.

More in-depth information on signs, symptoms and

Definitions for the terms:
- symptom,
- manifestation,
- syndrome
- comorbidity,

are provided on page 41.

comorbidities of hypermobile Ehlers-Danlos syndrome and its management can be found in Chapters 2 & 3. The 2017 International Classification diagnostic criteria for hypermobility hypermobile Ehlers-Danlos syndrome can be found in Chapter 3, page 121.

Box 1.

Additional observations:

Injuries may cause immediate 'acute' pain and can also lead to longer-term 'persistent pain', which can be severe and widespread. Whilst the majority of hypermobile people do recover from an injury (though this may be slower than normal), others only partially recover, or continue to repeatedly injure various parts of their body.

Experts, such as Dr Clair Francomano, propose that structural defects in the body's connective tissue proteins allow micro-traumas, which are often not visible on tests such as MRIs, to occur repeatedly in the same area of connective tissue without completely healing (Francomano C. 2011).

The skin and internal organs may be affected, as connective tissue is found in all areas of the body. For some, this can cause additional problems involving the gastrointestinal system, the autonomic nervous system and bladder function.

Severe fatigue that persists despite management, rest or a proper nights sleep, is another common symptom for those with hEDS. In addition, early muscle fatigue may be caused by muscles having to work hard to stabilise joints. Fatigue in hEDS can also easily be confused with a condition called chronic fatigue syndrome. It is important that the right diagnosis is made, as the approach to treatment such as physiotherapy and occupational therapy may be different.

The severity of symptoms, the joints that are affected and the level of pain / fatigue, experienced by those with hEDS/HSD, can vary greatly from day to day, or even hour to hour. These symptoms can interfere with daily activities of living, and/or schooling or work. The associated pain can become widespread and persistent, and might initially be diagnosed as, or confused with, another condition called fibromyalgia.

(Additional observations above: Francomano C. 2011; 3/ HMSA 2014 - Hakim A, Wicks D, Smith C.)

© Understanding hEDS and HSD by C. Smith

Genetics and hEDS

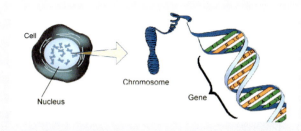

Terminology guide

In humans, most cells have 23 pairs of chromosomes of which 22 carry general genetic information, and 1 pair carry information about gender (called the sex chromosomes). One chromosome is inherited from each parent to make up each pair.

Each chromosome is made of huge amounts of DNA that is highly organised into structures that are called genes. Genes are the unique instructions which make us each individual. There are many thousands of genes, each carrying a different instruction. In decoding the information held on genes, the body is able to make all the chemicals and structures the body needs to function.

Every person has two copies of each gene; one copy of each pair is inherited from our mother, in the egg, and the other from our father, in the sperm. The copies sit side by side, one on each chromosome in a pair of chromosomes. Alleles are forms of the same gene but which have small differences in their structure between people. This is what gives each person their unique physical features, for example. Also, one copy of the gene pair may contain information that leads it to be expressed 'in favour of' or over-riding anything being expressed by its partner gene - this is called 'dominance'.

As discussed on pages 19 & 20, the features of hEDS suggest that there is a problem with connective tissues and possibly collagen, likely stemming from an alteration in a gene, or several genes, containing the instructions for making connective tissue (10/EDS Support UK). In a tiny minority of cases the genetic factors involved have been identified in families but, in the vast majority of cases, the exact cause(s) of hEDS is, as yet, unknown. Diagnosis of hEDS must therefore be made on 'clinical features' (signs and symptoms that can be assessed by a physician) as there are no laboratory tests available to confirm the diagnosis.

HEDS has traditionally been described using a 'classic' or 'simple genetics' model, where a parent passes a gene or trait to their children by one single genetic mutation. The clinical spectrum of hEDS is, however, so diverse in character that explaining it simply in terms of 'a single collagen gene mutation' is possibly an over simplification. Indeed, the causation of the wide range of manifestations seen in the whole spectrum spanning from joint hypermobility, through hypermobility spectrum disorders and hEDS is likely to be far more complex than that.

Over coming years, many genetic subtypes are likely to be discovered within the hEDS spectrum and, rather than being considered one single disorder, hEDS itself will likely be broken down into multiple subtypes, forming a 'family of disorders' resulting from differing gene mutations or combinations of gene mutations, the expression of which may be influenced by multiple factors including environmental and constitutional factors. More information on the multiple factors that can influence hypermobility can also be found on page 33 'Why are people so differently affected.'

Patterns of genetic inheritance in hEDS

Hypermobile Ehlers-Danlos syndrome appears to be passed on by various patterns of inheritance. In many families hEDS appears to follow a pattern called autosomal dominant inheritance; in others hEDS appears to be passed on in an autosomal recessive or De Novo gene mutation pattern (see explanations below).

<u>What does autosomal mean?</u>
Autosomal means a trait(s) can be passed on by both females and males, and can affect both female and male offspring. Many studies now point out that, in the adult hEDS population many more females are affected than males. The reason for this bias is not yet fully understood, but it is believed to relate to the greater influence of female sex hormones on hypermobility (Wolf J.M. 2009 / Shultz S.J. et al 2012 / Boyan B.D. et al 2013). More information on hormones and hypermobility can be found in 'Biological Sex' on page 35.

Autosomal dominant inheritance
The term 'dominant' is used when an abnormal gene from one parent causes disease even if the matching gene from the other parent is normal i.e. the abnormal gene dominates.

In an autosomal dominant inheritance pattern, if someone with hEDS has a child they will pass on one copy of the gene associated with hEDS to their child, either the altered or unaltered copy. Therefore, in each pregnancy there is a 50% (1 in 2) chance of a child inheriting the altered copy of the gene. Equally there is a 50% (1 in 2) chance of a child getting the unaltered copy of the gene and not inheriting the condition (10/EDS Support UK) (See **Box 2**, 1a).

Although it is only necessary for *one* parent to contribute the autosomal dominant gene mutation in order for the child to inherit the condition, if *both* parents are affected their child could inherit a copy of the defective gene from each parent (see **Box 2**, 1b). In this instance, the condition may be more severe (Pauker S.P. et al 2014). This could be due to each

Inheritance patterns of hEDS

1) Autosomal dominant inheritance
Only one copy of a disease allele is necessary for an individual to be susceptible to expressing the trait.

a) If only one parent has the dominant gene then, with each pregnancy:

- there is a 50% chance that the child will inherit the disease allele and express the phenotype to some degree*.
- there is a 50% chance the child will inherit no copies of the disease allele and will not express the phenotype or be a carrier.

b) If, however, *both* parents have one dominant gene then, the chance of the child inheriting the disease allele increases. With each pregnancy:

- there is a 75% chance that the child will inherit the disease allele and express the phenotype to some degree*.
- there is a 25% chance with each pregnancy of having a child unaffected by the disorder.

2) Autosomal recessive
Two copies of a disease allele are required for an individual to be susceptible to expressing the trait. Usually, the parents of an affected individual are not affected but are, instead, gene carriers.

a) With each pregnancy of carrier parents:

- there is a 25% chance the child will inherit two copies of the disease allele and will therefore express the phenotype to some degree*.
- there is a 50% chance the child will inherit one copy of the disease allele and will be a carrier.
- there is a 25% chance the child will inherit no copies of the disease allele and will not express the trait or be a carrier.

Box 2.

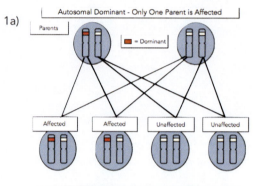

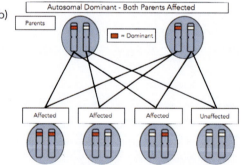

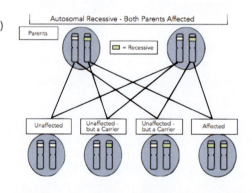

* Please also see 'Biological Sex' on page 35.
  Please also note - In the 'Genes and Inheritance' section of www.hypermobility.org, Dr Alan Hakim offers reassurance to those with hEDS who are thinking of starting a family, explaining that, if a child does appear to have inherited hypermobility, this may still turn out to be of no medical consequence at all. Even infants and toddlers without the hypermobility gene are naturally flexible/hypermobile and this may or may not lessen as the child grows. He suggests the most practical thing to do is to be alert to the fact that the child is hypermobile and, if they seem to be developing problems (for example: delay in their 'developmental milestones;' crawling, walking, clumsiness, joint pains, perhaps poor hand-writing skills at school, bruising or scarring easily), then ask a doctor whether the presence of hypermobility might be related to, or causing, the problem'.

© Understanding hEDS and HSD by C. Smith

parent passing on a different set of characteristics (see page 34, **Box 5**) thus compounding the effect on the child (Murray K & Woo P. 2001).

Autosomal Recessive

In autosomal recessive inheritance, two parents who are both 'carriers' of the recessive gene, and show no signs and symptoms of the disorder themselves, would, *each*, have to pass on a copy of their recessive gene mutation in order for the child to inherit the condition. If only one parent passes on a recessive gene mutation, and the other parent passes on an unaffected gene, then the child would not display characteristics, but would instead be a '*carrier*' of the disorder (see **Box 2, 2a**).

De Novo gene mutation

It should be noted that it is also possible for a child to be born with EDS as a result of a 'de novo gene mutation' (Levy H.P. 2004). This means that an alteration in a gene(s) is present for the first time in one family member (there may be no previously affected family members). This can be as a result of a mutation in a germ cell in the egg or sperm of one of the parents, or by a mutation in a germ cell in the fertilized egg itself. The proportion of EDS cases caused by De Novo mutations is unknown.

Complete or incomplete penetrance?

If a genetic disorder is described as having 'complete penetrance' it means that the percentage of people with the gene mutation, who then go on to exhibit some signs and symptoms of the disorder, would be 100%.

In disorders where some people with a genetic mutation do *not* develop signs and symptoms of the disorder, the condition would then be said to have incomplete or, in some cases, variable penetrance.' In hEDS penetrance is believed by many to be variable.

Variable expressivity

Some genetic disorders exhibit little variation, but most have signs and symptoms that differ among the individuals affected. This variation in signs and symptoms is called 'variable expressivity' (1/ghr.nlm.nih.gov).

HEDS is described as having variable expressivity (Castori M. 2012/ Syx D. et al 2015), referring to the range of signs and symptoms that can occur in different people with the same genetic condition. In hEDS, the observable features vary widely, both in terms of the severity of the joint hypermobility itself and also the

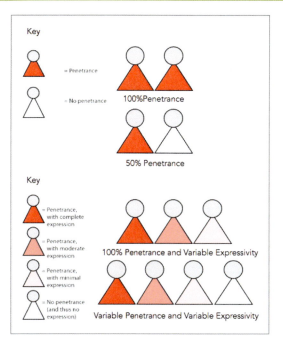

range and severity of associated symptoms such as gastrointestinal dysfunction, easy bruising and other skin signs (Bird H. 2007) - some people have only mild signs and symptoms, while others have signs and symptoms that are far more complex and debilitating (Hakim A. J. 2013c). Even within the same family, it is common to see members who develop a variety of signs and symptoms that are complex and debilitating, whilst other hypermobile members of the same family may be only mildly affected or have no problems at all (Hakim A. J. 2013c).

The future

There is a great deal of work to be done before complete genetic analysis of EDS can become routine. However, many of the tools needed to achieve the work now exist and, slowly, progress is being made. It is hoped that the creation of an international registry for Ehlers-Danlos syndrome will help accelerate research and, in the future, lead to the discovery of the genetic mutations involved in the wide range of manifestations seen in the spectrum of hEDS. More information on the proposed registry can be found on page 29.

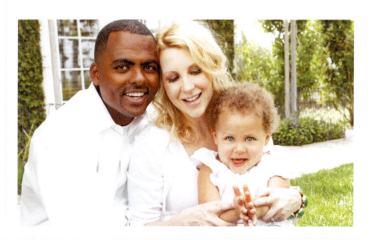

Box 3.

Joint hypermobility syndrome - where does it fit into the picture?

Around 20 years ago, two different medical specialities identified characteristics of, what are now considered by many experts to be, different parts of the same disorder. Experts in rheumatology identified the set of musculoskeletal characteristics they observed, as '(benign) joint hypermobility syndrome.' At the same time, experts in genetics, seeing the wider genetic multi-systemic manifestations, were re-defining what is now seen as a continuum of the same condition - Ehlers-Danlos syndrome hypermobility type (the old name for hEDS) (Grahame R. 2012c). The connection between the two disorders was not made at the time, and different diagnostic criteria that shared many of the same indicators were created. For many years, (benign) joint hypermobility syndrome (JHS) has been the medical diagnosis given to those with symptomatic hypermobility that was considered to have mainly rheumatological signs and symptoms, predominantly affecting the musculoskeletal system.

While it is true that its predominant clinical characteristics *do* typically affect joints, over the years, clinical evidence has led experts to believe that in many cases, the condition (that until recently has been known as JHS) actually involves, or sits on the periphery of, a much wider spectrum with several features corresponding with the criteria for hypermobile Ehlers-Danlos syndrome.

Writing on this subject in 2012, Marco Castori explained that, because of the advancement in research and understanding, clinical research on JHS was gradually moving from rheumatology (the study of disorders of the joints, muscles and ligaments), towards clinical genetics (the study of heredity and the variation of inherited characteristics). Varicose veins, rectal and uterine prolapses, recurrent urinary tract infections and myopia were all beginning to be recognised as being more common in patients with JHS, indicating a widespread anomaly in the structure of connective tissue rather than a limited involvement of the musculoskeletal system as previously thought (Soyucen E.& Esen F.-2010).

Research by Trinh Hermanns-Le et al (2012) also led to the increased recognition of JHS sharing the same spectrum as hEDS. The team carried out research into the fine structure of the dermal layer of the skin in those diagnosed with JHS, hEDS, and controls. Their findings showed key changes in collagen fibrils of those with JHS and hEDS. Using an electron microscope, they were able to see that, rather than having 'normal' round collagen fibrils of uniform size and spacing (see **1A**), those with a diagnosis of JHS or hEDS had irregularly spaced collagen fibrils, some of which looked smaller and some of which looked 'flower-like' in shape (see **1B**). They also found alterations in the elastic fibres of the collagen. The study concluded: '*We support the concept that JHS represents a mild variant of Ehlers-Danlos hypermobile type*' (Hermanns-Le T. et al 2007 & 2012a). Other changes to the dermal layer of those with hEDS include granular thread-like deposits and the presence of large rosette shaped hyaluronic acid-like globules (Pierard G.E. et al 1998).

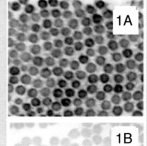
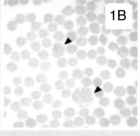

In recent years, several proposals have been put forward as ways to try to distinguish the differences between JHS and hEDS. At one stage, it was thought that the 'normal' skin in those with JHS, compared with the mildly stretchy skin found in those with hEDS, could be used to differentiate between the two, but experts such as Prof. Rodney Grahame no longer believe that this distinction is absolute.

Others had tried to separate JHS from hEDS by pointing to findings laid out in reports by Arendt-Nielsen L. in 1990 and 1991 (whereby researchers found that those with hEDS did not receive the full benefit of local anaesthetic, and therefore stood apart from those with JHS). It has since become clear that some patients with JHS also experience problems with anaesthetic and, according to one large survey, were three times more likely to report the poor effectiveness of local anaesthetic compared to people without JHS (Hakim A.J & Grahame R. 2003 & Hakim A. J. et al 2005).

On this subject, Rodney Grahame wrote:

'Unfortunately, the criteria for selection in the study (by Arendt-Nielsen) were not documented clearly. In particular, it is not clear how the patients with Ehlers-Danlos syndrome type III (hEDS) were distinguished from the hypermobility patients. In the intervening seven years this work has neither been confirmed nor refuted. Were it to be repeated, this time with rigorous attention to clinical selection, it could, perhaps, carry the key to the solution...'

As research and understanding has increased, experts in heritable disorders of connective tissue, such as consultant rheumatologists, Professor Rodney Grahame and Dr Alan Hakim, and chartered physiotherapist, Rosemary Keer, have led the way in raising awareness of JHS as a pathological entity similar to, or the same as, hEDS, potentially forming part of the existing family of conditions known as heritable disorders of connective tissue

'It (JHS) is not a trivial articular problem occurring in healthy individuals, it is now recognised as a multi-systemic disorder and a major source of chronic widespread pain, dysautonomias, and gastrointestinal dysmotility. It is a neglected area within rheumatology' (Fikree A. et al 2013).

So, why has so much confusion continued to exist within the medical community regarding JHS/hEDS?

Despite many papers having now been published by leading professionals, explaining that the disorders formerly known as hEDS/JHS are both considered multi-systemic, 'overlapping' conditions, for many years the message failed to get through.

Doctors who graduated medical school some years ago may be out of touch with current thinking in respect to hEDS/JHS, relying instead on information provided during their original training; much of which would be considered out-dated by today's experts in the field. At best, these practitioners may have a vague memory of being shown pictures of a patient with one of the rarer forms of Ehlers-Danlos syndrome during their training, one who could perhaps stretch their skin out like elastic on either side of the neck or bend themselves into extreme contorted shapes. The patient they see in front of them in their surgery, complaining of pain, fatigue, gastrointestinal issues or other body-wide manifestations does not 'fit the picture' they have of hEDS/JHS. Even in today's media it is often only the most extreme cases of EDS that are featured. This reinforces the belief that that *all* types of Ehlers-Danlos syndrome are extremely rare, and many healthcare professionals think they are unlikely to see a case in their lifetime.

Names originally allocated, such as 'benign joint hypermobility syndrome (BJHS), have further increased misunderstanding within the medical community. The name 'joint' hypermobility syndrome may give the impression that only the joints are affected, when, in a significant amount of cases, many other areas of the body that involve collagen/connective tissue are affected, including blood vessels and skin. The name 'benign' joint hypermobility only serves to confuse people even further, implying that the condition causes no other problems. The word 'benign' is, after all, most commonly used to explain that a lump, you thought might be serious is, in fact, nothing to worry about and needs no treatment. Patients who experience what can be persistent, debilitating and, in some cases disabling manifestations may, understandably, not feel 'benign' is an accurate description of their condition but, instead trivialises it in the mind of the medical practitioner.

Where do things stand now?

To date, the decision of whether to diagnose hEDS or JHS, and the interpretation of the diagnostic criteria used, has been left to a medical professional's personal preference or belief, which may well be influenced by whether they come from a rheumatological or genetics background. Many have simply chosen to use the terminology with which they are most familiar.

In March 2017, however, the International Consortium on Ehlers-Danlos Syndrome, proposed a new unified classification; one that, where specific

...continued

criteria are met, formally recognises the hypermobile type of EDS and joint hypermobility syndrome as being indistinguishable from each other (please see 'A unified set of diagnostic criteria is presented', Page 28) (Tinkle B. et al 2017).

The new terminology proposed in the classification and its implications for both new patients and those with an existing diagnosis are discussed over the next few pages. The related diagnostic criteria mentioned above, can be found in Chapter 3, pages 121-122).

EDS Classification history

What do we mean by classification?

The classification of medical diagnoses (also known as nosology) is a core group of well-integrated, up-to-date, clinical terminologies, put together by a group of experts in order to serve as a backbone of clinical information about a particular disorder or group of disorders.

A classification helps to provide a compilation of internationally consistent data to which healthcare professionals can refer, and can also be used to facilitate the comparison of health-related data within and across populations over periods of time.

All classifications have their limitations however, and it is often impossible to make the features of a disorder sit perfectly within individual boxes. In the case of Ehlers-Danlos syndrome, this is certainly true - there is still so much be to be learnt, and a great deal of overlap is observed among the phenotypes, sometimes making absolute clinical diagnosis of one particular 'type' difficult (Kakadia N. et al 2011 / Grahame R. 1999).

Although no single classification document is likely to have the depth and breadth required to represent the spectrum of features seen in Ehlers-Danlos syndrome, the creation of a medical classification does go some way to providing a 'broad description' of features for each type.'

Classification history of Ehlers-Danlos syndrome

Categorisation of the Ehlers-Danlos syndrome first began in the late 1960s. Some twenty years later, the first formal classification took place in Berlin and has subsequently been updated twice. The history of these classifications is provided below:

Berlin Classification

Following the identification of specific mutations in the genes encoding collagen types I, III, and V, as well as several collagen-processing enzymes, a meeting was held by the branch of medical science who deal with the classification of diseases (Berlin 1986) and a proposal was put forward to formalise a properly defined system of names, terms and features that would allow medical professionals to more easily distinguish between the main types of Ehlers-Danlos syndrome. This classification was published by Beighton et al., in 1988, describing a narrowed EDS classification of six distinct clinical syndromes, with emphasis placed on the molecular basis of each form.

Villefranche Classification

During the following decade, research into the biomechanical and molecular basis of EDS moved on sufficiently to enable experts to clarify the types of EDS further and, in 1997, experts met again (in Villefranche) to update the previous classifications. This time, they based the classification on the 'cause' of each type of EDS, and set out the major and minor criteria for each, along with, wherever possible, any laboratory findings.

In 2017, the Villefranche Classification was superseded by the 'International Classification 2017.' Below we will look at this in more detail:

International Classification 2017

Since the Villefranche Classification, many rarer types of EDS have been identified, and the clinical description of some types in medical literature have expanded considerably. The clinical description of the hypermobile type of EDS in particular has grown extensively, now encompassing features such as persistent pain, persistent fatigue, cardiovascular autonomic dysfunction and anxiety amongst other associated symptoms (Castori M. et al 2017).

'...a lot of knowledge (has been) gained since the 1997 Villefranche Criteria and an expanded classification was needed to reflect new information about the genetics and clinical manifestations of the syndromes. The 1997 criteria offered a general description of what these were but they remained open to interpretation which

UNDERSTANDING

has not been helpful. ... patients are not being managed and quality of life is not what it could be because of the lack of credibility associated with EDS.' (3/Ehlers-Danlos Society)

With this in mind, in 2012 an initiative to found the 'International Consortium of Experts on Ehlers–Danlos Syndromes' was set in motion by a group of world leading experts, with the aim of updating the classification and diagnostic criteria for the hypermobile form of EDS, along with all other existing and newly defined subtypes.

In 2016, the Ehlers-Danlos Society, with support from EDS Support UK and Ehlers-Danlos National Foundation, facilitated this initiative to come to fruition and, in May 2016, a group of around 250 world renowned experts met in New York with the primary goal of redefining the diagnostic criteria for all the types of Ehlers-Danlos syndrome, and developing best practice clinical guidelines for diagnosis and management.

During this process, a systematic review of available data relating to all the symptoms and conditions that arise either as direct complications of hEDS or which might have direct associations with hEDS was carried out. This, combined with clinical experience accumulated by participating experts such as Castori, Hakim, Seneviratne, Francomano, Malfait, Tinkle, Chopra, Levy et al, as well as many 'patient experts', depicted the hypermobile type of Ehlers-Danlos syndrome (known synonymously as joint hypermobility syndrome), as being a more complex clinical picture than had previously been described in preceding classifications, with *'reverberations in practically all organs and systems.'*

A unified set of diagnostic criteria is presented

In March 2017, the International Consortium on Ehlers-Danlos syndrome, formally recognised the hypermobile type of EDS and joint hypermobility syndrome as being part of the same clinical spectrum (Castori. M et al 2010 / Tinkle B. et al 2017). They proposed a new, unified set of diagnostic criteria, designed to enable more precise diagnosis and lead to better treatment for patients (3 Ehlers-Danlos Society 2017). The Consortium advised that where this criteria is met by new patients, or by patients with an existing diagnosis of EDS-H/hEDS/BJHS/JHS who are being re-evaluated, (and where all other differential diagnoses have been considered and excluded), the term 'hypermobile Ehlers-Danlos syndrome (hEDS) be used (Tinkle B. et al 2017).

These new hEDS criteria, which can be found in Chapter 3 (page 121), are clearer and stricter than those formulated within the old Villefranche classification and the Brighton criteria and evidence of a 'syndrome' being present is emphasized - i.e. a group of symptoms consistently occurring together (Castori M. et al 2017). The criteria is intended to define a more uniform set of observable characteristics shared among patients, and to more accurately reflect the original description of the disorder within the Classification (Castori M. et al 2017 / Tinkle B. et al 2017).

'In being more clear about the diagnosis and how it is made in individuals, we are better able to draw together groups of people with similar aspects to their condition, and undertake studies that look at the cause of the condition and the response to treatment. We have been consistent with other areas in medicine in aiming to better

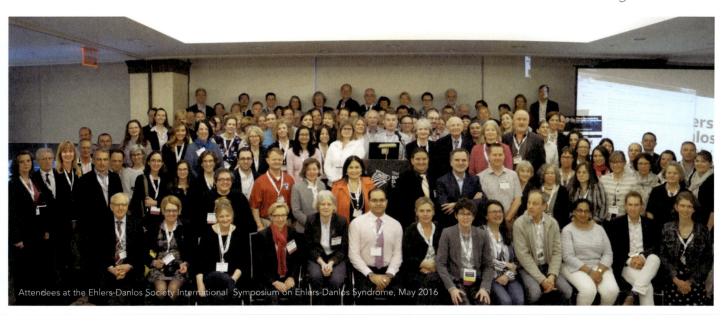

Attendees at the Ehlers-Danlos Society International Symposium on Ehlers-Danlos Syndrome, May 2016

define subgroups of people with similar concerns.' (3/Ehlers-Danlos Society 2017)

Associated disorders - the disparity between what we 'know' and what we can actually *prove* at this time

Whilst many advances in classification were undoubtably made, and an *'association'* with hEDS and a number of disorders was evidenced both through clinical experience and the systemic review of available literature, insufficient research currently exists to prove that these disorders are *directly caused* by having hEDS. Also, for a number of them it has not yet been shown exactly how common they are in the whole hEDS population compared to the general population, or other groups of people with chronic medical conditions (6/HMSA 2017). More funding and research is urgently required in order to evidence beyond doubt the multi-system manifestations that experts are recognising daily in their patient clinics, i.e there is a significant difference between what we *'know'* and what can actually be *proved*.

This disparity means that, for now at least, some disorders, which many had hoped to see included, will not form part of the criteria for hEDS, although their *'significant association'* is recognised in the classification papers, which are to be reviewed every two years and updated where necessary. These disorders include, but are not limited to:

- Functional gastrointestinal disorders
- Cardiovascular autonomic dysfunction (including postural orthostatic tachycardia)
- Sleep disturbance
- Fatigue
- Anxiety and depression
- Tethered cord and chiari malformation
- Mast cell activation syndrome

'All the evidence and expert opinion was gathered to determine whether any of these features (e.g. fatigue, cardiovascular autonomic dysfunction, bowel pain, etc.) might form part of the criteria. At present there is insufficient evidence to add these to the criteria, but we recognise that they are present in some people with EDS and that health care professionals should be looking for them.'
(3/ Ehlers-Danlos Society 2017)

Details of symptoms and manifestations that are included in the six most common types of EDS, including hEDS, are shown in Chapter 2, page 42, **Box 1**.

Highlighting the 'gaps' in research data is a small step forward in itself, as it assists researchers to target specific areas of interest/uncertainty. The evidence based signs and symptoms included in the classification will ensure an enhanced level of credibility and understanding of hEDS going forward, and enable progress to be made in research and management (3/Ehlers-Danlos Society).

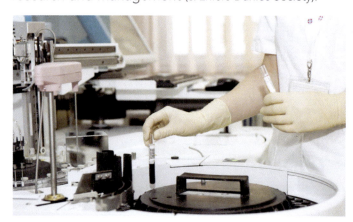

The need for an International EDS Registry

At the time of writing, the Ehlers-Danlos Society are planning an International EDS Registry. Creating such a registry is a huge undertaking and will take time to build and be universally agreed-upon. When complete, it will help identify the global EDS population for the purpose of raising awareness, standards of care, clinical trials, facilitating scientific identification of the underlying genetic cause(s) of hEDS and, in the future, a treatment or cure.

Introducing 'hypermobility spectrum disorder'

Whilst the new term 'hypermobile Ehlers-Danlos syndrome (hEDS)' would cover all those previously diagnosed with JHS or EDS-H whose symptoms were felt to meet the new criteria (following the 2017 EDS International Classification), the Consortium needed to consider what would happen to those who do not meet the new criteria (both existing and future patients). These individuals, many of whom are significantly affected by hypermobility related disorders arising through various causations (see page 31 'Aetiology'), need equal access to treatment and management; but how should their condition be defined? The 2017 international classification was designed to address this, giving clarity to the spectrum. The term JHS has been dropped (6/HMSA 2017). Those individuals with hypermobility-related problems that do not meet the criteria for hEDS or any other heritable disorder of connective tissue, are now given the diagnosis of hypermobility spectrum disorder (HSD) (Tinkle B. et al 2017, Castori M. et al 2017).

So what is HSD?

When symptomatic joint hypermobility is experienced, but the symptoms do not meet the diagnostic criteria for defined syndromes or disorders that feature hypermobility (such as those described on page 18) a patient may be given a diagnosis of 'hypermobility spectrum disorder (HSD).

HSD is a group of four different categories, created to better identify subtypes of symptomatic hypermobility within the single continuous spectrum that ranges from asymptomatic joint hypermobility at one end through the various hypermobility spectrum disorders, to hypermobile Ehlers-Danlos syndrome at the other extreme (see box below) (Castori M. et al 2017).

> The single continuous spectrum that ranges from asymptomatic joint hypermobility at one end through the various hypermobility spectrum disorders, to hypermobile Ehlers-Danlos syndrome at the other extreme:
>
> GJH (Asymptomatic generalised joint hypermobility)
> PJH (Asymptomatic peripheral joint hypermobility)
> LJH (Asymptomatic localised joint hypermobility)
>
> G-HSD (generalised hypermobility spectrum disorder)
> P-HSD (peripheral hypermobility spectrum disorder)
> L-HSD (localised hypermobility spectrum disorder)
> H-HSD (historical hypermobility spectrum disorder)
>
> hEDS (hypermobile Ehlers-Danlos Syndrome)

The four different HSDs which may be identified are:

- Generalised (joint) hypermobility spectrum disorder (G-HSD): G-HSD is diagnosed where generalised joint hypermobility has been assessed using the Beighton score (shown on pg.122) and a patient is also affected by one or more secondary musculoskeletal manifestation (see bullet point list - next column).
- Peripheral (joint) hypermobility spectrum disorder (P-HSD): P-HSD is diagnosed where joint hypermobility is limited to hands and feet, plus one or more secondary musculoskeletal manifestation (see bullet point list - next column).
- Localised (joint) hypermobility spectrum disorder (L-HSD): L-HSD is diagnosed where joint hypermobility is found at single joints or group of joints, plus one or more secondary musculoskeletal manifestation

regionally related to the hypermobile joint(s) (see bullet point list below).

- Historical (joint) hypermobility Spectrum Disorder (H-HSD): H-HSD is diagnosed when symptoms of symptomatic generalised joint hypermobility are reported historically / self-reported by the patient; the joint(s) having, perhaps, stiffened with age or having been affected by surgery or disability. The Beighton score is negative, and the patient is affected by one or more secondary musculoskeletal manifestation (see below) (Please note: a 5-point questionnaire re: historical joint hypermobility can be found on page 122, Box 3, point ii).
(All above: Castori M. et al 2017)

As mentioned in each of the descriptions above, in symptomatic hypermobile patients, a series of secondary musculoskeletal manifestations that result from their mobility are evaluated for as part of the diagnostic process (5/Ehlers-Danlos Society 2017):

- Pain
- Musculoskeletal / soft tissue trauma
- Degenerative joint and bone disease
- Disturbed proprioception
- Other musculoskeletal / orthopaedic traits

Examples of these can be found in Chapter 3, Page 122, **Box 3** (point **i**).

(Castori M. et al 2017 / 5/Ehlers-Danlos Society '17)

It should be noted that these musculoskeletal concerns fall within a wide range of severity (both in terms of the physical signs and severity of symptoms), and, as with hypermobile Ehlers-Danlos syndrome, individuals with HSD may also be affected by one or more of the comorbid disorders commonly associated with joint hypermobility such as postural orthostatic tachycardia, fatigue, functional gastrointestinal disorders, pelvic and bladder dysfunction etc. Indeed, the 2017 International EDS Classification specifically highlights these disorders as being associated with both HSD and hEDS. However, overall, their diagnosing physician decides that their symptoms do not meet the criteria for a recognised, well-defined syndrome. (6/HMSA 2017, Castori M. et al 2017). Please note, more in-depth descriptions of signs, symptoms and associated disorders are provided in Chapter 2.

'These patients do indeed have real medical needs even if they do not meet criteria for hEDS or another syndrome, and there is need for a logical framework of diagnostic terms to adequately describe their manifestations.' (Castori M. et al 2017).

According to Dr Marco Castori, the spectrum of clinical implications of hypermobile joints, even outside rare and well-defined heritable disorders of

© Understanding hEDS and HSD by C. Smith

connective tissue, actually seems to be even wider than previously expected (Castori M. 2012 / 2011b).

Is hEDS worse than HSD?

Not necessarily. *'Both sit on a vast spectrum and can cause the same symptoms. The spectrum acknowledges that there can be severe effects on lives, whether they're the direct result of joint hypermobility, or because they are known to be associated with having joint hypermobility. What is important is that the problems that arise, whatever the diagnosis, are managed appropriately and that each person is treated as an individual. Both disorders can be equal in severity but, more importantly, both need similar management, validation and care'* (3/ & 6/Ehlers-Danlos Society 2017). Please also see the post-it note, opposite.

Aetiology

It is thought that hypermobility spectrum disorder can arise from various aetiologies (originating causes). In many cases, these may have a genetic influence, being inherited as a genetic trait(s) in the same way as an individual inherits the traits for eye colour, body type or height. However, HSD can also be 'acquired.'

Inherited genetic traits

Research has not, as yet, progressed sufficiently to establish the molecular basis on which this inherited hypermobility takes place. HSD running through a family, may suggest it has a heritable / genetic basis, but then again it may not (3/Ehlers-Danlos Society 2017). In some families, cases may occur in scattered or isolated instances, segregate within families as single gene traits, or they may cluster in families as traits controlled by multiple genetic and/or environmental factors and constitutional factors (Castori M. et al 2017). More information on the multiple factors that can influence hypermobility can also be found on page 33 'Why are people so differently affected?'

Acquired symptomatic hypermobility

Symptomatic hypermobility can be 'acquired' in various ways. For example some individuals acquire symptomatic hypermobility through:

- Injury - for example, dancers, gymnasts and sports people put themselves through grueling workouts in order to produce graceful, flowing movements and may over-stretch joints, muscles and ligaments when trying to create the lines that are desirable.
- Overuse - e.g. massage therapists may acquire problems in their finger and thumb joints triggered by applying repetitive pressure through their joints.
- Malalignment - e.g. those with asymmetrical hip rotation, flat feet or unequal leg length may find that otherwise asymptomatic hypermobile joints become symptomatic over time.
- Physical weakening of tissues due to surgery resulting in symptomatic joint laxity.
- Musculoskeletal malalignment or malformation
- Pharmacological (medicine/drug) interference with collagen biosynthesis can increase joint laxity.

(Refs: Beighton P., Grahame R and Bird H. '89 & '99 / Oliver J.'05)

Certain medical conditions can also cause an individual to acquire symptomatic hypermobility, these include lupus and rheumatoid arthritis, which are autoimmune diseases. In these conditions, otherwise healthy connective tissue is attacked by the body's own immune system, causing it to be defective (Punzi L. et al 2000).

'Whenever symptoms commence, and irrespective of the cause of the hypermobility, the term "hypermobility syndrome" [now know as hypermobility spectrum disorder] *is used to describe the condition. Even hypermobility in a single joint can cause pain and/or instability in that joint; the diagnosis may still be a hypermobility syndrome* [hypermobility spectrum disorder] *if there are other symptoms and signs.* (Grahame R. 2012a)

Information on diagnosing HSD can be found in Chapter 3, pages 120 - 125.

Concerns arising from the 2017 Classification

Is it necessary to obtain a new diagnosis if I already have an existing diagnosis of EDS-H or JHS?

At the time of writing, the recommendation is that diagnoses made before the publication of the 2017 criteria do not need to be changed unless a patient decides to participate in new research or needs to be reassessed for some other reason. As discussed on page 29, an international registry for Ehlers-Danlos syndrome is planned, and researchers will want confidence in the data on the registry, particularly when using the information provided to identify subgroups of people for future studies. The Ehlers-Danlos Society advises that before an individual has their

© Understanding hEDS and HSD by C. Smith

UNDERSTANDING

Box 4.

In the 2017 Classification/criteria, the International Consortium on Ehlers-Danlos syndrome attempt to better define the signs and symptoms of hEDS, and to address the key problem of distinguishing hEDS from symptomatic hypermobility.

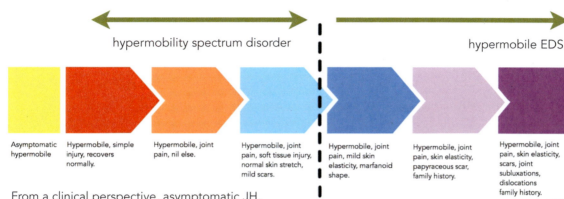

From a clinical perspective, asymptomatic JH, HSDs, and hEDS can all be brought back to a single continuous spectrum ranging from isolated JH to hEDS passing through the various HSDs. As you travel left to right in the examples it becomes more and more possible to consider hypermobile Ehlers-Danlos syndrome as a diagnosis.

Above Image based on information provided by Dr A. Hakim in the HMSA Statement of Position February 2017

Important: Where a patient is placed within the spectrum does not necessarily represent the 'severity' of symptoms experienced, it represents the 'range' of symptoms experienced. Indeed, one person's hypermobile Ehlers-Danlos syndrome joint pain may be less severe than another's hypermobility spectrum disorder joint pain. The overall spectrum isn't strictly linear; from least to most severe, it represents the range of symptoms seen in patients; from single joint issues through to the 'syndrome of disorders' seen in hEDS. Symptoms of both disorders can be equal in severity and, importantly, need similar management, validation and care (see more on page 134). (Wicks D. and Hakim A.J. 2017)

details placed on the registry a prior diagnosis of hypermobile EDS should be checked against the 2017 criteria for hEDS, thus ensuring the registry contains the most up to date and accurate information possible (3/Ehlers-Danlos Society 2017).

Can one family member be diagnosed with HSD and another with hEDS?

Each person should be assessed as an individual but their family history also be taken into account:

'The new criteria recognises there may be members of a family who are hypermobile and well, or who have HSD, within a family where there are also individuals with hEDS. Such presentations might suggest the same underlying genetic trait with variable expression. However, from a classification perspective, the diagnosis of hEDS is established only when the patients signs and symptoms meet the criteria for hEDS...'
(Tinkle B. et al 2017).

This means that there might be a scenario where the diagnosis of HSD is given to an individual with a family history of hEDS (i.e. relatives with an independent diagnosis of hEDS) (3/Ehlers-Danlos Society 2017).

In the 2017 classification papers, Castori et al suggest that for some patients with HSD, who come from families with other relatives with a previous diagnosis of hEDS (according to the new criteria), a 'relaxed' follow-up in clinical genetics services may be scheduled due to a potential future revision of the diagnosis to hEDS or potentially another JH-related syndrome (Castori M. et al 2017).

Will my benefits and insurance codes be affected?

Efforts are being made by many organisations, including the Ehlers-Danlos Society and the Hypermobility Syndromes Association, to ensure that benefit providers, healthcare professionals and insurance companies are aware of the changes, and that, regardless whether a patient is diagnosed with HSD or hEDS, the recommended management is offered and patient care pathways are in place.

Why are people so differently affected?

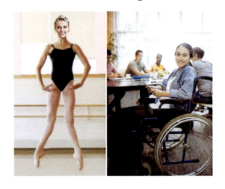

At the beginning of the section on genetics, we noted that describing the inheritance patterns of hEDS using what is known as a 'classic' or 'simple genetics' model is probably too simplistic. In fact, to fully understand the whole range of variations seen in the spectrum spanning joint hypermobility, through hypermobility spectrum disorders and hEDS, it is likely that geneticists will need to look towards a slightly more complex model, which allows for the expression of the single or multiple gene mutation(s) to be further influenced by other genetic, environmental, or constitutional factors.

The Threshold Model

The potential influence of genetic, environmental or constitutional factors may be better explained using the 'Threshold Model' - whereby a single, highly penetrant, dominant, inherited gene mutation is considered to increase risk, but is not necessarily sufficient for the disorder to be expressed (for symptoms to show). The underlying connective tissue variant seen in the hEDS/HSD spectrum can vary in severity and is not always sufficient per se in causing the disorder outright but, when other genetic, environmental, or constitutional factors are added, the combination may be sufficient to reach the threshold for disease expression in a hypermobile person. These factors impact on how specific segments of the genetic code are turned on or 'expressed' and whether, when, and how the process happens (Castori M. 2011 / Rothstein M. et al 2009).

Examples of environmental and constitutional factors include:

- An individual's ethnicity
- Their biological sex
- Age(ing)
- The combination of hypermobility types inherited (see **Box 5**, page 34)
- The physical character of an individual (build, strength, general health etc.)
- Psychological characteristics
- Sports activities they may pursue
- Dietary habits
- Traumas and/or surgeries they undergo
- Periods of temporary immobility
- How well an individual's brain interprets proprioceptive feedback

(See more examples in **Box 6**)

In this section, we will take a look at some of the factors, which may contribute to the variation in manifestations and severity, in more detail.

Ethnic background

People of different ethnic backgrounds have differences in their joint mobility, which may reflect differences in the structure of the collagen proteins. Hypermobility is more common in those from Asian backgrounds, African Black populations (Birrel F.N. et al 1994) and those from Indian heritage, than in white Caucasians. For example, people from the Indian sub-continent often have much more supple hands than Europeans (1/Arthritis Research UK).

Bony, collagen-related, and neuropathic hypermobility

There are three main types of hypermobility, namely bony hypermobility, collagen-related hypermobility and neuropathic hypermobility (see **Box 5**), and each type has its own characteristics (Knight I. 2011 / Celletti C. et al 2013a). Any one person will have varying combinations of these types, but one type may predominate (Bird H. 2007).

Muscle tone

Muscle 'tone' refers to the muscles' ability to resist stretching while in a passive, resting state. Without us being aware of it, muscle tone keeps our muscles in a partially contracted state, which helps maintain posture, protects against injury, and declines during REM sleep. The more relaxed our muscles are, the more movement we have in our joints (1/Arthritis Research UK). Poor muscle tone results in decreased stretch reflex responses, and the limbs' resistance to passive movement being decreased (Boundless.com 2015 / NHS Direct Wales 2014). Those with HSD, and hEDS, need to try to retain or increase their muscle strength and tone as much as possible in order that their muscles can compensate for the effects of defective connective tissue in other supporting structures such as ligaments.

Box 5.

The Three Types of Hypermobility - by Prof. Howard Bird 2007 / Beighton et al 1989)

A) Bony hypermobility – characteristics
• Shallow joint sockets that may dislocate easily.
• Less hypermobility overall, but profound at a smaller range of joints.
• Involves the joint articulating surfaces.

B) Collagen-related hypermobility - characteristics
• More likely to be hormonally dominant – for example more likely to dislocate during progesterone changes in menstruation in females.
• Stretchy skin.
• May be more likely to have problems with other collagen structures, e.g. bladder (weakness),lungs (asthma), bowels (IBS).

C) Neuropathic hypermobility - characteristics
• Late walkers, problems in maintaining core stability, clumsy gait.
• If linked to the bony type of hypermobility, it is possible that some of the bones of the spine may be abnormal.
• Sometimes linked to proprioceptive defect and new research is highlighting problems with the reflex arc (how well an individual's brain interprets proprioceptive feedback) (Ferrell W. and Ferrell P. 2010).

Age

Age, and the stages of aging, appears to have an influence on hypermobility. For example, children (and in particular infants and toddlers) are, in many cases, naturally hypermobile. The hypermobility may or may not lessen as the child grows (Hakim A. 2013a).

At the age of puberty, symptoms can worsen, particularly in females, due to hormonal effects (for more on the effects of hormones see **Box 5**b and also page 35).

Menopause is another milestone where symptoms may be affected. Muscle strength decreases with the onset of menopause, and it is thought that oestrogen may have a negatively inotropic (weakening) effect on muscle strength (Dieli-Conwright C.M. et al. 2009 / Greising S.M. et al. 2009), which may

UNDERSTANDING

render a female's muscles less able still to compensate for already lax tendons.

As a hypermobile person moves into later life, collagen fibres in the ligaments tend to bind together more, and some (but certainly not all) people find they become less hypermobile as a result (1/Arthritis Research UK / 1/EDNF.org, Uptodate.com). It should be noted, however, that the 'associated symptoms' often worsen (Hakim A. 2011); for example 'stiffening' does not always bring less pain, it can bring more (Gurley-Green S. 2001).

It would seem then, that although the vast majority of individuals diagnosed with laxity of the joints describe an onset of symptoms before the age of 15, symptoms arising from joint hypermobility can begin at any age (Beighton P. et al 1998). Indeed, the 1967 study by Kirk et al described a group of patients in whom the age for initial onset of symptoms varied significantly - ranging from age 3 to age 55.

Sense of joint movement (proprioception)
Some people find it difficult to interpret the proprioceptive feedback involved in controlling the increase, decrease and balance of muscle tone. This makes it harder to sense the position and motion of a

Box 6.

Examples of other environmental and constitutional factors

Injuries, a change of job, or a sudden change from an active to less active lifestyle can all trigger the onset of pain and musculoskeletal manifestations (Grahame R. 2012a). Problems with biomechanics and posture can also play a part, over the long term; creating stresses on ligaments, muscles, joints, discs, and spinal nerves. Alternatively, symptoms could become more prominent after a patient undergoes surgery.

Some may acquire problematic symptoms of hypermobility through 'overuse' of particular joints. For example, massage therapists may develop symptomatic hypermobility in their thumbs, fingers or wrists from the repetitive motions or poor technique employed when giving deep tissue massage.

Continued...

...continued

Athletes, such as dancers and gymnasts may also be affected by overuse injuries (Briggs J. et al 2009). Excessive joint loading, faulty technique, anatomical factors and muscle imbalance can all exacerbate damage that will occur as overuse injury, premature degeneration or mechanical failure (Archambault J. et al 1995 / Briggs J. et al 2009). Once a hypermobile dancer, or athlete, is injured, the likelihood of future injury is high (McCormak M. et al 2004).

joint, and may make them more likely to develop, or exacerbate, joint hypermobility by over-stretching joints without realising it (more information on proprioception can be found in pages 57 and 140).

Biological Sex

As discussed on page 22, hEDS is inherited in an autosomal manner (i.e it is carried on the chromosomes that do not determine biological sex). On this basis, science tells us that each child of an individual with hEDS has a 50% chance of inheriting the gene alteration(s) regardless of its sex . Therefore, males and females should be equally affected. Perhaps confusingly then, such an expectation is not confirmed by what is generally found in clinical practice - where the predominance of patients who meet the criteria for hEDS are females (Remvig L. et al 2007/ Castori M. 2010). Not only that, the clinical experience of experts also suggests that hEDS often has more severe clinical expression in females than males.

This 'seeming bias' towards expression of symptoms in females has not been well studied, but might be explained by considering innate differences between males and females, for example:

- Tolerance and perception of pain Studies, such as that carried out by Paulson P.E. 1998 and Fillingim et al., 2009, have found gender differences in both the perceptual and neurophysiological response to pain, which appear to demonstrate that male and female subjects differ in their response to painful stimuli.

- Inherent joint stability Inherent joint instability, particularly at the knee, in females as compared to males, is frequently described in research (Rozzi S.L et al 1999). In fact, both muscle tone and

tendon and ligament stiffness are significantly influenced by biological sex. These factors cooperate to contribute to greater joint stability in men (Kubo K. et al., 2003 / Blackburn J.T et al., 2009 / Castori M. 2010).

- Effects of the sex hormones Women tend to be more supple than men of the same age and are therefore more likely than men to have hypermobile joints (1/Arthritis Research UK). Hormonal fluctuations at key points in females lives, such as puberty, hormonal contraception usage, or the peri-menopause can trigger symptomatic hypermobility (see **Box 7**). It is also now widely recognised that, for many women, symptoms also significantly increase at certain points during their monthly menstruation cycle. In men, it is thought that their increased ability to build more muscle mass and the presence of testosterone offers a larger degree of protection (Bhasin S. et al 1996 / Bird H. 2013)

(For more information about the influence of hormones on hEDS & HSD, see **Box 7**).

It would seem then that, although *on the surface* expression of the phenotypic manifestations of hEDS seem to be higher in females than males, it may actually be that a milder expression of symptoms in males is there in many, but is being missed. Indeed, Castori writes that, when he interviews the parents, siblings and other close relatives of females he identifies with hEDS, he often detects additional undiagnosed mutation carriers, including males who have never been considered affected simply because they do not display the more overt debilitating manifestations (Castori M. 2010a). In addition, males are also often less vocal on forums, and statistically less likely to visit their GP to pursue treatment or a diagnosis, and may, therefore, be under-represented in statistics.

Box 7.

Hormones which are relevant to hypermobility:

Metabolic Steroids:
Metabolic steroids, such as cortisol, 'tone up' organs during the daytime and allows them to rest while we are asleep.

Continued...

...continued

Effect on hypermobile joints:
In both males and females the 24 hour changes in metabolic steroids may produce cyclical symptoms of pain and stiffness over a 24 hour period in joints, but this is normally a minor problem.

Sex hormones:
Sex hormones, are divided into three types; androgens (mainly in males); oestrogens and progestogens (mainly in females).

Effect on hypermobile joints:
In males, the predominant androgen hormones (such testosterone) probably have very little effect on collagen, though they may increase muscle bulk around the joints which is likely to be helpful as the increased muscle power more than outweighs any effect on the collagen structure. In females, it is quite a different story. The balance between oestrogens and progestogens, which is constantly changing, controls the 28-day menstrual cycle in the female (in whom these hormones are almost absent prior to puberty and tail off after the menopause). Although oestrogen tends to stabilise collagen, progestogens loosen it.

Many hypermobile females, though not all, first notice the onset of, or an increase in, symptoms at puberty. This would suggest a hormonal influence, though growth spurts that might have occurred about the same time could also be contributing. Many females report noticing a worsening in symptoms, more pain in the joints, clumsiness or a greater tendency to dislocate in the five days leading up to menstruation and in the few days after menstruation. This is exactly the time when the progesterone compounds far exceed the stabilising oestrogen compounds. This effect is most pronounced when the joint hypermobility is due mainly to collagen structure (see **Box 5B**, page 34) - the clue here is that all joints are almost equally lax throughout the body. Where the hypermobility is a marker of unusually shaped bony surfaces at the joint however (see **Box 5A**, page 34), typically these individuals have very pronounced hypermobility at only a small number of joints, and the effect of hormones is much less pronounced.

Those females whose joints become worse at the time of menstruation often note that if their periods become irregular, for whatever reason, joints not only become worse but are worse for longer. This may be because, in these patients, progesterone is present in high concentrations at times when it would not normally be present.

Above extracts taken, with permission, from 'Hormones and Hypermobility' by Professor Howard Bird at www.hypermobility.org

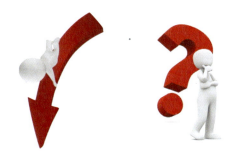

Are hEDS or HSD progressive?

'...(hEDS & HSD) *are non-progressive, non-inflammatory connective tissue disorders. For most people significant improvements can be achieved through lifestyle modification, an appropriate exercise regime and joint protection.*' (Grahame R. et al 2000 / Gedalia A. et al 1993a & 1993b / Russek LN. 2000, Castori M. et al 2017)

So how can the deterioration of physical health, mobility and wellbeing that occur over time in some people with hEDS or HSD be explained?

When patients live with hEDS or HSD, and see their symptoms getting worse as time goes on, it can be understandable that they describe their condition as progressive. '*Patient speak*' and '*medical speak*' are, however, two different languages, and words such as 'progressive' can represent different concepts in the different contexts.

Image attribution:
Down arrow Stuart Miles - Freedigitaldownloads.net
Man with questionmark - Freedom Wiki

© Understanding hEDS and HSD by C. Smith

A member of the Team Inspire forum explains: *'If you are a doctor, then 'progressive' is a label applied to conditions that are known to have a standard set of stages or phases, with a somewhat predictable timeline. Generally all patients with such diagnoses follow a recognisable path, as far as what problems crop up or get worse in what order, and how long plateaus can be expected to last.'* Duchenne Muscular Dystrophy is one example of a truly progressive disorder, as is Parkinson's and certain cancers too. With these conditions, diagnosis is often made possible by recognising which stages have occurred. Some of the other, rarer forms of Ehlers-Danlos syndrome are also considered progressive, such as the severe 'kyphoscolisosis type' which may leave people unable to walk once they reach their 20s or 30s (due to increasingly severe scoliosis).

In hEDS or HSD, on the other hand, the range and severity of symptoms manifest themselves uniquely in every patient; there are no common stages. The defective nature of the collagen involved in hEDS, and HSD, does not accelerate - it doesn't change, it is what it is. However, aggravating factors, such as injuries, hormonal changes, reduced fitness levels, lifestyle, kinesiophobia (see Chapter 3, page 42), weight gain, secondary and co-morbid conditions that occur and most importantly, how they are managed by the individual and the medical professionals supporting them, can play a significant role in the increase or decline of symptoms and levels of disability (See **Box 8**).

Worsening of symptoms caused inadvertently by a physiotherapist, surgeon or other healthcare professional as a result of inappropriate diagnostic or therapeutic procedures can all contribute to short, or long term deterioration. Prolonged periods of inactivity following surgery can cause muscle weakness that triggers joint problems in other areas of the body; and certain medications are known to cause side effects that cause problems in the stomach and bowel. Stiffening, and the potential for osteoarthritis caused by wear and tear on lax joints, may also bring about increasing levels of pain as age advances. Without proper, informed treatment or management, it is easy to see how symptoms can spiral downwards.

For many adults, lack of guidance and poor levels of medical intervention and management in the past, has already left them with significantly disabling symptoms. However, the news for today's children is better according to Ellie Haggard, highly specialist physiotherapist in paediatric rheumatology at Great Ormond Street Hospital. She writes *'the prognosis for today's children is far brighter, with big advances in paediatric physiotherapy transforming the prospects of children with hypermobility. If they get the right targeted intervention they shouldn't have the problems their parents may have had'* (The Chartered Society of Physiotherapy).

The successful management of patients with hEDS or HSD requires early recognition of joint laxity being related to the symptoms, *before* the symptoms become chronic and perhaps disabling. Appropriate advice needs to be provided to parents, in order that they know how to best support their hypermobile child; education needs to be provided for healthcare professionals, schoolteachers and sporting coaches who can play a critical role in improving symptoms and allowing more gradual rehabilitation and return to full activities (or to modified activities that are less likely to lead to recurrent joint injury). Appropriate intervention with physiotherapy and occupational therapy can be important for the optimum management of problems, as can psychological support or counselling if the individual has developed a chronic pain syndrome. (Murray K.J & Woo P. 2001)

Self management techniques taught by the Hypermobility Syndromes Association, at UK-wide hypermobility masterclasses and events such as the HMSA Family Programmes, can be of great value. Such techniques, if implemented early enough, can play a significant part in breaking the cycle of symptoms that affect so many people with a hypermobility syndrome.

More information on self management can be found in Chapter 3, page 150).

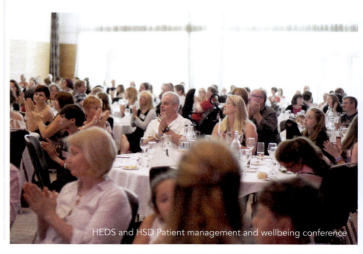

HEDS and HSD Patient management and wellbeing conference

Box 8.

Case studies, demonstrating the significant part that aggravating factors can play in the increase or decline of symptoms and levels of disability:

Outwardly, it would appear that the girls in the following examples have a 'progressive' condition, but their collagen defects have not actually progressed in any way. What has changed is their bodies; they have been affected by a chain of events, including a lack of appropriate medical advice and advice on self-management, which have led to their symptoms worsening.

Case study 1: It was always clear to Amy's family that something was not quite right – she was slow to walk, and preferred to sit in the "W" position (in some cases, a child's way of compensating for the poor balance associated with weak core muscle strength). As she grew older, her parents noticed that she experienced easy bruising and poor wound healing, and would carry out 'party-tricks' with her bendy fingers, but they never understood the cause.

In the absence of an obvious family history, and with no symptoms such as dislocations having occurred, it is perhaps understandable that no underlying HDCT was checked for. It is, after all, notoriously difficult to diagnose hEDS or HSD in young children, as most children are flexible in their early years. From puberty, however, symptoms became far more apparent; she experienced pain, joint instability and autonomic dysfunction, particularly around her time of menstruation. Despite repeated trips to their GP, no diagnosis was made and, although pain killers were prescribed, no appropriate management plan was implemented.

As is the case for many, the lack of awareness within the medical community meant that Amy was not diagnosed until later in life, by which time unexplained injuries, chronic long term pain, fatigue and anxiety had become commonplace for her.

Case study 2: Here, we consider Harriet, who is hypermobile, but went through childhood untouched by any negative hypermobility symptoms (i.e. she was asymptomatic).

Harriet's ballet teacher spotted her potential early on, as hypermobility allowed her to achieve the desired ballet positions easily. Out of the blue, at age 17, Harriet twisted her ankle during a dance routine and the injury refused to heal; she began to walk with a limp, causing a knock on effect to her knee and hip and the physical strain on her joints from relying on crutches soon caused further problems in her wrists and left shoulder.

Within months; this once asymptomatic young woman found herself in a downward spiral as her body became deconditioned and pain and muscle fatigue became a daily occurrence.

Important Note:

The remainder of the content in this book, including signs, symptoms comorbidities, and management are of equal importance to those with hEDS, and HSD. For those who are hypermobile, but experience no symptoms, the content may also be of interest with a view to preventing injuries from occurring in the future.

'Both HSD and hEDS sit within a vast spectrum and can cause the same symptoms. What is important is that the problems that arise, whatever the diagnosis, are managed appropriately and that each person is treated as an individual. Both can be equal in severity, but more importantly, both need similar management, validation and care' (3/ Ehlers-Danlos Society 2017)

© Understanding hEDS and HSD by C. Smith

Chapter 2
Symptoms & Comorbidities

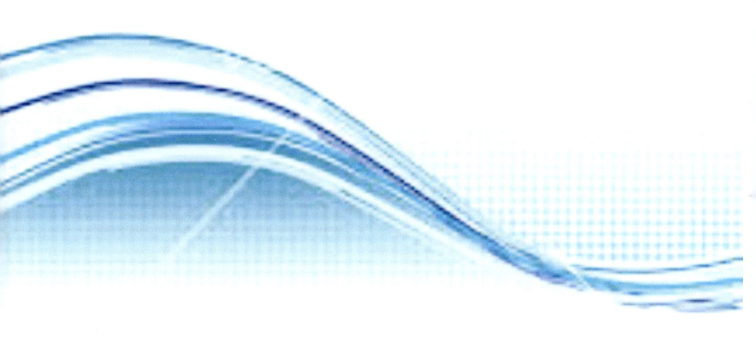

What are symptoms, manifestations, syndromes and comorbidities?

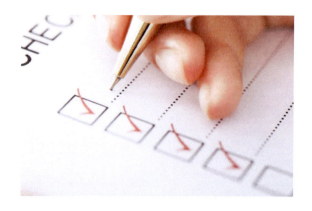

What is a symptom?
The word symptom is used to describe what the patient is experiencing, and may indicate a condition or disease. Symptoms are often subjective; for example, anxiety, pain, and fatigue are all 'symptoms' - only the patient can perceive them, they are not visible to others.

What is a sign or manifestation?
A manifestation (sign) can also indicate a condition or disease but, in contrast to symptoms, manifestations are objective; they can be observed by a physician during clinical examination. For example, hyperextensible skin, bruising and scoliosis are all manifestations which can be observed through clinical examination.

What is a syndrome?
A syndrome is a group of symptoms which consistently occur together; at least one of which is known or thought to be causally related. For example, hEDS is classed as a syndrome because it is a disorder identified by an established group of manifestations and symptoms which appear causally related. The presence of joint hypermobility in combination with secondary musculoskeletal symptoms alone would not usually suffice for delineation of a syndrome (see Box 4, page 32) (Francomano C. & Bloom L. 2017).

Comorbidities
Put simply, comorbidities are two or more conditions that occur together. They may each be common in their own right and therefore appear together often. Sometimes a direct link between them can be established. Sometimes they are things that are seen more times than can be coincidental, but, as yet, there has not been enough funding or documented research to categorically prove the link. In hEDS there are several comorbidities such as bowel and autonomic problems that appear alongside the joint and skin problems. Research is beginning to demonstrate that these are linked to hEDS and not just arising independently of each other.

Important
This chapter aims to cover many of the symptoms and manifestations directly related to hEDS or HSD, and to also highlight the wide range of disorders frequently described as having 'an association' with joint hypermobility (wherever possible, explanation has been provided as to they ways in which it is thought these signs, symptoms and manifestations are linked to hEDS or HSD or, in the case of comorbidities, how it is hypothesized that they *may* be associated). This is an extremely complex subject, but the author has done her best to cover as many as possible, using information from the most recent nosology papers, academic research, medical literature, and from trusted charities, resources, and professional colleagues.

Please note:
- As stated in Chapter 1, a hypermobile person may have any combination of the conditions listed or, indeed, may never develop these problems.

- Due to the complexity of signs and symptoms seen in those with hEDS/HSD, the list contained in this chapter cannot be exhaustive and will, likely, be updated in future editions as advances in research occur, and revisions to the classification are made.

- It is beyond the scope of any one publication to provide details on diagnostic methods and treatment for each individual condition but, in the case of some of the larger comorbidity topics (e.g. cardiovascular autonomic dysfunction, mast cell activation syndrome etc), some information linked to diagnosis and management has been included at the end of the relevant sections in chapter 2. Chapter 3 then goes on to provide more detailed information regarding diagnosis and general management related to hEDS and HSD specifically. (NB/Please see post-it note opposite).

© Understanding hEDS and HSD by C. Smith

Box 1.

A) Symptoms and manifestations that can arise as a direct complication of hEDS

- Hypermobility of the joints.
- Skin - stretch marks, hyperextensibility, atrophic scarring, bilateral piezogenic papules of the heel.
- Pelvic floor - Pelvic floor, rectal, and/or uterine prolapse in children, men or nulliparous women without a history of morbid obesity or other known predisposing medical condition.
- Dental crowding or narrow palette.
- Arachnodactyly - as defined by the Steinberg signs and Walker signs (tests is used in clinical evaluation).
- Arm span to height ratio equal to or greater than 1.05.
- Mitral valve prolapse.
- Aortic root dilation.
- Musculoskeletal trauma / soft tissue trauma (macrotraumas such as dislocations, subluxations; damage to ligaments, tendons and muscles; loss of joint function; microtraumas too small to be noticed as they happen).
- Pain (acute, chronic, neuropathic, myofascial)
- Disturbed proprioception.
- Other musculoskeletal traits - flat feet, misaligned bones in the elbow or big toes, mild to moderate scoliosis, kyphosis, upper spine lordosis.

(Malfait et al 2017, 4/ and 5/Ehlers-Danlos Society - 2017, Hakim A.J 2017c, HMSA)

B) Symptoms and manifestations that can arise as a direct complication of HSD

- Hypermobility of the joints.
- Musculoskeletal trauma / soft tissue trauma (macrotraumas such as dislocations, subluxations; damage to ligaments, tendons and muscles; loss of joint function; microtraumas too small to be noticed as they happen).
- Pain (acute, chronic, neuropathic, myofascial).
- Disturbed proprioception.
- Other musculoskeletal traits - flat fee, misaligned bones in the elbow or big toes, mild to moderate scoliosis, kyphosis, upper spine lordosis.

(Malfait et al 2017, 4/ and 5/Ehlers-Danlos Society - 2017, Hakim A.J 2017c, HMSA)

C) Comorbidities - which may be associated with hEDS and HSD (this list is not exhaustive)

For some, these conditions may be more debilitating than the joint symptoms / musculoskeletal symptoms, they often impair functionality and quality of life, and should always be determined during clinical encounters, and treated (Malfait F. et al 2017).

- Sleep disturbance.
- Fatigue.
- Cardiovascular autonomic dysfunction - including postural orthostatic tachycardia syndrome.
- Functional gastrointestinal disorders.
- Depression
- Mechanical and neuropathic bowel dysfunction (e.g. hernia, reflux sluggish bowel and constipation).
- Chronic bowel inflammation (inc. mast cell activation.
- Chiari type 1 malformation.
- Tethered cord syndrome.
- Craniocervical instability.
- Anxiety disorders
- Myopia.
- Astigmatism.
- Poor response to anaesthetic.
- Pelvic floor weakness.
- Chronic bladder inflammation (inc. mast cell activation.
- Earlier than 'normal' onset of osteoarthritis.
- Influence of progesterone - worsening musculoskeletal symptoms.
- Heavy and painful menstrual cycle.
- Musculoskeletal and pelvic complications in pregnancy.

(Malfait et al 2017, 4/ & 5/Ehlers-Danlos Society 2017, Hakim A.J 2017c, HMSA)

Readers are urged to take appropriately qualified medical advice in all cases. The information in this book is intended to be useful to the general reader, but should not be used as a means of self-diagnosis, or for the prescription of medication. Practitioners must check clinical procedures and always rely on their own experience and knowledge of their patients to make diagnoses and in evaluating and using any information, methods, compounds, or experiments described herein, and to take all appropriate safety precautions.

Symptoms and comorbidities

Part 1 - Widespread symptoms & comorbidities

Widespread symptoms & comorbidities

Some symptoms seen as direct complications of hEDS or HSD, or comorbidities associated with hEDS and HSD are 'widespread.' They affect the person as a whole, or have the potential to affect multiple areas of the body. Examples would include fatigue, dislocations, skin involvement and cardiovascular autonomic dysfunction. The following list should not be considered exhaustive.

Widespread symptoms

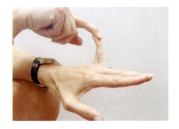

Joint hypermobility

A hypermobile joint is one with a range of movement that exceeds the norm, taking into consideration age, sex, and ethnic background.

In those with laxity of the connective tissue (as seen in hEDS and HSD), joint hypermobility is part of a their genetic make up and, like the myriad of other symptoms frequently experienced, is likely caused by a defect in their fibrous protein genes that encode collagen, elastin and fibrillin. The laxity found in ligaments and other joint structures can allow joints to rest in extreme positions and to rely on the stretched structures for support instead of using muscle strength and controlled movement to provide stability to the body. (Melson P. & Riddle O. 2010)

The range of movement that a joint is capable of is determined by four factors, which each affect people to varying degrees:

1) The extent of ligament laxity that is experienced:
Ligaments are supposed to be restraints that control motion between individual bones and groups of bones by reciprocal tension. They connect the bones within a joint to each other and to the rest of the body. They are made up of several types of protein fibre including elastin and collagen.

It is thought those with hEDS, and HSD, have weakened collagen fibres and more elastic ligaments, causing weakness and a reduced ability to adequately keep the joint within a stable range, with extra-muscular effort required to create stability before it is moved.

2) The shape of the joint sockets:
If the socket of a joint is particularly shallow, the range of movement within the joint will be greater than usual and a person may have a greater risk of pain and dislocation and increased wear and tear.

3) Proprioceptive feedback:
Proprioceptive feedback is used by the body's central nervous system to understand the position and movement of the body and limbs, allowing it to process information from special receptors in the skin, joints, muscles and tendons to provide knowledge about the body's position in space. For example, even with their eyes shut, an individual should know whether their arm is bent or straight. Those affected by poor proprioception find it difficult to sense the position of their joints; in the case of joint hypermobility, making it harder to sense when a joint is overstretched.

4) Muscle tone:
Muscle tone is the term used to describe the 'always at the ready' state of partial contraction in our muscles which maintains balance and posture, and it also functions as a safety mechanism that allows for a quick, subconscious muscle reflex reaction to any sudden muscle fibre stretch. The tone of the muscles is controlled by the nervous system. The weaker or more relaxed the muscles are, the more movement there is likely to be within a joint. (Points 1-4 1/Arthritis Research UK by Prof H. Bird)

As explained in previous sections, joint range can sometimes be increased into the hypermobile range by those who are *not* born hypermobile, by overuse, injury, or purposely through training. For example, ballet dancers who are not inherently lax jointed need to acquire hypermobility in certain joints to perform their art. (Grahame R. 1999).

Important note: Please note that, where used throughout this book, the term 'overuse' does not mean doing too much activity overall, but rather overusing a specific tissue or a structure to the point that it becomes injured.

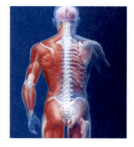

Recurrent musculoskeletal disorders

The term musculoskeletal disorders (MSDs) refers to physical symptoms that concern or involve the body's movement or musculoskeletal system (i.e. muscles, tendons, ligaments, nerves, discs, blood vessels, etc.). MSDs are common in the general

© Understanding hEDS and HSD by C. Smith

population, but in those with hEDS or HSD, the degree of joint laxity and the associated clinical features are a major contributing factor behind many of the multiple and recurring MSDs they experience, with injuries such as ligament and muscle tears happening with increased frequency (Murray K.J. & Woo. P. 2001). The severity of MSDs can vary, but for some, pain and discomfort may interfere with everyday activities. In Stanitski et al's study into the orthopaedic manifestations of Ehlers-Danlos syndrome (2000), it was found that the hypermobile type of Ehlers-Danlos syndrome was the most debilitating form with respect to musculoskeletal function. Common contributing factors include repetitive or sustained awkward postures, forceful exertion of the muscles in response to heavy loads, and high repetition tasks.

Common examples of MSDs seen in hEDS and HSD, include ligament sprains, pulled tendons, tendon tears, (Hakim A.J. 2014b) tendonitis, bursitis and plantar fasciitis (Graham R. 1999; Beighton P. Grahame R. & Bird H. 2012; Castori M. 2012).

Bursitis
A bursa is a small, fluid-filled, balloon-like sac that can be found around joints and other moving parts of the body, such as the shoulder, elbow, foot, hip, knee and ankle. Inflammation of the fluid-filled sac within a joint is called bursitis.

These small balloon-like sacs (bursae) have a small amount of lubricating fluid within them known as 'synovial fluid'. This fluid allows a bursa to act like a cushion while also reducing friction between sliding tendons and bones. When joints are loose and friction occurs, a bursa can be subjected to ongoing stress or a sudden trauma. When this happens, it usually results in an inflamed bursa that fills with fluid. This condition is known as 'bursitis' and can be the cause of considerable discomfort and pain. The most common sites for bursitis to occur are the hips, shoulders and elbows (13/NHS.uk).

Sprains
Sprains occur when the joint twists, rolls in or out, or is forced into an abnormal position, causing the ligaments that connect the bones to tear or stretch (livestrong.com). Instability arises when the injured ligament fails to regain its structural elasticity, or has too much anatomic elasticity due to defective tissue proteins (as in hypermobility), causing the joint to move in atypical ways. Chronic low-grade swelling and pain may also be noted. Once sprained, the

WIDESPREAD SYMPTOMS & COMORBIDITIES

frequency of future sprains may increase if long-term weakening of the joints' structures occur and go untreated.

Tendonitis, tendonopathy and tendon ruptures
The term 'tendonitis' is usually used for tendon injuries involving acute injury accompanied by inflammation. The term 'tendonopathy' is used when it is unclear whether the symptomatic tendon is actually inflamed or not. Whether the symptoms are classed as tendonitis or tendonopathy, the most likely causes of injury are having poor control over one's joints when carrying out tasks, and overloading/ overuse, caused by activities such as carrying heavy shopping bags, repetitive movements at work or while playing sport (10/Patient.co.uk). These kinds of activities can result in small micro-traumas (tears) occurring in the tendon and, if the rate of these micro-tears is faster than the rate of recovery, it can lead to the prolonged inflammation known as tendonitis. Untreated, this can result in tendon scarring or degeneration which may be classed as a tendonopathy i.e. the tendon is no longer inflamed but there is pain, stiffness and limited ability to load the tendon to perform tasks.

Tendon ruptures are uncommon, but may cause severe initial pain and bruising, and lead to permanent disabling symptoms if untreated. They are usually graded according to their degree of severity, and management may be surgical or non-surgical depending on the site and severity of the rupture, and the clinical features and disability caused.

Plantar fasciitis
Plantar fasciitis is the most common cause of heel pain. The plantar fascia is the flat band of tissue (ligament) that connects the heel bone to the toes. It supports the arch of the foot. When strained, the plantar fascia gets weak, swollen and inflamed (webmd.com 2013).

Muscle Spasms
Spasms of skeletal muscles are associated with many chronic pain conditions, including hEDS and HSD. Spasms can affect many different types of muscles in the body, leading to different symptoms and presentations. Spasms occur abruptly, are painful and, although the spasm itself may be short-lived, may occur repeatedly. They can be caused by muscles tightening reflexively, guarding a painful area, nerve irritation or generalised tension, and can be more painful than the original injury (4/ ednf.org). Other causes of muscle spasms can include dehydration and electrolyte abnormalities.

© Understanding hEDS and HSD by C. Smith

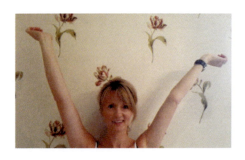

Hyperextended alignment of joints

Hypermobile people experience the ill-effects of malalignment caused by hyperextension, or, for example, asymmetrical hip rotation, flat feet or leg-length inequality far earlier than people who are not hypermobile (Oliver J. 2005).

When muscles and ligaments are lax, a person's joints can extend into a range that is greater than considered 'normal'. However, just because someone with hypermobility *can* bend his or her joints further than normal doesn't mean that it is a good idea to do so. In an individual with lax muscles and ligaments, the body will opt for the most efficient way of obtaining stability. This can be seen in children (or adults) when they choose to sit in the W-position, or when people stand with their knees locked in hyperextension, because they find the position more stable than standing with the knees in a neutral position.

W sitting position

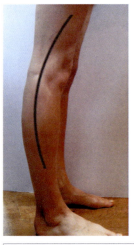
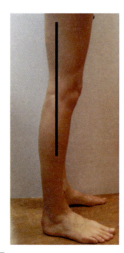

Image left: Knee hyperextension

Although hyperextended alignment of joints in individuals with hEDS is their 'normal', allowing joints to be used in day to day activities whilst in hyperextension can put stress on the connective tissues around the joint.

Standing with one's knees in hyperextension has also been shown to affect control over postural stability (Siqueira C.M. et al 2011), causing knock on effects throughout the body.

Exercises focusing on improving proprioception and building strength can be beneficial. When carrying out physiotherapy or exercise programmes, some experts believe that patients should refrain from allowing their joints to extend beyond what is classed as normal, whilst others argue that studies show it is just as effective, easier, and causes no detrimental symptoms to allow patients to use and exercise into their full range (Pacey V. 2013 & Pacey V. et al 2014). The children's rehabilitation programme for those with symptomatic hypermobility at Great Ormond Street Hospital includes carefully prescribed, graded exercises, which patients build up gradually to keep muscles strong throughout their *entire* range of motion (including into the hyperextended range), in the hope that the increased strength in, what is, after all, *their* 'normal' range of motion, will offer some protection when the child naturally slips into what we consider to be 'extended range' during their day-to-day activities (Maillard S. in person 2012).

This practice appears to be backed up by the 2014 study by Pacey V et al that states: '*Even if advised to avoid the hypermobile range, it is likely a child with JHS* [HSD] *will inadvertently use their knee joint hyperextension when walking. If the treating clinician incorporates proprioceptive training within a treatment programme for a child with JHS* [HSD], *this training should not be limited only to neutral knee extension.*' (This subject is also discussed in 'Physiotherapy' - Chapter 3 - page 139)

Image attribution (page 48): Bandita - Creative Commons Licence

© Understanding hEDS and HSD by C. Smith

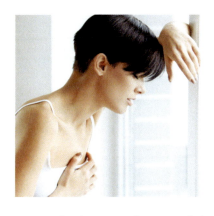

Pain

Pain, which is usually one of the first symptoms to occur in hEDS and HSD, may be widespread in the body or localised to one region such as an arm or a leg (Chopra P. et al 2017). In one study, the prevalence of chronic pain was 90% in patients with various types of EDS, with the highest scores on severity of pain found in the hypermobility type (Voermans N.C. et al 2010 / Shirley E.D. et al 2012). It can be experienced both as a result of acute injuries (dislocations, tendonitis etc) and in the form of chronic pain (now frequently referred to as 'persistent' pain).

As is the case with many other symptoms of hEDS/HSD, pain rarely fits neatly into a single category. For many, it is a combination of both 'chronic' pain and 'acute' pain, or is, perhaps, a hybrid of both.

'It often starts as occasional/recurrent joint pain facilitated/triggered by joint instability, dislocations and sprains, but subsequently it becomes diverse in character, frequently manifesting in the form of widespread myalgias and arthralgias and often with neuropathic features' (Castori M. 2012). For many with hEDS, and HSD, musculoskeletal pain can play a major role in the deterioration of quality of life (Castori M. 2012)

Unfortunately, the causes of pain (other than that arising as an initial acute response to injuries such as dislocation), are not currently fully understood by experts, leading to much misunderstanding in the medical community and often leaving patients feeling isolated and confused (Tinkle B. 2010 / Berglund B. 2000). It is likely, however, that it is caused by a combination of excessive movement within the joints - increasing stress on joint surfaces, ligaments and neighbouring structures (Simpson M.R. 2006); a complex mixture of nociceptive, myofascial, and osteoarthritic pain factors, and because of an impaired connective tissue function (as suggested by the discovery of small fibre neuropathy in adults with classical, hypermobile, and vascular types of EDS).

© Understanding hEDS and HSD by C. Smith

WIDESPREAD SYMPTOMS & COMORBIDITIES

Types of Pain

In hEDS and HSD, several types of pain are recognisable. These mechanisms can combine, overlap and interact forming a pain 'syndrome'.

Acute pain

Acute pain is defined as 'pain that lasts for a specified time-frame for a given condition' (Bonica J. 1990). Acute pain often originates from nociception. Nociceptors are a kind of sensory receptor found all over the body, which are responsible for detecting, transmitting and processing potential damage to the nervous system (Basbaum A.I. et al 2009). It is usually directly related to an obvious cause, such as an injury, and is immediate, sudden and new. With painkillers, acute pain will usually get better fairly quickly.

Acute pain is generally considered '*useful*' because it serves a purpose, signaling damage or a potential injury. It is also considered '*time limited*', because, once the tissue damage heals, the pain typically resolves.

Persistent (chronic) pain

Persistent pain in hEDS and HSD is a serious complication and can be both physically and psychologically disabling, interfering with socialisation and activities of daily living. (Levy H.P. 2012, Chopra P. et al 2017). The onset often begins in a gradual, subtle way, but with harmful effects. It doesn't necessarily keep to the areas of the body that might be expected, or need to relate to a specific injury.

Persistent pain is defined as pain that continues beyond the time one would expect normal healing of an injury to take (Bonica J. 1990), but it can also be experienced when there is no clearly identifiable pain generator to explain the pain.

Unlike acute pain, persistent pain is not warning the patient of bodily harm and, unless it persists as a result of an injury / symptom that has not healed or has not be properly diagnosed, persistent pain serves no useful purpose (Winterowd C. 2003).

In such cases, instead of regulating pain, the central nervous system may actually be:

- Amplifying pain - intensifying the volume of the original pain messages as they are sent

Continued...

from the source to the brain

- Maintaining pain - continuing to send signals even after the initial injury might have healed
- Generating pain - sending pain signals even though there is no tissue damage.

In simple terms, the nervous system itself is actually misfiring and creating the pain. What started out as a useful warning signal becomes a 'fire alarm' relentlessly ringing. In such cases, the pain itself is the disease rather than a symptom of an injury and needs to be treated as the primary pathology (1/ Spine-health.com).

'Chronic pain can utterly disrupt and damage one's life, ...making it hard to enjoy even the simplest daily activities, and certainly making it a challenge to carry out an exercise routine and other healthy activities' (2/Spine-health.com).

Neuropathic pain

Neuropathic pain is experienced as the result of a malfunction, or injury, in the peripheral or central nervous system. It can be placed in the chronic pain category, but has a different 'feel' than chronic pain of a musculoskeletal nature (1/ Spine-health.com). Neuropathic pain is often described with the following terms: severe, sharp, lancinating, lightning-like, stabbing, burning, cold, and/or ongoing numbness, tingling or weakness (Richeimer S. 2000). For some, even stimulus such as a light touch can cause pain (Hakim A.J. 2013c). It may be felt travelling along the nerve path from the spine down to the arms/hands or legs/feet (1/ Spine-health.com). Some examples of neuropathic pain include: neuralgia, complex regional pain syndrome / causalgia (nerve trauma) and entrapment neuropathy (e.g., carpal tunnel syndrome) (Richeimer S. 2000)

It has been suggested that neuropathic pain in hEDS and HSD may result from direct nerve impingement e.g., by subluxated vertebrae, herniated discs, vertebral osteoarthritis, or peripheral joint subluxations. Although this seems possible, the hypothesis is, so far, unproven. Unfortunately, traditional methods of diagnosing neuropathic pain in those with hEDS or HSD may be of little value, as the pain often arises even in the absence of evidence of nerve abnormality (entrapment) and in the absence of endocrine or metabolic disorder (Castori M. et al 2010). Diagnostic testing, such as nerve conduction studies, usually does not provide enough evidence for a diagnosis

and, although skin biopsy may reveal a reduction in or absence of small nerve fibres, they often come back 'normal' (Levy H.P. 2012). There may be mild-to-moderate nerve compression within areas of myofascial spasm, but, again, this possibility has yet to be evaluated clinically (Levy H.P. 2012).

Neuropathic pain has different treatment options to other types of pain. For example, NSAIDs such as ibuprofen, COX-2 inhibitors, or opioids (such as morphine) are not usually effective in relieving neuropathic pain, whereas treatments including certain medications such as Gabapentin, or nerve "block" injections may provide relief (1/Spine-health.com).

Myofascial pain

Myofascia is a web of connective tissue fibres, primarily collagen, which form sheets beneath the skin to attach, enclose, and separate muscles, bones, internal organs, blood vessels and nerves, in a similar way to wrapping something in cling film, thus providing stability and support. Myofascia is one continuous structure that exists from head to toe without interruption. Its interconnected nature means that, by way of the myofascia, everything in the body is connected to everything else (selfcare4rsi.com, 7/HMSA 2013).

Although possibly one of the least well known, myofascia is in fact our richest sense organ. It has the ability to contract independently of the muscles it surrounds, and it responds to stress without conscious command (EDSInfo.org 2013). Chronic joint instability makes it difficult for the body to protect itself against changing forces and leads to reduced body stabilisation and support. This has a knock on effect, which results in poor posture and imbalances in the musculoskeletal system, which it is thought can lead to myofascial pain. Areas of tightness and restriction cause the myofascia to become less pliable and more rigid, creating pulls, tensions, and pressure that do not show up in many of the standard tests such as x-ray or MRI (Chopra P. 2013b).

Myofascial pain exists as part of many soft-tissue conditions including hEDS and HSD, but the causation has not been systematically studied (Levy H.P. 2012). It is often described as aching, throbbing, or stiff in quality, and therapists can detect palpable muscle knots and trigger points.
'The result of an overly-stretchable fascia can be

WIDESPREAD SYMPTOMS & COMORBIDITIES

literally body-wide because it is wrapped around nearly everything. In addition, every time a joint slips or dislocates, the soft tissue connected to that joint (i.e. tendons, ligaments, muscle, fascia, blood vessels) all stretches.' (Quote: Dr A Hakim 2013e)

Please note: Treatment and management of pain are discussed in Chapter 3, pages 148, and 151-153.

Osteoarthritic pain:

For some, osteoarthritic pain may develop later in life (but earlier than usually seen in the general population) and typically presents as aching pain in the joints, frequently associated with stiffness. It is often exacerbated by stasis (motionlessness) and by resistance and/or highly repetitive activity. (Levy H.P. 2012)

The experience of persistent (chronic) pain

Persistent pain is a personal experience and cannot be measured like other problems in medicine. It is influenced by many factors, such as ongoing pain signal input to the nervous system even without tissue damage, physical deconditioning due to lack of exercise, a person's thoughts about the pain, as well as emotional states, such as depression and anxiety. Each experience we have in life, including that of pain, causes a pathway to form to our brain. If you have a good, bad, or traumatic experience in relation to your pain, that experience will also become a part of your pain pathway.

Pain is detected by nociceptive receptors located in the peripheral nerves, muscles, tendons and internal organs. These fibres send pain signals to the spinal cord. The pain signals then travel up the spinal cord via 'pathways' and reach an area of the brain called the thalamus. Once in the thalamus, the signal is processed and then relayed to several other areas of the brain, where memories thoughts and emotions are processed (Winterowd C. 2003). The body releases certain chemicals associated with emotions, thoughts and feelings; some can calm down the system, but others can excite it (Chronic Pain AU).

The brain has an effect on the pain signal, and should exert a modifying or controlling influence on it, but in those whose pain pathways have been adversely strengthened by negative factors such as repeated injury, it can have an 'amplifying' influence on pain signals instead.

Robyn Hickmott, Physiotherapist, explains: 'It is likely that for those with EDS/JHS [EDS/HSD], nociceptive input from over-stretched joints, feeds the hypersensitivity to pain in the form of central sensitisation, in response to repeated tissue damaging events. In many, the stimulus may be something that does not normally provoke pain in others' (Hickmott R. 2013). Prof. Rodney Grahame writes: '(people with hEDS/HSD) may also have a fault in the way their pain signals are picked up for onward transmission to the brain, where they reach consciousness. Research work is in progress to try to sort out this enigma. Much more needs to be done.'

'Contrary to popular belief, all pain is real. This may seem like an obvious statement, but people with chronic pain are sometimes treated as if their chronic pain is either imaginary or exaggerated. Unfortunately, some doctors still practice in this manner, having no appreciation for the unique problem of chronic pain, newer theories about chronic pain, and the many factors that influence a chronic pain problem' (2/spine-health.com).

People show and feel pain in different ways depending on a number of factors such as:

- The situation in which an individual finds themselves when the pain happens.
- Whether we know the cause of the pain.
- Whether we feel we have coping strategies to control some of the pain.
- A person's stage of development i.e. baby, school age child, teen or adult.
- Gender scientists have known for a few decades that men and women feel pain differently, although the reasons are unclear.
- Genetics - researchers have found that some genes are linked to a higher predisposition for pain.
- The kind of thoughts a person has about about the pain, such as "this is nothing serious" versus 'this pain could be a sign that something is really wrong.'
- Cultural influences determining whether a person is to be more stoic or more dramatic in showing pain to others.
- Emotions associated with the chronic pain, such as depression and anxiety versus hopefulness and optimism.

continued...

- Fear of pain, which can lead to a patient not moving (especially when a certain movement caused pain in the past).
- Dwelling on pain - inability to stop thinking about one's pain and characterising it as unbearable, which may increase activity in areas of the brain related to pain anticipation.

While the experience of pain can vary from person to person, in hEDS and HSD it is frequently described in ways such as the following:

- Pain in single or, more commonly, multiple joints.
- Daily pain that gets worse with activities and worsens still throughout the day (Tinkle B. 2010).
- Pain that occurs after sleep - many wake up in the morning with an aching and tightness in the muscles and joints throughout the body that can hinder movement and range of motion. Dr Brad Tinkle says 'This muscle joint stiffness can subside fairly quickly or can last for hours'; he describes the pain as being akin to an activity-related or pain 'hangover' (Tinkle B. 2010).
- Pain that is variable in age-of-onset (as early as adolescence or as late as the fifth or sixth decade), number of sites, duration, quality, severity, and response to therapy (Levy H.P. 2012).
- Severity that is typically greater than expected based on physical and radiologic examinations.
- Severity that sometimes has a connection with degree of joint instability and with sleep impairment [Voermans et al 2010a / Levy H.P. 2012].
- Headaches, of which migraine appears to be the most common form (Sacheti A. et al 1997 / Jacome D. 1999). Triggers for other forms of headache disorder include hypermobile joints in the cervical spine and temporomandibular joint dysfunction (Pocinki A. 2010 / Levy H.P. 2012).
- Pain with daily tasks. For instance, people with hEDS / HSD can have trouble with their finger joints causing difficulty with 'fine' skills such as using pens and pencils (because holding tightly to something so thin becomes painful) chopping vegetables, doing up buttons etc. Not infrequently, pain and fatigue in the hand, wrist or lower arm are noted, particularly by teachers, who may also note that unusual or bizarre hand postures are assumed for writing tasks, with the relatively less stable, hypermobile hand (Murry K. J. Woo P. 2001). Painful joints in the knees, shoulders, spine, hips etc., may cause pain when walking, washing and bathing.
- Back pain, due to laxity of the spinal ligaments, scoliosis, or hyperlordosis (deep lumbar area) caused by lumbar disc problems (Bravo J. 2013).
- Pain in the abdomen due to gastrointestinal dysfunction (Hakim A 2013d).
- Muscle stiffness and tightness caused by imbalances in the joints, postural issues and the extra work muscles have to do to try and keep a hypermobile person's joints stable. Muscles may tighten reflexively; guarding of a painful area, nerve irritation or generalised tension may occur (Chopra P. 2013b).
- Muscle spasms and knots - most persistent (chronic) pain conditions are associated with muscle spasms. According to leading pain expert, Dr Pradeep Chopra, these muscle spasms are more painful than the original pain. Muscle spasms or muscle knots develop to compensate for unbalanced forces from the joints .
- A feeling akin to having gnawing toothache within single or multiple joints of the body.
- Diffuse pain all over - patients often state 'I just hurt.'
- Fibromyalgia type pain (EDS Support UK).
- Complex regional pain syndrome (see page 53) a co-morbidity of patients with hEDS, and HSD (Castori M et al 2012a).

It is apparent that the sensory experience of pain, both in those with hEDS and in the population in general, cannot be separated from an individual's emotional experiences (Turk D.C.1983). Pain is, therefore, considered a subjective experience, primarily involving the senses, but also involving emotions, thoughts and behaviours. (Winteroud C. 2003)

'If pain truly has a subjective component, then perhaps the best definition of pain is what patients tell us it is!' (Winteroud C., Beck T. and Gruener D. 2003)

Dr Alan Hakim explains:

'Pain is something we feel. Even if it has a physical cause, as it undoubtedly has in the JHS/EDS-H [hEDS and HSD], it is still a subjective experience. It is often accompanied by an intense sense of exhaustion. The severity of the pain we feel is greatly influenced by our state of mind. If we are upset or agitated it tends to increase. If we are content, relaxed or just happy it tends to diminish to some degree. Those with JHS/EDS-H [hEDS or HSD] are often in the former category, and for good reason - lack of understanding of the condition[s] is widespread, and this, coupled with failure to receive adequate treatment for relief of symptoms, leads to frustration, resentment, anger (and lots more emotions which I could list but readers know them all only too well!) and, ultimately depression.'

Communicating about pain

Like many with chronic pain conditions, patients with hEDS, and HSD, often find it difficult to express their experience of pain.

'Because each person's pain is unique with different underlying causes, effective communication is crucial to achieving proper pain management. Yet many patients and their healthcare professionals encounter barriers that interfere with open and honest dialogue, such as difficulty in finding the right words to describe pain and limited time during medical appointments.'
(Partners Against Pain)

When asked about their pain levels, patients may not give their *actual* level of pain because their pain is chronic, and they are, therefore, *used to a certain level of pain*, and have grown to accept that as 'normal' for them. But remember, the word 'normal' in this situation does not mean 'fine', in the way that it might when describing the results of an X-ray. In this instance, it means 'usual / common'; it means '*this is what I put up with on a daily basis*'.

When asked to rate their pain using a traditional pain scale chart, someone who has chronic pain will often struggle to pinpoint the correct level and may only give you a correct pain level when:

- they have some form of acute pain,
- their 'normal' level of pain, which they live with daily, changes,
- they experience pain that now feels different (i.e., 'burning' instead of 'aching', 'shooting' instead of 'throbbing'),
- they are asked directly about their current levels of both acute and chronic pain.
  (Chronic Pain AU)

Managing pain

In addition to medication (see Chapter 3, page 148, a variety of techniques are now used to help manage persistent pain, which may provide significant benefits. These include physiotherapy,

WIDESPREAD SYMPTOMS & COMORBIDITIES

Different types of pain scale chart

Pain charts that offer descriptive option choices (see **B**) are becoming more widely used as they may help elicit more reliable responses than the traditional, purely numerical models (see **A**):

A

B

pain management classes, and behavioural and complementary therapies, all of which can help equip patients with long-term coping strategies to live better with their pain. The topic of pain management is discussed in more depth in Chapter 3, page 151-153.

© Understanding hEDS and HSD by C. Smith

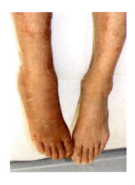

Complex regional pain syndrome

Complex regional pain syndrome (CRPS), also known as reflex sympathetic dystrophy, is ranked as the most painful form of chronic pain that exists today by the McGill Pain Index.

CRPS is a disorder of a body region, usually affecting an arm, leg, hand or foot. It frequently begins following an injury such as a bone break or sprain, or after surgery, and the area of pain is normally larger than the primary injury.

Symptoms
Signs and symptoms of complex regional pain syndrome can include:

- Constant pain is often felt even at rest, with intermittent exacerbations.
- Continuous burning or throbbing pain.
- Pain or sensitivity even to light touch.
- Sensitivity to cold.
- Range of motion may be limited.
- Changes in skin temperature - at times the skin may be cold; at other times it may be sweaty.
- Edema (swelling) of the painful area.
- Changes in skin colour, ranging from white and mottled to red or blue.
- In some, there may be trophic changes to the limb such as changes in skin texture (which may become tender, thin or shiny in the affected area), rapid or coarser hair growth, distorted or rapid nail growth.
- Joint stiffness, swelling and damage.
- Muscle spasms, weakness.
- Atrophy (muscle loss).

Symptoms may change over time and vary from person to person and, as with many chronic pain conditions, may be worsened by emotional stress.

Most commonly, pain, swelling, redness, and noticeable changes in temperature and hypersensitivity occur first. Over time, the affected limb can become cold and pale and undergo skin and nail changes as well as muscle spasms and tightening.

Individuals with CRPS show signs of peripheral nerve abnormalities, which involve the small nerve fibres that carry pain signals and messages to blood vessels. It is thought that these small nerve fibres become injured in some way, triggering the pain and other different manifestations seen in CRPS. The nerve fibres also appear to become hyperactive, secreting molecules that are thought to contribute to blood vessel abnormalities and inflammation.

Swelling is common in the affected limb, caused by dilation or leakage of blood vessels (Eorthopod.com). Underlying tissues and muscles can receive insufficient nutrients and oxygen, which can cause pain in the joints and muscles. At times, instead of dilating, the blood vessels may constrict tightly causing the skin to become cold, white, or bluish in colour (1/Mayoclinic.org).

The tissues of some people with CRPS have been found to contain high levels of inflammatory chemicals called cytokines, which indicates that the immune system can also be affected by CRPS (Alexander G.M. 2012).

CRPS may occasionally spread from its source to elsewhere in the body, such as to the opposite limb. In rare cases it can spread to areas such as the trunk, spine, abdomen and perineum (Chopra P. 2013a / Schwartzman R.J. 2009). In some people, signs and symptoms go away on their own. In others, signs and symptoms may persist for months to years, or become permanent.

CRPS and hEDS/HSD
CRPS has been described as a complication of both the hypermobility and classic forms of EDS (Stoler J.M. & Oaklander A. 2006 / Castori M. 2012 / Goldschneider K. 2013) and at some levels, seems to share similar features such as the potential for systemic autonomic dysfunction; musculoskeletal, endocrine, or dermatological manifestations; and changes in urological or gastrointestinal function (Schwartzman R.J. 2012). It has also been linked to Mast cell activation syndrome (MCAS); another comorbidity of those with hEDS, and HSD, with a study from the Netherlands showing significant levels of tryptase (contained in mast cells) in the involved extremity. The study concluded that mast cells are involved in the inflammatory reactions (possibly including

WIDESPREAD SYMPTOMS & COMORBIDITIES

central sensitisation) in CRPS Type 1 (Huygen F.J. 2004).

Contributing factors to CRPS in those with hEDS, and HSD, are thought to be one or more of the following:

- Stretch injury to the nerves that traverse hypermobile joints, increasing fragility of nerve connective tissue.
- Nerve trauma from more frequent surgery.
- Possible fragility of nerve connective tissue which may render them less able to protect the axons (the long thread-like parts of a nerve cell along which impulses are conducted from the cell body to other cells) within from trauma (Rothblum K. et al 2004 / Stoler J.M. 2006).

It is recommend that physicians caring for CRPS patients consider the possibility of an underlying disorder of the connective tissue (such as hypermobility spectrum disorders, Ehlers-Danlos syndrome, Marfan syndrome etc.) in patients with histories or examinations revealing joint laxity (Stoler J.M. 2006). Further studies are needed into the association of this condition with those who are hypermobile.

Diagnosis

A diagnosis of CRPS usually requires the presence of regional pain and a history of sensory changes following an injury or trauma to the limb. The pain is of a severity greater than that expected of the injury that triggered it and is often associated with such findings as abnormal skin colour, temperature change, abnormal sudomotor activity, or edema (Uptodate.com)

Two types of CRPS have been recognised:

- Type I (the form also known as reflex sympathetic dystrophy) corresponds with patients with CRPS without a definable nerve lesion and represents about 90 percent of clinical presentations.

- Type II was formerly termed causalgia and refers to cases in which a definable nerve lesion is present.

Treatment

In the initial states of CRPS, it is the nerves that are affected but, without early intervention, the problem very quickly moves from the nerves into the surrounding Glia cells that constitute 70-80% of all cells in the central nervous system and immune system. When these Glia Cells are activated, they release inflammatory chemicals in the affected limb and, at that stage, nerve desensitisation medications become ineffective. Consequently, alternative treatment, which can reach the Glia cells, may need to be considered. When treatment is given early enough, improvement and even remission are possible for some, but there is no specific cure for CRPS (1/mayoclinic.org).

Treatment centres around relieving the painful symptoms and restoring as much function and quality of life as possible. Therapists use a variety of techniques to do this, of which physiotherapy is probably the single most important. Other widely used techniques include mirror image therapy desensitisation practice, relaxation, stress management and body perception awareness therapy. Most will begin very gently to avoid a flare-up of symptoms, and need to be gradually built up in duration and intensity, even if progress seems slow at times. Several different classes of medication, including some types of tricyclic antidepressants and anticonvulsants, have been shown to be effective for CRPS, particularly when used early in the course of the disease (14/ www.nhs.uk).

Image attribution:
Page 53: Timsong311 2013
Page 54: Golan Levin, Creative Commons Licence

© Understanding hEDS and HSD by C. Smith

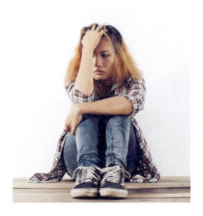

Fatigue

Fatigue associated with both hEDS and HSD appears to fall into two main categories:

- that which is caused by early muscle fatigue
- that which is more akin to the symptoms found in conditions such as systemic exertion intolerance disease (previously known as chronic fatigue syndrome) and fibromyalgia. Known in hEDS and HSD as 'Persistent Fatigue.'

Early muscle fatigue

In those with hEDS, and HSD, it is thought that the collagen-related areas of the body, such as the tendons, are repeatedly stretched beyond their capabilities, causing micro-traumas to occur. It is hypothesized that these plentiful, reoccurring, micro-injuries, which can only be seen using high resolution MRIs, don't have the opportunity to successfully heal, thus causing pain degeneration and physical fatigue (Francomano C. 2011, Järvinen M. et al 1997, Cheung J.P. 2010, Rees J.D. 2006).

When sufficient support and structure is not provided by the ligaments, the muscles are forced to compensate by taking on part, or all, of the work. Unless the body's muscular system is strong, it is likely that a person with hEDS or HSD will struggle to control the hypermobility of their joints (Hows J. 2000). The increase in workload and strain will cause the muscles to fatigue far more easily and more quickly than those in someone who is not hypermobile, leading to an overall feeling of weakness and fatigue. There is some evidence to suggest that the muscles of those with hEDS, and HSD, have to work harder and use a different strategy to stabilise the joints than those of non-hypermobile people, just to achieve the same tasks. In a condition where functional deconditioning due to injury, hospitalisations and chronic fatigue is common, it is vital that an appropriately graded exercise programme is introduced as part of a long-term management plan (see Chapter 3, pages 136-138).

Persistent fatigue

The exact cause of persistent (chronic) fatigue in hEDs and HSD is not fully understood. It is, however, recognised to have a more prominent association with hEDS than with Ehlers-Danlos syndrome classical type (Tinkle, B. 2010). Another condition which is more prominent in the hypermobile type than the classical type is autonomic dysfunction, such as orthostatic intolerance and postural orthostatic tachycardia syndrome. This increased prevalence of autonomic dysfunction may provide clues as to some of the symptoms of fatigue in hEDS, and HSD. More information on postural orthostatic tachycardia can be found in later in this chapter (page 69), and in Chapter 3, page 142).

> 'A careful search for hypermobility and connective tissue abnormalities should be part of the evaluation of patients with system exertion intolerance disease (also known as chronic fatigue syndrome and orthostatic intolerance syndromes).'
> (Rowe P.C. 1999).

Persistent fatigue is often felt as both physical and mental fatigue, like wading through treacle, and is said to be overwhelming, or to be like no other type of fatigue. It can vary in its severity (from mild to moderate) on a daily, weekly or monthly basis and can affect every aspect of daily life (Wicks D. 2015). It can come on without warning and prevent plans from being able to be carried out. It is not fully alleviated by rest or sleep and is not due to, or like, tiredness following over-exertion. It is not due to muscle weakness (although the individual may feel weak) and is not linked to a loss of motivation or pleasure which occurs in people who are depressed. The physical and mental effects can feel overwhelming (2/ Patient.co.uk).

> '(Those affected) report difficulties with simple everyday tasks such as brushing hair, washing their face or lifting a kettle. They may experience exhaustion after having a shower and feel overwhelmed by the idea of planning, preparing and cooking a simple meal.
>
> It is not necessarily just a physical experience. Concentration is a huge problem for people with severe persistent fatigue. Many people describe it

as 'brain fog'. A person can struggle to stay focused, to participate in a conversation or follow simple instructions. Persistent fatigue can also influence a person's ability to recall information (ARC, 2014).

The fatigue impacts not just on one's ability to self-care but also on your ability to maintain relationships, a social life, attend school, or go to work (Wicks D. HMSA 2015).

Fatigue versus persistent (chronic) fatigue

Fatigue:
- Being overtired
- Temporary
- Usually has an identifiable cause and remedy
- Not the same as sleepiness
- May be physical and/or mental

Persistent (chronic) Fatigue:
- Lasts longer and is more profound
- Constant
- Develops over time
- Diminishes your energy and mental capacity
- Impacts emotional and psychological well-being

Source: Ehlers-Danlos National Foundation Conference - August 2013 - Dr A Pocinki

---

Autonomic dysfunction and fatigue

The autonomic nervous system regulates all body processes that occur automatically, such as heart rate, blood pressure, breathing and digestion. It is believed that much of the cardiovascular autonomic dysfunction seen in hEDS, and HSD may stem from increased venous pooling (too much blood collecting in over-stretched veins) instead of being pumped back to the heart, which leads to many symptoms including fatigue. Although research on this is scarce, this would seem a plausible mechanism (Schondorf R. et al.1999 / Hakim A.J. 2017a). The body reacts to the venus pooling by releasing adrenaline (also called epinephrine), a hormone secreted by the adrenal glands, in order to force the blood up to the heart. Once released adrenaline produces a variety of effects on the body, including increased heart rate; a symptom frequently described both by those with hEDS and HSD, and

WIDESPREAD SYMPTOMS & COMORBIDITIES

cardiovascular autonomic dysfunction (Hakim A.J. et al 2017a). Unfortunately, the more tired a person becomes, the more adrenaline the body makes in order to keep going. Dr Pocinki explains:

'If you get too tired, your body responds by making more adrenaline, so you keep going, not realising how tired you really are. It appears that as you get more and more run down, your body gets more sensitive to adrenaline, so the small amount you have left can produce the same response a larger amount used to, so you still don't feel tired even when you are. Even when you do feel tired, you may continue to "push through" the fatigue, collapsing when the adrenaline wears off. Years of not feeling, ignoring, or pushing through fatigue may be one factor in the development of illnesses like chronic fatigue syndrome' (Pocinki A.G. 2010).'

The subject of cardiovascular autonomic dysfunction and the processes believed to be involved in hEDS, and HSD, are discussed in detail on page 136.

Sleep problems

Hypermobile people often struggle to sleep due to the pain they experience and/or an inability to get, or stay, comfortable. Appropriate pain medication at bedtime may need to be considered, in order to achieve a restful night's sleep. Stimulated adrenaline caused by anxiety, stress, pain and autonomic dysfunction can also have a detrimental effect on sleep. Writing on this subject, Dr Alan Pocinki says:

'If they (people with hEDS or HSD) are able to fall asleep, they may continue to make too much adrenaline overnight, giving them a shallow, dream-filled sleep, so that they wake feeling unrefreshed. Pain further stimulates adrenaline, making restful sleep even more difficult. When studied in the sleep lab, they often have a relative and sometimes complete lack of deep sleep, and/or an increased number of sleep-disrupting "arousals." Poor sleep can cause irritability and fatigue, which in turn can trigger more adrenaline (to try to overcome the fatigue), which in turn can make sleep worse. This vicious cycle can eventually cause serious disability.' (Pocinki A.G. 2010)

According to Dr Pocinki, data, collected from heart-rate-monitoring, lends weight to this theory. Results showed increased fluctuations and occasional sudden increases in heart rate that correspond with arousals and awakenings in patients. He has also observed that medication to block or offset extra adrenaline help many patients get a better night sleep.

Authors of the 2012 study, 'Prevalence of sleep disorders in Ehlers-Danlos syndrome', found that the most frequent complaints revolved around the difficulties of actually maintaining sleep, with pain and anxiety likely influencing sleep disturbance. They concluded that insomnia should be considered as a criteria symptom amongst patients with hypermobility type EDS. Sleep disturbing restless leg syndrome also seems to be more frequent (see Page 111) in those with hEDS, and HSD. (Metlaine A. 2012)

Practicing good sleep hygiene techniques may be beneficial for those experiencing fatigue associated with sleep disturbance. These techniques are discussed in Chapter 3, page 154 - 155.

Overview

Fatigue can occur as a result of multiple factors including dysautonomia, muscle weakness, micro-injuries, traumatic injuries (dislocations etc), poor sleep, insomnia, over use of (or side affects from) analgesics, malabsorption in the intestines, and reactive depression/anxiety, many of which are frequently found in those with hEDS, and HSD. It is also important to remember, however, that having hEDS or HSD does not exclude a person from having other unassociated medical complaints, the possibility of which should be ruled out before assuming that fatigue is caused by hEDS or HSD (see box below) (Wicks D. HMSA 2015).

Please note: It is important that all other differential diagnosis be excluded or investigated further if thought to be present, before diagnosing persistent fatigue associated with EDS or HSD:

- Chronic infection (e.g., hepatitis, tuberculosis, brucellosis, endocarditis, Lyme disease).
- Endocrine disorders (e.g, diabetes, thyroid disease, adrenal insufficiency).
- Autoimmune inflammatory conditions (e.g., joints, skin, bowel, liver, and renal disorders).
- Cardiorespiratory disease.
- Sleep disordered breathing.
- Neurological disorders (e.g., myasthenia gravis, multiple sclerosis).

(Hakim A.J. et al 2017b)

Proprioceptive Dysfunction

What is proprioception?

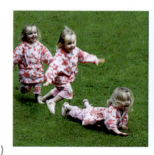

'Proprioception is the term used to describe the body's ability to transmit a sense of position, analyse that information and react (consciously or unconsciously) to the stimulation with the proper movement' (Houglum P. A. 2001 / Tarrant M.L. 2003).

Many structures of the body have specific receptors that supply the brain with sensory information. This 'proprioceptive feedback' is used by the body's central nervous system to understand the position and movement of the body and limbs and lets us know when and how far we stretch our muscles. It allows us to process information from special receptors in the skin, joints, muscles, tendons and connective tissues, which sense the body's position in space, and help us hold and maintain our postural muscles and responses, giving safety and stability during movement. In its most basic form, proprioception allows us to scratch our nose without needing to check where our nose is by looking in the mirror, or walk down a staircase without having to look at each step.

What is proprioceptive dysfunction?

Proprioceptive dysfunction is the term used to describe problems with sensory proprioceptive feedback. Diminished responses to incoming sensory stimuli can have an effect on balance, fluency of movements, the body's ability to maintain and hold posture, or to walk through a doorway without bumping the sides, the ability to know how much pressure to apply when gripping objects or how much force will be needed to pick something up (Tarrant M.L. 2003). It affects motor planning - the body's natural ability to register, plan for and then perform a movement correctly and then be able to remember this feedback in order to adapt movements in the future.

What causes proprioceptive dysfunction?

Joint proprioceptive dysfunction is documented in a variety of musculoskeletal conditions including osteoarthritis, ligament and meniscal injuries, and individuals with increased hypermobility, such as those with Marfan or Ehlers-Danlos syndrome (Smith T.O. et al 2013).

In the general population, impairment of proprioception can arise as a result of medical conditions such as multiple sclerosis, epilepsy or migraine, through injury to, or overuse of, joints, and at times of rapid growth spurts (particularly during adolescence). It can also occur temporarily in those that gain new levels of flexibility, stretching and contortion, for example through dance training or yoga, until their bodies adjust.

Both children and the elderly are more prone to injuries during proprioception activities. In childhood and adolescence, the central nervous systems are not fully developed and information may not be relayed fast enough to provide the necessary protection against excessive body stresses. In older adults, the impulses that transmit vital information to and from the central nervous system tend to slow down and the onset of osteoarthritis may impair joint proprioception further. Both groups may also be affected because they tend to have less muscular strength than adults (Tarrant M.L. 2003).

When a structure such as a ligament or muscle is injured, the proprioceptive sensory receptors may also be damaged. Receptors in the body's ligaments should inform the brain of a joint's position and the potential danger of it extending or rolling too far. In a split second the brain should then respond by contracting the appropriate muscles to bring the joint to a proper position. But, if that ligament lacks tensility due to defective collagen, the brain will not receive the normal sensory information it gets from the joint in the event that it starts to flex, hyperextend or roll. The result is that the body's joints not only lack fully supportive ligaments, but also have a proprioceptive deficit, making it more likely that injuries will occur more easily, even while just carrying out routine daily tasks (footjax.com).

It is perhaps not surprising then, that those with conditions such as hEDS or HSD, whose connective tissue lacks tensility, and whose feedback-producing tissues (that surround the joints, tendons, ligaments, muscle, fascia and blood vessels) stretch every time a joint slips or dislocates, should be affected by proprioceptive dysfunction. Limited research is available, but in 2013, Smith et al carried out a systematic review and metanalysis to try and

WIDESPREAD SYMPTOMS & COMORBIDITIES

establish whether those with HSD have reduced joint proprioception. They found that those with HSD showed significantly poorer lower limb joint position sense and threshold detection to movement than those without HSD. The evidence relating to upper limb proprioceptive difference was less clear, with no difference shown between the cohorts for shoulder positioning sense, but a statistically significant difference in finger joint position sense was found (Smith T.O. et al 2013).

It is thought that when a limb moves beyond the normal range of motion, proprioception is affected and the brain may momentarily lose a sense of where the limb is in relation to the body. Even a slight, or momentary, lack in proprioceptive feedback could trigger subluxations, dislocations (Hefti F. 2007), instability and falls. This 'reduced sensory feedback' may also lead to biomechanically unsound limb positions being adopted, mechanical stress, poor posture (Clayton H.A. 2013), over-pronation of feet and ankles, muscles becoming overactive whilst others become under-active, causing pain and excessive strain on joints, and the increased potential for development of overuse injuries and muscle strains.

Early studies by researchers such as Hall et al (1995) gave rise to this hypothesis. They found that, within their study participants, adults with hEDS, and HSD, had reduced knee joint proprioceptive sensitivity at their 'end of joint movement range', compared to peers who weren't hypermobile. They hypothesized that this may contribute to recurrent joint injuries and instability.

Further investigation is still needed, however, to fully understand how proprioception is affected by range of movement in the joints, especially as a recent study by Pacey et al (2014), involving child participants, found that there was no significant difference between knee joint proprioceptive acuity, either in full hypermobile range or early flexion, when measured by a functional, active, weight-bearing test.

It is likely that various contributing factors are actually at play, such as:

- the effect of reduced mobility due to lifestyle, injury or surgery - evidence currently suggests that proprioceptive acuity is use-dependent (Muaidi Q.I. et al 2009).

- the involvement of kinesiophobia (a well documented disorder in physiotherapy, where a person believes that movement can cause more injury and pain) See Chapter 3, page 142.
- in the knees; the role of the hamstrings in knee extension control - stretching of the hamstrings and quadriceps may diminish sensitivity to knee movement (Pacey V. et al 2013) Streepey J.W 2010).

Interestingly, a study by Clayton H.A. et al, in 2013, found that the degree to which the body is hypermobile is directly related to the overall degree of proprioceptive impairment. The study found that EDS patients showed significantly larger uncertainty ranges (i.e. less precision) at peripheral reference marker locations compared to control subjects. These uncertainty ranges significantly correlated with patients' Beighton scores, to the extent that those who were the most hypermobile were the least precise when estimating the position of their unseen hand.

Overall, it would seem that hypermobility in those with hEDS or HSD leads to mild impairments in proprioception, and the conclusion that the peripheral proprioceptive signals from the controlling muscles are disrupted by disturbances that interfere with their normal flow.

The effect of pain on proprioception

The brain's ability to process proprioceptive information can also be significantly reduced by pain. The pain signals distract the brain, crowding out other incoming sensory information. Pain also tends to make people reduce the amount of movement they carry out, which means the amount of proprioceptive feedback transmitted to the brain is also less, limiting the opportunity for reinforcement of the 'normal' sensory pathways that are necessary to establish good quality proprioception and co-ordination (Hargrave T. 2008).

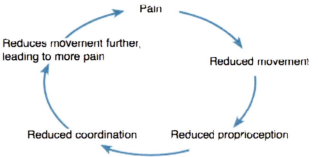

Proprioception and arthritis

It is hypothesized that defective proprioceptive mechanisms may be associated with acceleration of degenerative joint conditions such as osteoarthritis, and may account for the increased prevalence of such conditions seen in hEDS and HSD patients.

Some studies have suggested that reduced proprioception may be responsible for initiation or advancement of degeneration of joints (Hall M.G. 1995 / Koralewicz L.M. 2000). Others suggest that mechanisms such as laxity of the joint capsule and ligaments, and the release of lytic enzymes (triggered by inflammation) may damage the receptor end organs (specialised nerve endings devoted to detection of stimuli) within the joint capsule, decreasing proprioceptive perception (Barrett D.S. et al 1991). As yet, no studies have shown with certainty whether loss of joint position sense *'causes'* osteoarthritis or *'occurs as a consequence of it'* (Barrett D.S. et al 1991 / Kumar A. 2012).

Photo attribution (page 57) - Jamie Campbell - Creative Commons Licence

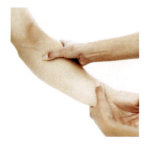

Muscle stiffness and tightness

We usually associate hypermobility with flexibility, but some hypermobile people may not present as particularly flexible, and may complain of stiffness and tightness. This is often because muscles are not working in an efficient way; they are, instead, having to work overtime to try to stabilise and support the joints, causing them to go into a state of extreme muscular tension.

Many people also find they wake in the morning with severe stiffness, which often takes until around mid-day to dissipate (Tinkle B. 2010). This can occur as a result of factors such as the amount or type of exercise a person has carried out the previous day, restless sleeping, or sleeping so heavily (possibly with the aid of medication) that their joints remain in one position for too long, or are relaxed into hypermobile range throughout the night.

Once a person has developed tight muscles, spasms and pain often follow, the brain anticipates that the muscle will go into spasm if moved too quickly and responds by slowing down movement to prevent this. 'The key is to release the muscles that are gripping, while training others to kick in for support' (Rotstein R. 2012). In combination with the appropriate strengthening physiotherapy, therapies known to be effective for the relief of stiff muscles such as gentle massage therapy and Pilates, may be of benefit to some individuals (see Chapter 3, page 157). Such manipulations may help to re-educate the brain to realise that, once appropriate strength has been regained, it is 'safe' to move freely and let go of protective muscular tension. These forms of therapy are only likely to be truly effective if the practitioner understands and addresses the underlying physical causes of muscle stiffness and tightness in hEDS and HSD.

When carrying out stretching exercises, it is important that we aim to lengthen our muscles and not our ligaments. Here 'Restorative Exercise Specialist' Jenni Rawlings, explains why:

> 'When muscles stretch, they return to their original length after the stretch is released - a tissue property called elasticity. But when ligaments stretch, they behave elastically during just the first tiny bit of the stretch, and if they're stretched beyond that point, they will permanently stay at that new length and are referred to as 'lax'. Lax ligaments can no longer stabilise our joints for us and are a source of chronic pain and injury for many people. Over stretching our ligaments is therefore decidedly uncool.' (Rawlings J. 2014)

(Please also see 'Chronic Neck Strain' on page 87).

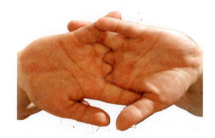

Habitual 'cracking' of joints

Many hypermobile people habitually 'crack' their joints, particularly those in their knuckles fingers and spine. The cracking noise heard is believed to be due to cavitation - the formation of an empty space within body tissue (Protopapas M.G.et al 2002). As a joint is stretched, the volume of the joint space increases slightly as the joint surfaces separate, which causes a drop in joint pressure resulting in the formation of a small bubble of CO_2 (DeWeber K. et al 2011). The action of 'cracking' the joint temporarily lengthens and stretches all of the soft tissue in the area (ligaments, muscles, and nerves), which accounts for the relief from stiffness or aching that may be felt.

It typically takes at least 15 minutes for the joint to be able to be cracked again due to the time required for the microscopic bubbles to fully dissolve into solution and for the joint space to retract back to its resting position (Unsworth A. et al, 1971). The amount of force required to crack a knuckle has been shown in in-vitro studies to exceed the energy threshold that can lead to articular cartilage damage (Watson P. et al 1989) and it would, therefore, seem logical to theorise that habitual joint cracking might lead to gradual thinning of articular cartilage and eventual clinical osteoarthritis. However, this claim remains unsubstantiated in medical literature. Adverse effects of joint cracking were cited in 1990 by Castellanos et al, when their study revealed that habitual knuckle crackers did show signs of some damage, including soft tissue damage in the joint capsule and a decrease in grip strength. However, it is now thought that the damage described most likely arose as a result of the rapid and repeated stretching of the ligaments surrounding the joint. Most studies find that habitual 'cracking' of joints is usually harmless to the joint (Protopapas M. et al 2002). This view has been further established in a more recent study, by DeWebber 2011, which concluded that a history of habitual knuckle 'cracking' did not seem to be a risk factor for hand osteoarthritis.

It should be noted, however, that when an individual experiences involuntary joint clicking combined with grinding or crunching, or accompanied by pain and/or swelling, it can be a sign that conditions representing a more serious joint status, such as crepitus or degenerated cartilage from osteoarthritis are involved (healthline.com), and the appropriate investigations should be carried out.

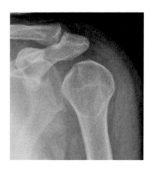

Frequent dislocations or subluxations

Joint dislocations occur when the normal alignment of a joint is separated abnormally. The term subluxation describes an incomplete or partial dislocation of a joint. In those with hEDS or HSD, either can happen with or without trauma, and sometimes occur spontaneously. Research carried out into the manifestations of hEDS, by Marcos Castori et al, found 85.7% of 21 patients formally assessed as having hEDS, suffered frequent dislocations. The ankles and temporomandibular joints were found to be the most commonly dislocated joints.

Dislocations and subluxations in hEDS and HSD are usually linked to an abnormality in the shape of the joints, ligament looseness (laxity), and muscle tension (Mehta N.R. 2013). A dislocated joint will need to be moved back into place. Some people with hEDS or HSD may be able to put their joints back into place themselves, but some experience profound dislocations and are unable to do so, instead requiring frequent medical intervention. General recommendation would be that you should always seek medical attention if you have dislocated a joint (2/Mayo Clinic 2015).

Other than the ankles and temporomandibular joints, other common dislocations and subluxation sites include the knees, elbows, shoulders, fingers, wrists and hips (Castori 2010) and so-called 'pulled-elbow' which is actually a subluxation of the radial head from the annular ligament (Kaplan R.E et al 2001).

Areas which many clinicians would think were 'very unlikely' or 'impossible' to dislocate, are frequently mentioned by those with hEDS/HSD, for example, wrists that dislocate and vertebrae that sublux. Rib subluxations are also often described (including those that move out of position from front to back as well as inwards and outwards - inspire.com/EDNF), but there is still a surprising lack of scientific evidence supporting the existence of such a phenomenon. Whilst ribs are not generally thought of as 'joints', they rely on the same problematic ligaments, tendons and cartilage that affect other areas of the body, so it may be feasible that they can be affected in the same way. Please note, each area of the body mentioned in this section is discussed in more detail later in this chapter.

Osteoarthritis

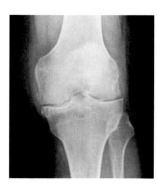

Recurrent injury or abnormal wear and tear of joints caused by impaired proprioception and chronic joint instability, might contribute toward the development of osteoarthritis. One epidemiological study in rheumatology clinics evaluated 130 consecutive new patients with joint hypermobility (Bridges A.J. et al 1992). They found that musculoskeletal problems were the main reason for referral, and there was a statistically significant association between widespread joint hypermobility and osteoarthritis, supporting the hypothesis that joint hypermobility predisposes those affected to musculoskeletal disorders (particularly osteoarthritis) (Bridges A.J. et al 1992 / Beighton P. 2012). However, there is currently no hard evidence to confirm this data, and further clarification is required to establish whether joint hypermobility is a significant risk factor in the development of osteoarthritis.

Those with hEDS or HSD who do develop osteoarthritis at a younger age than normally seen have typically overworked these joints very hard and for a long time e.g. through dance, gymnastics, manual labour etc. Unbeknown to them, their inherent joint laxity/instability may have resulted in increased stress on the joints from a very early age (Hakim A.J Clinician's Guide to JHS 2013c).

Osteoarthritis typically presents as stiffness and aching pain in the joints, which is often made worse by resistance and/or highly repetitive activity.

Osteopenia

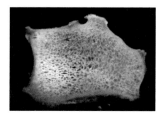

Osteopenia is the name given to low bone density. Bone density is a measurement of how strong and dense the bones are. Reduction in bone density occurs naturally in many people as they reach and pass middle-age. This is because existing bone cells start to be reabsorbed into the body quicker than new bone can be made. However, in some individuals, bone density reduces to levels that warrant a diagnosis of osteopenia. A diagnosis of osteopenia means there is a greater risk that, as the person ages, they may develop osteoporosis (bone density that is very low compared to normal at that age).

Osteopenia is not one of the principle features of EDS and was not listed in early reports, but it would seem from studies such as those carried out by Coelho P. (1994), Deodhar A. (1994), Dolan A. (1998) and Theodorou S. (2012), that bone density may be reduced in those with EDS. Any increased risk of osteopenia in EDS is likely to involve a number of factors, including: an inheritance of a hereditary defect of the connective tissue that may lead to weakened bone structure, the bone density reducing effects of extensive periods of reduced mobility or reduced exercise due to pain and/or fatigue, and reduced exposure to sunlight (due to confinement) which is needed for the production of vitamin D (Dolan A.L. 1998 / Castori M. 2012). The influence of exercise-induced loading on the development of bone mass has been shown to be at its optimum in early puberty which is, for many with hEDS, and HSD, exactly the time when mobility-reducing symptoms such as pain, fatigue and dislocations first appear (Janz K.F. 2010 / Gunter K.B. 2012).

Unfortunately, the small sample sizes, and a possible bias in referral and selection for these studies, limited the interpretation of their findings. There is, however, an awareness that those with osteopenia in childhood may be at greater risk for adult-onset osteoporosis as they enter adulthood with a lower bone mass than would otherwise be anticipated (Colì G. 2013), and it is hoped that more research will be carried out into the association between genetic disorders and osteopenia in the near future.

Osteoporosis

If the early signs of bone loss seen in osteopenia worsen (see previous column) it may progress to become osteoporosis, where the reduction in bone mass is so significant that it leads to increased risk of fractures. Work by Coelho P.C et al (1994) appears to demonstrate that where osteoporosis is found in those with EDS, the cancellous bone found in the vertebrae in the spinal column is more likely to be affected than other areas in the body.

As with osteopenia, research into a potential link between osteoporosis and hEDS has been limited. To date, the few, relatively small studies that have taken place have usually concentrated predominantly on EDS classical type and/or have provided contradictory evidence. For example, Gulbahar et al's (2006) research into JHS [HSD] and osteoporosis reported bone density reduction among pre-menopausal women with HSD, whereas six years earlier, Carbone et al found no difference in bone density between women with hypermobile EDS compared to age and sex matched controls.

Writing for Ehlers-Danlos Support UK, Dr Atul Deodhar says that *'theoretically, we can postulate that some forms of EDS with type 1 collagen defects could be associated with osteoporosis* [NB/ the collagen type linked with hEDS is a yet unknown]'. He goes on to explain that in another, closely related heritable disorder of connective tissue, called Osteogenesis Imperfecta (OI), osteoporosis has been associated with defects in the structure or synthesis of type 1 collagen and he states: '*In some types of EDS, defects at the molecular level have been identified and include similar abnormalities [as seen in OI] in the synthesis and processing of types 1 and 3 collagens.*' (7/EDS Support UK).

Image attribution: Pages 61 & 62
(shoulder): Hellerhoff - Creative Commons Licence
(osteoarthritis) by Pexels.com
(osteopenia): wardel - Creative Commons Licence

Skin Involvement

While one of the 'characteristics' of the hypermobile type of EDS is considered by many to be the *'lack'* of observable features in the skin, it is actually a common sites of mild abnormalities which, when recognised by medical professionals, and put together with the myriad of additional features of hEDS, can aid early diagnosis and management of potentially dis-abling complications in the future (Castori M. 2012). Observable features of the skin are discussed below.

Slow wound healing / scarring

The skin is more fragile in hEDS than normal, but much less so than in the other types of EDS (Tinkle et al 2017). A history of slow wound healing is a feature (Ainsworth and Aulicinio 1993, Tinkle B. 2010, Castori M 2012), with minor healing defects and capillary fragility being the most frequently reported. Healing defects may present as mildly atrophic, nonpapyraceous, wider or more sunken scaring scars, compared to the hemosiderotic and/or papyraceous cigarette-paper' scars

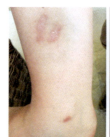
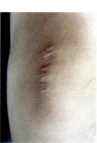
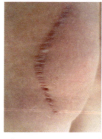
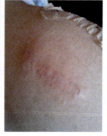

Above images - examples of scars in an individual with hEDS

observed in other EDSs (Castori M. 2012 / Tinkle B. et al 2017). It is thought these defects may form as a combined result of minimally delayed wound repair and fragility of the skin at areas of the body exposed to repeated traumas, for example the elbows and knees. When considering surgery in those with hEDS, often no changes in treatment are necessary, but larger wounds may need more support such as different stitches (Tinkle 2010). See Chapter 3, page 165 'Surgical issues'.

Easy bruising

In EDS, the term 'easy bruising' relates to the breakage of blood vessels under the skin that then leak, forming dark patches of discolouration either spontaneously, or with little (or no) apparent cause. This feature is seen in varying degrees of severity in all subtypes of EDS and bruising tendencies in the hypermobility type are present but quite variable in severity (EDNF.org). Adib N. (2005) and Ainsworth S.R. (1993), report that up to 75% of patients with hEDS self-reported easy bruising, but that excessive bruising is usually considered more consistent with the classical type of EDS.

The easy bruising seen in EDS is caused by capillary fragility, resulting from defects in the structural integrity of skin and blood vessels. (Anstey A. 1991). It has been hypothesized, in other disorders of connective tissue, that bruising may be caused by the blood platelets failing to interact adequately with the abnormal collagen in the walls of the blood vessels (Åström E. 2011).

In children with EDS, excessive bruising is often the first symptom noticed by medical professionals. If pronounced, it can be confused with a malignancy, a disease of the blood, or even suspected to be the result of child abuse (De Paepe A. 2004). In order to distinguish between a heritable disorder of connective tissue and other causes of bruising, it is therefore very important that careful evaluation of the medical and family history, and rigorous clinical examination for subtle skin features of EDS, are carried out (De Paepe A. 2004).

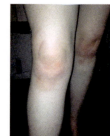

Bruising in an individual with hEDS

Texture of the skin

Evaluation of skin signs in EDS are best carried out by somebody who is familiar with heritable disorders of connective tissue (B. Tinkle 2010), and this is particularly the case when looking at the texture and hyperextensibility of the skin.

The texture of the skin in those with hEDS is generally described as soft and smooth with only mild hyperextensibility compared to classical EDS (Castori M. 2012). The abnormal underlying connective tissue structure may also lead to skin being described as 'doughy', or '*skin you love to touch*' (EDNF.org / Tinkle B. 2010), but there is little diagnostic information available to measure these descriptions against, meaning it can be very subjective. For example, one clinician's perception of 'soft' skin could be very different from another's; it is down to their discretion. Even experts can disagree, as seen when considering Beighton's 1998 study - he describes the skin of those with hEDS as smooth and '*velvety*', compared to Susan Pauker's findings in 2014, where she describes the skin in those with hEDS as soft and smooth but says it should *not* be described as 'velvety.'

Skin hyperextensibility

Hyperextensibility is defined as 'skin that can be stretched beyond normal limits and immediately return to its original state without forming transient redundant folds' (Castori M. 2012). In the hypermobility type of EDS, only mild hyperextensibility is evident, if present at all (Pauker S.P. et al 2014). As is the case with the evaluation of skin 'texture' in hEDS, skin 'extensibility' evaluation is largely left to a practitioner's experience as there is a lack of standardised methodology. Skin hyperextensibility should be tested at a site that is not subjected to mechanical forces or scarring, such as the mid-forearm (Tinkle B. 2012). It is measured by pulling up the skin until resistance is felt. Where there is even limited hyperextensibility, the skin should extend easily and snap back after release (De Paepe A. 2004).

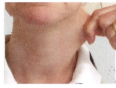
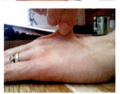
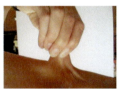
Mild skin hyperextensibility in and individual with hEDS

Stretch marks

Stretch marks (striae), often appear between the ages of 11 and 13 years when adolescent growth begins. In the general population, striae are typically found on the hips, thighs, abdomen and buttocks, with females having a tendency to develop them around the breasts, and males having a tendency to develop them toward the low back, arm pits, upper arms and low back. In hEDS however, stretch marks can appear from an early age and at less commonly affected areas such as the elbows, chest, under the arms, and on the inner thigh (Hakim A.J 2013g / Castori M. 2012).

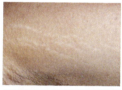
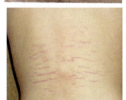
Striae (stretch marks) underarm and lower back

The layer of skin beneath the epidermis consists of connective tissue and cushions the body from stress and strain. Impaired stiffness of this dermal layer, caused by defective collagen fibrils, can allow stretch marks to develop. It is seen to varying degrees of severity in EDS, and to a lesser extent in Marfan syndrome.

Varicose Veins

Varicose veins develop when the small valves inside the veins stop working efficiently. In a healthy vein, the blood is prevented from flowing backwards by a series of small valves that open and close to let blood through. When weakened or damaged, the blood in these valves is able to flow backwards and can collect in the vein, which eventually causes it to swell and become varicose (NHS.uk). Dark purple or blue in colour, they can look bulging, lumpy, or twisted and, although any vein can become varicose, they are most commonly found in the legs (1/Arthritis Research UK). Symptoms may include:
dull aching, uncomfortable, heavy feeling legs, muscle cramps, and swelling in the ankles and feet.

Certain things may increase your chances of developing varicose veins, such as pregnancy, weight gain and ageing, but those with a disorder of the connective tissue may also be predisposed to weaker valves due to the structural make up of their collagen (Andreotti L. & Cammelli D. 1979 Chello M. 1994)

Keratosis pilaris

Keratosis pilaris seems more common in hEDS, but no systematic study assessing such an association has been carried out. It is considered a common and harmless condition where the skin becomes rough and bumpy, as if covered in permanent goose pimples. It primarily affects the back of the upper arms, and sometimes the buttocks and front of the thighs. Less often, the forearms and upper back may be affected.

There's no cure for keratosis pilaris, but there are things that can be done to improve the rash, such as using soap-free cleansers and gently exfoliating (removing dead skin cells from the surface of the skin). There's no real need to see a GP unless the condition is causing concern. It will usually improve with age and sometimes disappear completely in adulthood. There are also rare variants of keratosis pilaris which affect the eyebrows, face and scalp, or the entire body.

Piezogenic papules

Piezogenic papules may be seen in hEDS (Pauker S. P. et al 2014). They are small, fatty herniations caused by subcutaneous fat protruding through defects in the connective tissue of the layer of skin, called the dermis. They are most commonly found on the heels as well as the wrists and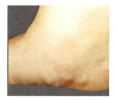
ulnar margins of the wrists (Castori M. 2012). Although Piezogenic papules are common in a healthy

population, the incidence is increased in disorders of the connective tissue such as Ehlers-Danlos syndrome (pcds.org.uk).

Perturbed perspiration

Perturbed perspiration means perspiration that is caused by an underlying disorder.

Many people with hEDS, and HSD, suffer from perturbed perspiration in form of:

- diaphoresis (sweating to an unusual degree as a symptom of disease or drug side-effect).
- hypohidrosis (diminished sweating in response to appropriate stimuli, which can lead symptoms such as elevated body temperature, heat exhaustion and heat stroke (Bravo J. & wolff C. 2006).

In the experience of Dr Marcos Castori, symptoms such as excessive sweating from the palms and soles is the most common presentation of exocrine dysregulation, which may relate to underlying dysautonomia, a common feature of those with hED, and HSD.

Local Anaesthetics

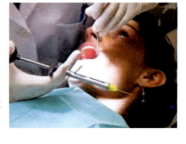

Some patients with hEDS, and HSD, report problems in obtaining sufficient relief from local anaesthetic and painkillers. They do not appear to experience the full anaesthetic affect of lidocaine injections when these are given for dental purposes and minor surgery, or for epidural anaesthesia (Hakim A.J. 2005 / Arendt-Neilsen L. 1990).

> '(In those with hEDS) *The present quantitative findings support clinical observations that long-lasting cutaneous* (skin) *analgesia is difficult to obtain for this group of patients.*' (Arendt-Neilsen L. 1990)

This finding is further bolstered by surveys carried out by the Hypermobility Syndromes Association, with one large survey finding that patients diagnosed with hypermobility spectrum disorders were three times more likely to report the poor effectiveness of local anaesthetic, compared to people without the condition. At the moment, the most reasonable hypothesis appears to be that the local anaesthetic solution diffuses away more rapidly from the microenvironment of the site of the injection because of the lax nature of the connective tissues. The same problem is reported by many in relation to topical analgesics such as EMLA cream and alternatives may need to be tried. Those undergoing epidural pain relief for surgery or childbirth (see page 104) may find they gain little or no benefit (Tinkle B. 2010. & 4/Hakim A. and Keer R. 2014). Many also find that painkillers, which would normally be expected to effectively stop pain, do not work well in people with hEDS or HSD. A patient should make their pain specialist or anaesthetist aware of any problems they may have had in the past.

Anaesthetic, and analgesic issues are also discussed in Chapter 1 (page 25), Chapter 2 (page 104) and Chapter 3 (page165).

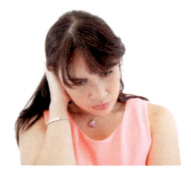

Anxiety

Anxiety can be experienced as a feeling of jittery shakiness which leaves an individual unable to relax. They may feel uneasy and restless and experience physical symptoms such as a fast heart rate, palpitations, nausea, tremor, dry mouth, sweating, headaches, chest pain, and fast breathing. When trying to calm themselves down, they may find they are unable to, which can cause anxiety levels to spiral out of control and may lead to panic attacks.

hEDS/HSD and anxiety

A significant association has been found between hEDS, HSD, and anxiety disorders, particularly panic disorder, agoraphobia and socialphobia in rheumatologic patients (Bulbena A. 1993, Bulbena A. 2011a, Hakim A. HMSA website, Bulbena A. et al 2017).

Of course, anxiety is normal in stressful situations and it is perhaps, to be expected that patients with chronic and/or complex conditions, such as hEDS or HSD are likely to experience feelings of anxiety, as

Photo attribution (this page):
David Castillo Dominici -FreeDigitalPhotos.net
Conor Lawless - creativecommons.org/licences

factors, such as the following, take their toll:

- Uncertainty about future health.
- Poor treatment by medical professionals who have little understanding of hEDS or HSD.
- Potential loss of earnings.
- Inability to plan because of unpredictable symptoms.

Sometimes, however, medical professionals can be too quick to assume that patients with hEDS or HSD are suffering from anxiety as a reaction to their circumstances, when instead, an underlying pathology is involved. Worse still, if the patient has yet to receive a diagnosis of hEDS or HSD, a doctor may jump to the conclusion that the anxiety a patient is displaying is *causing* their hEDS or HSD related symptoms, and an opportunity to diagnose the underlying disorder is then missed.

This latter assumption is easy to understand when considering a GP faced with a patient, who describes persistent fatigue, mysterious and persistent pain for which there is often no obvious cause, and a baffling array of other symptoms including rapid heart rate, sweating, and bowel dysfunction, all of which mimic those seen in generalised anxiety and/or depression. For the patient, it can lead to inappropriate medications being prescribed, their symptoms being dismissed as stress or hypochondria, and frustration that no one is listening.

Clearly, anxiety *can be* triggered by emotional stress, but it is important that medical professionals remember that many of the physical disorders associated with hEDS, and HSD, such as fatigue, pain, or dysautonomia are *also* potential causes of *anxiety-like* symptoms (Pocinki A. 2010). In such cases, patients need these underlying causes to be investigated and treated, rather than just being prescribed anti-anxiety medications.

'I have a right to be treated by medical professionals that do not solely focus on my psychiatric issues as being the source of my problems. EDS causes anxiety and depression, chronic pain causes anxiety and depression, POTS causes adrenaline rushes and tachycardia. It's all very complicated, and there are psychiatric issues, but they are symptoms of a bigger problem and should be treated as such. Don't dismiss me as anxious or depressed without treating my other problems too. (Quote: an_angel_with_wings - See more at: www.chronicpainpartners.com)

WIDESPREAD SYMPTOMS & COMORBIDITIES

Research going back as far as 1993, carried out by Bulbena A. et al, established that joint hypermobility syndrome (now known as hypermobility spectrum disorder - HSD) was found to be *16 times* more likely in patients with panic disorder than other patients - even after controlling for age and sex ([HSD] was found in 67.7% of patients with an anxiety-like disorder, but in only 10.1% of psychiatric and 12.5% of medical control subjects). Of the patients who suffered symptoms of anxiety, those who had HSD were younger and more often women, and had an earlier onset of the disorder than those without HSD.

Interestingly, although panic and anxiety-like symptoms were associated with HSD in this study (along with agoraphobia and simple phobia), neither depression or the more commonly seen form of anxiety in the general population, called generalised anxiety disorder (GAD), were. GAD is what many of us would associate with a diagnosis of anxiety; it is the ongoing, excessive, uncontrollable and often irrational worry or apprehensive expectation about events or activities. Although it is quite possible for someone to have separate diagnoses of both hEDS/HSD and GAD, it would seem that, for many with hEDS/HSD, it is the 'fight or flight' responses caused by underlying dysautonomia that are the cause of their anxiety-like symptoms (nausea, sweating, bowel problems, fatigue etc) rather than GAD.

'There is [now] *enough evidence showing that comorbidity of anxiety disorders and some medical conditions share a similar physiopathological mechanism mediated by the clinical features of joint hypermobility syndrome* [HSD]'. *(Bulbena 2011a)*

Unfortunately, this relationship between symptoms associated with anxiety disorders and hEDS/HSD, has since been neglected, despite subsequent studies confirming the findings (Gazit et al 2003 / Hakim A. 2004 / Eccles J. et al 2012 & 2015). This may be due, in part, to the fact that another finding in the same study, relating to Mitral Valve Prolapse, has not been replicated since, thus casting doubt on the remaining content.

Lines of research being explored in pursuit of a better understanding of anxiety and hEDS/HSD

It would seem that the links between hEDS/HSD and anxiety are far more complex than originally thought, and several lines of research are being explored in the pursuit of better understanding.

The first involves a branch of genetics concerned with the study of the structure and function of the cells and chromosones and considers the genetic predisposition to anxiety and the nature and extent of that contribution (Gratacos M. et al 2001 / García Campayo J. 2010 / Morris-Rosendahl D.J 2002 / Bulbena A. et al 2017) (see **1** below).

The second, and most well known, is looking into the significantly higher prevalence of autonomic nervous system symptoms (dysautonomia) in joint hypermobility patients as found by Gazit Y. 2003 (see **2** below).

The third involves findings which suggest that processes compromising function in neuro-developmental conditions may occur in individuals with hypermobility, seemingly enhancing their vulnerability to stress and anxiety (Eccles J. A.et al 2012) (see **3** below).

These three avenues are not clear-cut and, most likely, overlap in several areas. A brief explanation is give below:

1. Genetic predisposition

It has long been hypothesized that there is a common personality trait between both hEDS/HSD and anxiety since a predisposing disposition to feel stress, worry, and anxiety discomfort was found in subjects with hypermobility spectrum disorders in general population samples by Bulbena et al (Bulbena A. et al 2011a).

This hypothesis is supported by previous work carried out in 1998, when Martin-Santos M. et al., published the results of a series of family studies, revealing an unexpected comorbidity between panic disorder and benign joint laxity with hypermobility. They concluded that joint laxity is highly prevalent in patients with panic disorder, agoraphobia or both, and may reflect a 'disposition to suffer from anxiety'.

This group of geneticists found that, of the cohort studied, those patients who had both panic disorder and joint laxity had inherited a slightly longer arm of a chromosome known as chromosome 15, leading to three instead of two copies of about 60 genes in most cells. The patients came from families with multiple incidences of panic disorder and joint laxity, who had originally been recruited for a genome scan. Not only did the duplication segregate with panic/hypermobility spectrum disorders in the families, but also unrelated patients with panic disorder were much more likely to have the duplication.

The findings of this research by Martin-Santos et al was particularly interesting to researchers because panic and social phobias have generally been regarded as some of the least heritable psychiatric disorders, and the field of molecular genetics has been fairly unsuccessful in unravelling their origins (Martin-Santos M. 1998 / Collier D.A. 2002).

> '[The findings] *could have some advantages for diagnosis, because* [in the future] *patients with anxiety disorders could be classified on the basis of their genome. Importantly, it will necessitate a re-evaluation of the definition of anxiety disorders as it is now evident that panic, agoraphobia, social phobia and hypermobility can be manifestations of the same underlying genomic event. Genetic testing might also make patients feel better about their condition once they know that it has a biological origin* (Collier D.A. 2002).

When considering the implication of these findings on treatment, Collier goes on to stress that, just because a condition has been found to be genetic or genomic, it doesn't mean that it shouldn't be treated with cognitive therapy, as this form of therapy can help patients learn very useful coping skills. In fact studies, such as that carried out by Marks I.M. (1986), show that some phobias that appear to be highly genetic, still respond successfully to treatment using cognitive strategies.

Work continues to better understand the duplication of chromosome 15 and its association with panic disorders, anxiety and hypermobility.

2. Cardiovascular autonomic dysfunction and anxiety

The autonomic nervous system (ANS) is the part of the peripheral nervous system which controls visceral functions (those of the organs in the chest and abdomen). It is divided into two subsystems; the parasympathetic nervous system which deals with the functions of 'rest and digest' and the sympathetic nervous system which regulates processes such as tightening blood vessels and increasing heart rate when you stand up, and force of the heartbeat when you exercise (also known as "flight or fight" responses).

Cardiovascular dysfunction of the ANS is a commonly experienced comorbidity of hEDS, and HSD, (Gazit et al 2003 / 1)Patient.co.uk / Hakim et al 2017a), and is thought to either act as a trigger for anxiety (Eccles J.A. et al 2012), or to mimic symptoms frequently

© Understanding hEDS and HSD by C. Smith

associated with anxiety disorder (Pocinki A. 2010).

According to Dr Alan Pocinki, a leading expert in hEDS and HSD, many of the symptoms of autonomic dysfunction associated with hypermobility, are characterised by an 'over-response' to physical and emotional stresses, which often lead to fluctuations in heart rate and blood pressure, as well as respiratory and gastrointestinal symptoms. He explains that, in order to compensate for stretchy blood vessels and increased venous pooling (too much blood collecting in over-stretched veins), most people with hypermobility appear to make extra adrenaline and consequently suffer from chronic sympathetic nervous system overload. These symptoms of adrenaline highs and lows can also be mistaken for the mood fluctuations seen in bipolar disorder.

In an open letter for his hypermobile patients, Dr Pocinki stresses the importance of doctors recognising that the symptoms of anxiety, experienced by many hypermobile individuals, are a physical reaction and, as such, the underlying causes need treating and the usual treatment pathways, such as counseling, will often not be as effective in treating this type of anxiety.

HEDS and HSD, and their implications on cardiovascular autonomic dysfunction is discussed in greater detail on page 69.

3. Brain structure and joint hypermobility

In 2012, a study by Eccles J. et al. was published in the British Journal of Psychiatry. The study by the team was remarkable because, for the first time, they were able to present a neuroimaging study of hypermobility which examines the individual's ability to perceive and process bodily signals along with malfunction or faulty regulation in the involuntary nervous system. The authors tested for associations between regional cerebral grey matter and hypermobility in 72 healthy volunteers, using a neuroimaging analysis technique that allows investigation of focal differences in brain anatomy and provides photographic evidence of the outcome.

Findings included regions of gray-matter volume difference in hypermobile participants compared with the non-hypermobile group, and suggested that the same processes that compromise function in neuro-developmental disorders, may occur in individuals with hypermobility, and that this may

WIDESPREAD SYMPTOMS & COMORBIDITIES

enhance a person's vulnerability to stress and anxiety. The findings specifically link hypermobility to structural differences in key emotion processing regions of the brain, notably in bilateral amygdala volume. It also found decreased anterior cingulate and left parietal cortical volume, and that the degree of hypermobility correlates negatively with both superior temporal and inferior parietal volume (Eccles et al., 2012). From their observations, the team endorsed hypermobility as a 'multi-system' phenotype.

Addressing anxiety

Of course, just because an individual's life experiences or biological makeup leaves them *disposed* to anxiety, it does not mean that this must

be the outcome, or that nothing can be done if anxiety is experienced.

When anxiety is disabling, medications such as benzodiazepines and SSRIs, prescribed by a GP, may provide temporary relief, but they are not for everyone and do not necessarily address the underlying triggers. Research shows that the brain and body are always developing, never staying the same and, through guidance and appropriate intervention, can be taught to respond more appropriately to stressors, thus reducing or eliminating the symptoms of anxiety.

Promising new avenues to managing anxiety, which may help change even deeply ingrained thought and reaction patterns by encouraging the brain to make new neurons and synaptic connections between those neurons, include: Mindfulness meditation, cognitive behavioural therapy (CBT), and eye movement desensitisation and reprocessing (EMDR) - more information on CBT can be found in Chapter 3, page 153. Therapists can provide support, problem-solving skills, and enhanced coping strategies.

© Understanding hEDS and HSD by C. Smith

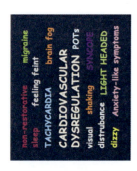

Cardiovascular autonomic dysfunction

Autonomic dysfunction is an umbrella term for various conditions in which the autonomic nervous system malfunctions.

The autonomic nervous system

The autonomic nervous system (ANS) regulates automatic (involuntary) bodily functions, controlling the activities of organs such as the heart, stomach and intestines, as well as the glands, smooth muscles and cardiac muscles. It is divided into three subsystems: the parasympathetic nervous system, the sympathetic nervous system and the enteric system. The actions of the parasympathetic nervous system can be summarised as the 'rest and digest' system, looking after functions like digestion and urination. The actions of the sympathetic nervous system regulates processes such as tightening blood vessels when you stand up, increasing heart rate, and the force of the heartbeat when you exercise. It is sometimes referred to as the 'flight or fight' system. The enteric system controls the workings of the gut.

Overall, the ANS affects functions such as heart rate, digestion, respiration rate, perspiration/temperature control, salivation and urination. When the ANS malfunctions, the organs it regulates malfunction. This is known as 'autonomic dysfunction'. When individuals suffer from autonomic dysfunction, they often present with numerous symptoms because the ANS regulates so many functions of the body.

Symptoms of autonomic dysfunction

The symptoms of autonomic dysfunction are numerous and vary widely from person to person depending on the organ system affected and the underlying cause. For example, while some people predominately experience symptoms associated with difficulty adapting to changes in posture (light headedness, rapid heart rate, shakiness), others suffer predominantly with digestive symptoms - many will experience multiple symptoms. Patients with dysautonomia can experience varying severity of symptoms, with some being only mildly affected, whilst others are disabled by their symptoms.

Primary symptoms of dysautonomia include:

- Lightheadedness or dizziness, often associated with orthostatic hypotension (abnormally low blood pressure on standing), sometimes resulting in syncope (fainting).
- Rapid heart rate / palpitations, or slow heart rate.
- Blood pressure fluctuations.
- Tremulousness (shakiness).
- Peripheral paraesthesia - transient or chronic skin sensations of tingling, tickling, pricking, burning or a feeling of something crawling over the skin.
- Abnormal dilation of the pupils, leading to blurry vision.
- Difficulty with breathing or swallowing.
- Excessive fatigue.
- Excessive thirst.
- Exercise intolerance.
- Slow digestion causing distention of the abdomen, nausea, loss of appetite, bloating, diarrhoea or constipation.
- Gastroparesis (delayed gastric emptying) with associated nausea, acid reflux and vomiting.
- Urinary problems can include difficulty starting urination, incontinence, and incomplete emptying of the bladder.
- Excessive sweating or lack of sweating due to problems regulating temperature control.
- Heat intolerance.
- Sexual problems including erectile dysfunction in men, and vaginal dryness and orgasmic difficulties in women.
- Non-restorative sleep / insomnia.
- Anxiety-like symptoms.

Cardiovascular dysautonomia and hEDS/HSD

In addition to more well known causes such as degenerative neurologic diseases or side effects from certain medications, autonomic dysfunction can also occur in association with inherited genetic disorders such as Ehlers-Danlos syndrome. Recent research in a number of areas suggests that many of the non-musculoskeletal manifestations of hEDS, and HSD, such as fatigue, poor regulation of circulation and blood pressure, irregular bowel habits, disturbed bladder function and disturbed sleep may actually be presentations of cardiovascular autonomic dysfunction (Gazit et al 2003 / 5/EDNF.org / Hakim A.J. et al 2017a).

Cardiovascular autonomic dysfunction such as orthostatic (upright) intolerance, orthostatic hypotension (low blood pressure on being upright), and postural orthostatic tachycardia syndrome is observed in a large number of hEDS and HSD patients (Hakim A.J. et al 2017a). .

Tests carried out by Gazit et al., 2003, found such conditions in over three-quarters of hypermobile patients, compared to just one tenth of controls. And a recent survey of 361 patients, carried out by Eccles et al., demonstrated that symptoms of autonomic dysfunction are not only higher in hypermobile patients, but also correlate strongly with the degree of hypermobility (number of joints affected). Overall, hypermobile patients were found to have higher mean autonomic dysfunction and orthostatic intolerance than non-hypermobile patients, and symptoms can be highly debilitating (Rowe P.C. et al. 1999 / Hakim A.J. & Grahame R. 2004 / Mathias C.J. et al., 2011 / De Wandele I. et al. 2014b).

The most common presentations (which are seen significantly more frequently amongst those who are hypermobile) are linked to the cardiovascular autonomic nervous system and include symptoms such as irregular heartbeat, palpitations and chest pain along with fainting or near fainting, gastrointestinal disturbances, fatigue and heat intolerance (Rowe et al., 1999 / Gazit Y. et al. 2003 / Hakim & Grahame 2004 / Mathias C.J et al. 2011 / Wallman D. et al. 2014 / De Wandele I. et al. 2014, 2016).

Postural orthostatic tachycardia syndrome (POTs)
POTs is a subset of dysautonomia and, in the general population, is classified as being either primary or secondary.

A diagnosis of primary POTs is given when the condition appears not to be associated with other disease processes, or when the causal factors are unknown. Secondary POTs is diagnosed when the condition *is* associated with other disease processes. Secondary POTs has been reported in conditions that cause damage of the nerves that usually control the redistribution of blood, such as Diabetes Mellitus or Amyloidosis. Secondary POTs is also seen in disorders associated with intrinsic abnormalities in the collagen structure of the blood vessels; for example the hypermobile type of Ehlers-Danlos syndrome.

POTS is poorly understood by GPs and other health care professionals (see 'Misdiagnosis' page 75), with many not knowing the appropriate diagnostic criteria, or believing this often debilitating condition is 'just' orthostatic hypotension.

In fact, POTs is distinct from the syndromes of autonomic failure associated with orthostatic hypotension and is distinct from orthostatic

WIDESPREAD SYMPTOMS & COMORBIDITIES

hypotension itself because, typically, there is **no** postural fall in blood pressure, although fainting (syncope) can occur. Some POTs patients do have a drop in blood pressure upon standing, but for most POTs patients there is no change, or they may even experience an increase in blood pressure upon standing (Grubb P.B. 2008 / Freeman et al., 2011 / Mar P.L 2014).

When clinical assessment does not show low blood pressure as being present, patients' symptoms may be dismissed as being caused by anxiety or hypochondria, or lead to patients being treated with inappropriate medications such as antidepressants, and the opportunity to further investigate and treat the underlying pathology missed. The chronic symptoms, and the frustration caused by the difficulty in obtaining medical help, can significantly lower the quality of life for those with POTs (Sheldon R.S.et al., 2015).

There is currently a great deal of debate about whether POTs is a systemic illness (affecting functions throughout the body). For example, the National Hospital for Neurology and Neurosurgery say POTs only causes orthostatic intolerance and palpitations; they propose that the rest of the symptoms individuals experience are due to secondary conditions such as EDS/HSD. Other organisations and consultants disagree (Castori M. 2011a / Kavi L. 2015), believing POTs to be multi-systemic with postural tachycardia being just one of several diagnostic criteria.

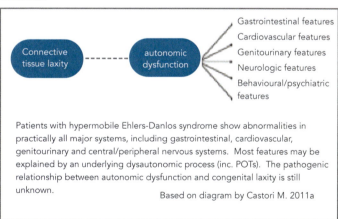

Patients with hypermobile Ehlers-Danlos syndrome show abnormalities in practically all major systems, including gastrointestinal, cardiovascular, genitourinary and central/peripheral nervous systems. Most features may be explained by an underlying dysautonomic process (inc. POTs). The pathogenic relationship between autonomic dysfunction and congenital laxity is still unknown.
Based on diagram by Castori M. 2011a

POTs predominantly affects females, most commonly between the ages of 15 and 50 years of age, and the symptoms mainly occur when the patient is standing upright, and are often relieved by sitting or lying flat. When someone stands up, blood automatically drops into their lower body (the abdominal cavity and their legs). The normal response would be for the brain to sense the sudden decrease in blood supply, and instruct the heart to beat a little harder and faster and the blood vessels in the lower legs to constrict, ensuring blood flow is appropriately distributed to the head and heart and the rest of the upper body. However, as a result of the various causes shown in **Box A**, this process happens less efficiently in those with POTs causing the symptoms listed below:

Symptoms of POTs
The symptoms associated with POTs can be divided into three major categories, those that occur when rising from lying to sitting to standing, those that are not associated with postural change and those that are systemic (Thierben M.J. et al., 2007):

- Weakness.
- Dizziness.
- Lightheadedness, near-fainting or, in some, fainting.
- Palpitations.
- Breathlessness.
- Shaking / tremulousness.
- Fatigue, which is above and beyond normal tiredness, and a strong desire for sleep.
- Sleep disturbance.
- Migraine headaches.
- Discomfort in the head and neck, such as headache and neck/shoulder pain.
- Nausea.
- Sweats and intolerance to heat and cold - patients describe intolerance to prolonged hot baths or needing to sit down after a shower.
- Raynaud's-like symptoms that happen not only with cold weather, but also with inactivity of the hands, due to poor blood circulation.
- Visual disturbances.
- Poor concentration - described as being like 'brain fog.'
- Bowel problems including many that are similar to those found in irritable bowel syndrome (bloating, nausea, diarrhoea, and abdominal pain).

Although POTs is not thought to reduce life expectancy, in some it can cause significant levels of disability, leaving an individual so badly affected that they become wheelchair users or are bedridden, with symptoms so severe that they may be equivalent to conditions like heart failure and chronic obstructive pulmonary disease (COPD) (Benrud-Larson et al 2002/ Dysautonomiainternational.org).

Box A, points 1-8 describe the various subsets of POTs including secondary POTs commonly linked to hEDS and HSD (see point 7).

© Understanding hEDS and HSD by C. Smith

Box A   **Subsets and causes of POTs**

Over the years, researchers have tried to separate POTs into various different types, to help identify the best methods of treatment. However, it is important to realise that the different 'types' of POTs are not *distinct* medical conditions and can overlap (Stars.org), with many POTs patients having several of the different characteristics present. For example, a doctor may find neuropathy, low blood volume and elevated norepineprhine in the same patient (Ref: Dysautonomia International).

1) Neuropathic POTs (also known as partial or restricted dysautonomic POTs)
Neuropathic POTs is thought to be caused by restricted autonomic neuropathy resulting in patchy or preferential (partial) loss of nerve supply in the sympathetic nerves supplying the lower body and legs. The ends of the longer nerve fibres are affected before the shorter ones (Schondorf R. 1993 / Thieben M. et al 2007).

To demonstrate this, consider the autonomic nerves that run along the small veins in the legs. These nerves help control blood pressure by telling veins to constrict when changing position from lying to sitting or standing. This instruction helps the body counter the effects of gravity on the blood, sending blood back up to the upper body. If those autonomic nerves are damaged, a person's veins won't be able to constrict very well. Gravity will pull the blood downwards into the abdomen, lower legs and feet, and the brain and heart will have trouble regulating blood pressure when they stand up. Autonomic nerves are also found in areas such as the bladder. If these nerves are damaged, a person's ability to hold urine and excrete it in a controlled manner may be impaired, leading to problems emptying the bladder, or infections.

When autonomic neuropathy occurs, the body's ability to properly regulate many of the functions of the ANS is impaired. The level of impairment depends on the severity of the autonomic neuropathy, and also on which autonomic nerves are damaged.

Neuropathic POTs is commonly described as having occurred following an initial catalyst such as infection, trauma, surgery, stress or pregnancy (Soliman K. et al 2010 / Mathias C.J 2011) and, indeed, in those who acquire the syndrome post-virally, serum

71

auto-antibodies have now been detected (Conner R. 2012).

2) Hypovolaemic POTs

Hypovolemia is an abnormal decrease in the volume of blood plasma. In these POTs patients, their kidneys fail to sense low blood plasma and therefore do not respond by appropriately increasing plasma renin activity and aldosterone. The knock-on effect is that salt and water retention is not increased and so the plasma volume is not increased (Dr Raj S. et al 2005). Some patients report being intensely sensitive to salt intake and can fine-tune their plasma volume and BP control with salt alone (Low P.A. 2009).

3) Central Hyperadrenergic POTs

This form of POTs is much less common than neuropathic POTs. It is characterised by an excessive increase of plasma norepinephrine (Jordan J. et al 2002) and large increases in blood pressure when a patient stands up, which indicates that baroreflex buffering is somehow impaired.

Hyperadrenergic POTs is associated with systolic blood pressure increases of more than 10 mm Hg while standing upright for 10 minutes and plasma norepinephrine levels of more than 600 pg/mL while standing.

These patients may have similar heart rate increment to nonhyperadrenergic POTS, but tend to have prominent symptoms of sympathetic activation (Jordan J. et al 2002) such as anxiety, shakiness and palpitations. In many cases the hyperadrenergic state of POTs is secondary to the neuropathic or hypovolaemia forms.

This form of POTs often runs in families (Sheldon R. S. 2015) although, to date, scientists have only managed to identify a specific genetic abnormality in one family with hyperadrenergic POTs. The abnormality is a single point mutation in the norepinephrine transporter (NET), which results in an inability to clear norephrinephrine sufficiently and produces a state of excessive sympathetic activation, in response to a variety of sympathetic stimuli. Although NET mutations are rare, it is important to be aware that many prescribed drugs inhibit NET and can mimic the symptoms or make them worse. e.g. Tricyclic antidepressants (POTs UK).

4) Developmental POTs

Developmental POTs is a second type of neuropathic POTs (see **1**). The majority of patients diagnosed with developmental POTs are young females, although males are also affected. The onset of symptoms in these young people often follows a period of very rapid growth, usually between the ages of 14 and 16 years. The cause is unclear, but appears to reflect a transient period of autonomic imbalance that occurs in rapidly growing adolescents (Grubb B. P. 2006). Many patients will have associated gastrointestinal and urinary problems as well (Ferrar et al 2012 for POTs.UK). The symptoms can be severe, with some being so badly affected that they are disabled with it, but this will normally slowly improve and resolve as they enter adulthood with around 80% of patients recovering by the time they are in their mid 20s (POTs UK).

5) Deconditioning POTs

Deconditioning relating to muscle disuse through pain, or fear of pain, is often present in patients with persistent (chronic) fatigue and fibromyalgia type symptoms. Studies have shown that POTs with deconditioning is similar to pure deconditioning and bed rest (Gazit Y. 2003).

The combination of hypervigilance in these patients raises the possibility that in at least some POTs patients there was an initial event or illness that evoked orthostatic symptoms and that the symptoms were then over interpreted and followed by reduced physical activity and deconditioning. However, this is open to debate as research is lacking and it is therefore impossible to be certain as to whether deconditioning is the cause of some forms of POTs or whether it is experienced as a consequence of having POTs (Hakim A.J. et al 2017a)

6) Hormones and POTs

According to the Santa Maria School of Medicine (2013), the menstrual cycle takes a toll on female patients with POTs, particularly during the actual 5-7 day bleeding phase when females feel the acute loss of blood volume. This results in them feeling drained, and an exacerbation of all of their usual symptoms - including, in particular, fatigue. According to Peggs et al (2012), patients with POTs report increased dizziness throughout the menstrual cycle, particularly during menses, compared to healthy controls.

In her 2015 study, Jessica Eccles explains that the gender differences in orthostatic symptoms associated with hypermobility may be explained to some extent, by the following hormonal changes:

The female hormone, oestrogen has an effect on blood volume (Pritchard J.A. 1965) as well as the renin-angiotensin-aldosterone system. Oestrogen therapy has, therefore, been used in post-menopausal women to improve regulation of the mechanism that regulates blood pressure changes via controlling heart rate (Hunt B.E. et al., 2001). Orthostatic intolerance has been found to improve half way through the latter phase of the menstrual cycle in postural orthostatic tachycardia syndrome patients (Fu et al., 2010), this may be caused by increasing levels of progesterone, which is at its highest during this phase and may upregulate renal-adrenal hormones (Stachenfeld N.S. and Taylor H.S. 2005).

7) Secondary POTs linked to hEDS/HSD

A large percentage of people with hEDS, and HSD, are affected by cardiovascular autonomic dysfunction, including orthostatic intolerance and orthostatic hypotension. POTs has however, been defined as *'the most specific form of cardiovascular autonomic dysfunction to affect those with [hEDs/HSD]'* (Rowe et al 1999). In those with hEDS, and HSD, experts suspect that POTs occurs due to abnormal connective tissue in the blood vessels, which permits veins to swell excessively in response to ordinary hydrostatic pressure and allows excessive amounts of blood to pool in the patient's abdomen and/or lower limbs when they stand. [Rowe et al. 1999 / Bohora, 2010 / Benarroch E. E. 2012 / Mathias C.J. 2012 / Eccles J. 2015). As a result, less blood is returned to the heart, and circulation in the brain is altered (see **Box B**.). The body tries to compensate by inducing tachycardia and, in some, excess adrenaline may be produced. It is postulated that the venous pooling can cause a secondary hyperadrenergic state (see **3**) or receptor dysregulation predisposing patients to autonomic dysregulation (1/ PoTSUK.org). Symptoms of altered blood flow to the brain include lightheadedness, fainting, personality changes and deteriorating cognitive ability, and autonomic overactivity, such as shortness of breath, tremulousness, palpitations, chest discomfort, bloating and diarrhoea. In those who also suffer the symptoms of migraine in connections with POTs, abnormal vascular reactivity within the cerebral vasculature is thought to be the cause.

Please note: The description above may sound similar to the one described in those who have POTs as a result of autonomic neuropathy (see **1**), but the causation factors are different i.e. in Neuropathic POTs *'nerve damage'* stops veins constricting effectively, whereas in hEDS/HSD POTs *'faulty collagen found in the connective tissue of the veins'* may render them less able to constrict effectively.

Another possible contributory factor to the association between hEDS/ HSD and POTs is 'excessive mobility in the neck', which was described by fibromyalgia researcher Andrew Holman in his 2008 study. Holman reported that 71% of the fibromyalgia patients and 85% of those with chronic

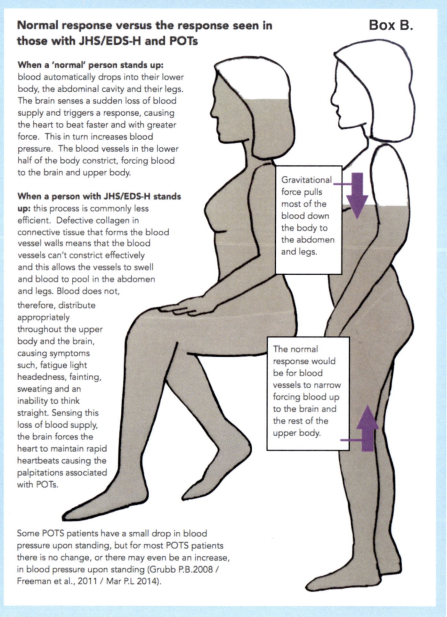

Box B.

Normal response versus the response seen in those with JHS/EDS-H and POTs

When a 'normal' person stands up: blood automatically drops into their lower body, the abdominal cavity and their legs. The brain senses a sudden loss of blood supply and triggers a response, causing the heart to beat faster and with greater force. This in turn increases blood pressure. The blood vessels in the lower half of the body constrict, forcing blood to the brain and upper body.

When a person with JHS/EDS-H stands up: this process is commonly less efficient. Defective collagen in connective tissue that forms the blood vessel walls means that the blood vessels can't constrict effectively and this allows the vessels to swell and blood to pool in the abdomen and legs. Blood does not, therefore, distribute appropriately throughout the upper body and the brain, causing symptoms such, fatigue light headedness, fainting, sweating and an inability to think straight. Sensing this loss of blood supply, the brain forces the heart to maintain rapid heartbeats causing the palpitations associated with POTs.

Gravitational force pulls most of the blood down the body to the abdomen and legs.

The normal response would be for blood vessels to narrow forcing blood up to the brain and the rest of the upper body.

Some POTS patients have a small drop in blood pressure upon standing, but for most POTS patients there is no change, or there may even be an increase, in blood pressure upon standing (Grubb P.B.2008 / Freeman et al., 2011 / Mar P.L 2014).

© Understanding hEDS and HSD by C. Smith

widespread pain exhibited compression of the cervical spinal cord, or that a disc was 'touching or resting against' the spinal cord, in extension views on MRI. This led him to hypothesize that chronic irritation in this region might give rise to dysautonomia as well as to widespread, referred pain. As both hypermobility of the neck and fibromyalgia are common among hEDS patients, many of whom need to brace their necks, or undergo surgery to stabilise them (6/ EDNF.org by Bianco A. 2010), it would seem fair to hypothesize that the same findings may apply to them.

Other plausible mechanisms in POTs/hEDS/HSD include:

- Deconditioning (see **5**).
- Hormones (see **6**).
- Side effects of mediations which may trigger or impair autonomic responses (Hakim A.J. et al 2017a).
- Low circulating blood volume also known as hypovolemia (Hakim A. J et al 2017a) - Raj. et al (2005) found that POTS patients had an average of a 12% deficiency in their plasma volume and/or a 27% deficiency of red blood cell mass. Patients who had both were found to have an average deficit of about 460 mL in total blood volume.
- Chiari malformations (see page 93) (Ireland P.D. et al 1996 / Milhorat T.H. et al 2007).
- Links with mast cell activation/excessive histamine release that are seen in so many with hEDS/HSD (see 'Mast Cells' page 77) (Louisias M.et al. 2013 / Frieri M. et al. 2013 / Cheung I. & Vadas P. 2015 / Hakim A.J. 2017a).

When patients have a combination of POTs *and* hEDS or HSD they tend to have earlier symptoms and have a significantly higher incidence of fainting and migraine (Grubb B.P & Kanjwal Y. et al 2006). Some are affected by their symptoms daily, but it is not uncommon for POTs to follow a relapsing-remitting course, in which symptoms come and go, and those affected frequently describe themselves as 'going through a 'POTsie phase', where they enter a period of increased brain fog, weakness and fatigue that may leave them debilitated and, in some case, unable to work or cope well with home life for hours, days, or weeks.

For many the symptoms associated with hEDs, and HSD such as tendonitis, dislocations, chronic fatigue, insomnia and gastroparesis, can make even the most basic self-management treatments for POTs (taking regular exercise, obtaining sufficient rest and eating regular meals) challenging.

WIDESPREAD SYMPTOMS & COMORBIDITIES

8) Secondary POTs linked to conditions (other than hEDS/HSD)
POTs-like symptoms have been reported in the context of other illnesses, including conditions that cause damage of the nerves that usually control the redistribution of blood, such as diabetes mellitus or amyloidosis.

Investigation and diagnosis:
According to the 2015 Expert Consensus Document, produced by Sheldon et al., the evaluation of a patient suspected of having POTs should include:

- A complete history and physical examination.
- Blood pressure and heart rate checks in both supine (lying face up) and then standing positions, and a 12-lead electrocardiogram (ECG).
- Selected patients might benefit from a thyroid function test, a full blood count, 24-hour holter, transthoracic echocardiogram, and exercise stress testing.

The clinical history should focus on defining the chronicity of the condition, establishing whether the patient has any existing medical disorders associated with secondary POTs, other possible causes of orthostatic tachycardia, modifying factors, the impact on daily activities, potential triggers, and family history. Those with POTs are likely to describe their symptoms as being exacerbated by dehydration, heat, alcohol, and exercise.

A full autonomic system review should assess symptoms of autonomic neuropathy. In his 2004 paper on hEDS, Dr Howard Levy states that when carrying out investigations, holter monitoring will usually show normal sinus rhythm, but sometimes reveals premature atrial complexes or paroxysmal supraventricular tachycardia. Halter monitoring should certainly be considered if there is clinical concern that an abnormality in the rhythm of the heart is present (Hakim A.J. et al 2017a).

If orthostatic vital signs are normal but the clinical suspicion of POTs is high and non-pharmacologic treatments have been ineffective, for most individuals a haematocrit, electrocardiogram, blood pressure monitoring, and echocardiogram are sufficient to screen for a POTs. If these tests are also normal but suspicion remains high, a tilt-table test might be helpful because it can provide continuous monitoring of heart rate and blood pressure, and over more prolonged periods than a simple stand test. During the test the patient lies flat on a special

© Understanding hEDS and HSD by C. Smith

bed, which is then tilted upright to around 60 degrees, and some patients may briefly faint. As previously discussed, in those with hEDS or HSD, it is common for symptoms of POTs to fluctuate. It can, therefore, be difficult to time such tests to coincide. Results may well be inconclusive during a period when symptoms are reduced. During investigations, patients may have other cardiology and neurology tests to rule out other conditions.

This minimal approach is considered sufficient to establish a diagnosis and initiate treatment in most people. However, for some, symptoms fail to improve despite treatment, and a more extensive evaluation including tests such as noting plasma epinephrine and norepinephrine levels when a patient is lying down and again when the patient is upright, thermoregulatory sweat testing, and a 24 hour urine sample collection to assess sodium intake is undertaken. An expanded approach to the evaluation could include a thermoregulatory sweat test to detect autonomic neuropathy (which manifests as abnormal patterns of body sweating), supine and upright plasma epinephrine and norepinephrine level tests, a 24-hour urine sample to assess sodium intake, and a psychological assessment. These tests should only be undertaken if clinically indicated.

- In those with POTs, a sustained increase in heart rate of over 30 beats per minute (or to higher than 120 beats per minute) within 10 minutes of standing or head up tilt can be seen, usually in the absence of orthostatic hypotension. In children and adolescents, a revised standard of 40 beats per minute or more increase has now been adopted (Freeman R. et al., 2011).
- Orthostatic tachycardia <u>must</u> be accompanied by symptoms of orthostatic intolerance and autonomic over-activity, such as palpitations, tremulousness, shortness of breath, chest discomfort and/or pain, and most symptoms <u>must</u> improve with lying down, and have persisted for at least 6 months.
- Symptoms must occur in the absence of conditions that cause orthostatic tachycardia.
- As mentioned earlier in this section, some POTs patients subsequently experience a drop in blood pressure upon standing, but for most POTs patients there is no change, or there may even have an increase in blood pressure upon standing (Grubb P.B. 2008 / Freeman R. et al., 2011 / Mar P.L 2014).

Misdiagnosis:
The diagnosis of POTs is often missed. The primary cause is that, in a clinical setting, patients are usually sitting down when their pulse is measured and the recordings taken may therefore be normal, even if they have POTs. Measurements of the sustained heart rate increases (which form part of the diagnosis for POTs) need to be taken not only in the sitting position, but also within 10 minutes of standing up or head up tilt (see the 'current diagnostic criteria' listed below. In addition, many doctors and nurses have not heard of POTs, and patients may not realise the significance of their own symptoms.

POTs may also be mistaken for other conditions with similar symptoms, such inappropriate tachycardia syndrome or other causes of low blood pressure, and phaeochromocytoma (adrenaline-producing tumour), chronic fatigue syndrome, panic disorders or anxiety. Patients with POTs are frequently labeled as having anxiety/neurosis or panic attacks (Soliman K. et al 2010) because doctors do not look for the diagnositic criteria and assume that the symptoms (palpitations, sweating, insomnia), which mimic those caused by anxiety, are caused by a psychiatric disorder or hypochondria. In fact, detailed psychometric and physiologic studies have shown that although anxiety is commonly present in POTs (as it is in many with long term health conditions), the heart rate response to orthostatic stress is not caused by anxiety, but is instead a response to an underlying abnormal functioning of the body (Masuki S. et al 2007).

Treatment:
Having POTs doesn't automatically mean that 'treatment' is required, particularly if it's relatively asymptomatic. Instead, many patients are taught self-management strategies which enable them to be re-assured and to manage it better (Hakim A.J. 2016a).

According to the 2015 consensus document written by Sheldon et al., there are no therapies that are uniformly successful. Dr Alan Hakim agrees, stating: 'Combinations of approaches are often needed - with some people requiring various combinations of non-pharmacological and pharmacological interventions.

As yet, there is also no consensus as to whether specific treatments should be used to treat the different subsets of POTs (**see Box A**) or whether a uniform approach should be used regardless of which subset is diagnosed.

Although medication can be prescribed to help alleviate the symptoms, the mainstay of treatment is achieved through self-management, with the main aim being to maintain blood supply to the heart and brain.

© Understanding hEDS and HSD by C. Smith

WIDESPREAD SYMPTOMS & COMORBIDITIES

The following measures are often found helpful:

• It has been reported that raising the head end of the bed will increase blood plasma volume in the morning (Low P. A. 2000).

• Dehydration reduces the volume of circulating blood. Increasing fluids helps many people with POTs to feel better. Many POTs patients report electrolyte solutions to be particularly helpful. It is important, however, not to drink excessive amounts of water because it can cause essential electrolytes to become diluted in the bloodstream, which may affect heart rhythm (Dinet.org).

• Try to eat frequent small meals instead of three large meals a day to reduce the amount of blood needed for digestion. It is also important to identify and avoid any food triggers, such as refined carbohydrates (Mathias C.J. 2000).

• Alcohol enhances peripheral venous pooling, which will exacerbate hypotension (Grubb B.P. 1999). Alcohol can also lead to a dehydrated state.

• Some patients are advised to increase dietary salt by 2-4 g per day because salt increases blood volume/ pressure. This should only be done on the recommendation of a doctor, as increasing salt is not suitable for some people.

• Taking a magnesium supplement has been anecdotally reported to be helpful by some patients with POTs and hEDS/HSD, but should be used carefully as it can lower blood pressure.

• Strenuous, exhausting exercise should be avoided, but it is important to avoid becoming deconditioned. Take regular, appropriate exercise. Initially, exercise should be restricted to non-upright exercises including (where suitable) the use of rowing machines, recumbent cycles, and swimming to minimise orthostatic stress on the heart. Increasing muscle strength is beneficial in fighting many of the symptoms associated with POTS; strengthening the calf muscles and tissues that surround the blood vessels helps to support them, reducing dilation / blood pooling in the legs and helping blood be pumped around the body more effectively.

• Try to get lots of rest. It has been reported that some POTs patients have significant sleep disturbances (Low P.A. 2000), so getting adequate rest is very important.

• Try to pace what you do in a day; planning activities in the afternoon as opposed to the morning may be helpful as many report symptoms are worse in the morning.

• Stand up slowly to give the body more time to adjust to upright posture.

• Avoid excessive standing and sitting.

• Climbing stairs, holding the arms in the air for long periods and lifting heavy objects are all anecdotally reported to increase symptoms.

• Bending up and down, as done when picking items up off of the floor, may increase symptoms. It is best to bend at the knee and squat down rather then to bend over forward at the waist.

• Do postural manoeuvres to avoid fainting/dizziness - e.g. lie down and elevate the legs if possible; otherwise, cross the legs and squeeze the thighs together and tightly clench the buttocks and fists.

• Avoid extremes of temperature. Heat enhances peripheral venous pooling (Grubb B.P.1999).

• Sit down when taking a shower instead of standing, and allow time for a rest after showering to recover from any symptoms triggered by the change in temperature.

• Drink water rapidly; two glasses of water drunk quickly has been shown to reduce heart rate in POTs (8/www.nhs.uk).

• Try wearing a compression device, such as an elastic abdominal binder and/or strong support tights; they have been shown to help reduce blood pooling in the abdomen and legs (Grubb B.P.1999).

• Cooling devices such as cooling vests may help patients tolerate hot environments.

• Consult your doctor about changing any current medication that may worsen symptoms (e.g. drugs that lower blood pressure).

Medication for POTs

Patients may be asked to try self-help treatments for 3-6 months. If unsuccessful, medications such as Fludrocortisone or Midodrine may be used, although few scientific studies have been performed to evaluate which treatment is best for which patient. At the time of writing, medicines for POTs are all unlicenced for use in POTs, which means that a GP is not obliged to prescribe them. GPs who agree to prescribe these medicines will probably need a recommendation from a hospital specialist. Patients with hEDS or HSD who feel they may be suffering from symptoms of autonomic dysfunction should visit their GP. They may find it useful to take supporting information on autonomic dysfunction and postural orthostatic tachycardia syndrome, to help explain concerns. Where possible, referral should be to a consultant with special interest in autonomic problems, who has an understanding of Ehlers-Danlos syndrome / hereditary disorders of the connective tissue.

© Understanding hEDS and HSD by C. Smith

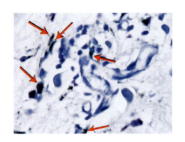

Mast cell activation syndrome

Introduction
Mast cell activation and a possible relationship with hEDS/HSD is a frequent topic of discussion on hypermobility-related forums and social media, and its wide-reaching manifestations are a debilitating phenomenon for many, with symptoms that include skin rashes, flushing, itching, nausea, headache, abdominal cramping, diarrhea, vomiting, respiratory symptoms, hypotension, tachycardia, unexplained arrhythmias, and neurological manifestations (Akin C. et al 2010). When it comes to identifying hard scientific evidence of a link between the two, however, it becomes apparent that research is still in its very early stages. In this section, we will look at mast cell activation and consider some hypotheses put forward by leading experts.

What are mast cells?
Mast cells are part of our immune system and are vital to our health. They play a protective role, defending our bodies against allergens and pathogens such as bacteria, viruses and parasites, that can cause disease or illness (Prussin C. & Metcalfe D. 2003). They also assist in wound healing (Jung M. 2013), accumulating in high quantities close by the site of injury and surrounding nerves.

Mast cells reside within connective and mucosal tissues located in the skin, respiratory system (mouth, nose and lungs), linings of the stomach, intestine and urinary tract, as well as near blood and lymphatic vessels, within nerves, and in the brain (Encyclopedia Britannica). They can tell the difference between different sorts of stimuli and, where necessary, respond accordingly by releasing pro-inflammatory mast cell mediators (frequently referred to as a kind of chemical 'alarm system'), including histamine, proteases, prostaglandins, leukotrienes and cytokines - a process known as degranulation.

The resulting inflammation is the body's protective response against allergy and infection. The 'chemical alarms' draw other components of the immune defence team such as immune cells, clotting proteins and signaling molecules, to areas of the body where they are needed (2/NIH). Histamine induces fluid secretion at the site of infection, in order to rid the body of infectious agents or allergens, and it causes the muscle walls surrounding blood vessels to relax allowing white blood cells to move easily to the site of infection (Pollock J. 2006). This process also causes less desirable manifestations that we commonly associate with allergic reactions, ranging from itching, sneezing and a runny nose, to flushing, swelling, hives, nausea, bloating, abdominal pain, and, in extreme cases, anaphylaxis (British Society for Immunology).

Systemic mastocytosis and mast cell activation syndrome
According to Dr. Andrew White, specialist in allergy and immunology, physicians usually think of mast cell mediator release as an 'all or nothing' phenomenon, in which mast cells are either resting quietly doing nothing, or are busy releasing high quantities of mediators in response to an allergic reaction. In his opinion, however, this is probably not the case. He explains: '...*mast cells are constantly interacting with the environment – sensing – reacting. And in some people, this process might not work correctly.*' Indeed, for reasons not yet fully understood, mast cells in some people can go into a state of *excessive* activity, reacting to things that they should ignore and releasing large amounts of chemicals (pro-inflammatory mediators) such as histamine, into the system, both spontaneously and in response to trigger stimuli (Moulderings G.J. 2011).

This excessive mast cell activity and mediator release is seen in a group of conditions known as mast cell activation disorders (see **Box 2**), of which mast cell activation syndrome is one. In order to understand mast cell activation syndrome (MCAS), we must first look a little more closely at a rarer, but perhaps, better known disorder called systemic mastocytosis (SM).

The clinical manifestations, shown in **Box 1**, have long been defined in literature as being associated with SM, a disorder in which symptoms are caused by an abnormal accumulation of malformed and functionally abnormal mast cells that gather in one or more organ system (Valent P. et al 2007). Recently, however, experts have identified another category of patients who share many similarities with those who have SM. They

Box 1.

Clinical manifestations of SM (and MCAS) include:

- Easy flushing from the chest upwards (triggered by certain foods, heat, stress etc).
- Dermatographia (ability to *write* on the skin with a light scratch that turns red in a minute).
- Chronic fatigue.
- Eyes that feel gritty, sore, watery, or have difficulty focusing.
- Hypotension (low blood pressure).
- Infections (bronchitis, rhinitis, and conjunctivitis).
- Anaphylaxis.
- Angioedema (swelling around lips or eyes).
- Bone pain, bone loss, osteoporosis, osteopenia, osteosclerosis.
- GI pain, bloating, cramping, gas, abdominal pain, gastroesophageal reflux.
- Malabsorption.
- Reactions to some local and general anesthetics (may include abdominal pain, diarrhea, vomiting, hives).
- Food and drug allergies or sensitivities (may be negative on IgE test but you still react, often increasing).
- Sensitivity or allergy to alcohol, especially red wine.
- Hives.
- Urticaria pigmentosa (reddish brown spots, ranging from the size of freckles to larger patches).
- Rashes (with or without itching).
- Muscle pain.
- Itching.
- Brain fog.
- Headaches.
- Oesophageal spasms.
- Wheezing, coughing, sudden congestion or sneezing, difficulty breathing.
- Nighttime waking.
- Sensory processing disorders.
- Anxiety and panic attacks - in order to counter-act the over production of histamine, the body may also react by producing adrenaline which helps to de-activate histamine. This can sometimes cause anxiety and panic attacks.

Symptoms of MCAS vary greatly from person to person. Some experience only one or two symptoms whilst others experience symptoms which are severely debilitating (Castells M. 2006)

Symptoms sources: Lee J.K 2008 / oreds.org / Castells M. 2006 / Pollock J. 2006 / Seneviratne S.L. et al 2017)

WIDESPREAD SYMPTOMS & COMORBIDITIES

present with the same classic signs and symptoms of episodic mast cell activation, but fail to meet the World Health Organisation's criteria for mastocytosis, because investigators have been unable to find any mast cell abnormality or external triggers that could explain these episodes (Alvarez-Twose, I. 2010 / Hamilton, M.J. 2011 / Alvarez-Twose, I. et al 2012 / Picard M. et al 2013).

It is instead hypothesized that, in *these* patients, their otherwise normal mast cells are hyper-responsive to everyday stimuli (Akin C. et al 2010). The term 'mast cell activation syndrome' has been introduced in order to provide a diagnosis for such individuals (Moulderings G.J. 2011).

Both SM and MCAS are capable of affecting functions in all systems, organs and tissues of the body; particularly the skin, gastrointestinal tract and the cardiovascular and nervous systems (Akin C. et al 2010 / Frieri M. 2013 / 7/Patient.co.uk).

Episodes of MCAS and SM can happen at any time, severely affecting a person's quality of life. Patients describe a 'minefield' of triggers and symptoms which significantly disrupt their lives. Valerie Slee, Vice Chair of the Mastocytosis Society agrees, saying: *"Living with Mastocytosis or MCAS can be very difficult, primarily because of the unpredictability of the symptoms. You can feel perfectly fine when you wake up in the morning, dress to go somewhere, then, just as you are going out the door you get chest pain or abdominal pain and your plans are waylaid.'*

Box 2.

Examples of mast cell activation disorders

- <u>Idiopathic MCADs</u> (there is no identifiable cause): Examples include **mast cell activation syndrome** and anaphylaxis.
- <u>Primary MCADs</u> (the result of a single primary cause): Examples include systemic mastocytosis, cutaneous mastocytosis, mast cell sarcoma, monoclonal-mast-cell syndrome and mast cell leukemia.
- <u>Secondary MCADs</u> (caused by another condition): Examples include drug reactions, allergies and some types of chronic infection or autoimmune dysfunction.

The disorders within this group differ in their severity and can involve various organ systems

(Akin C. 2014).

© Understanding hEDS and HSD by C. Smith

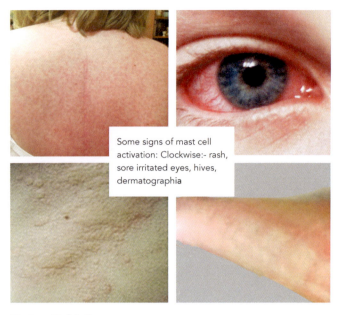

Some signs of mast cell activation: Clockwise:- rash, sore irritated eyes, hives, dermatographia

Potential triggers:

Some of the many 'normal' stimuli that can trigger episodes of MCAS include:

- Foods and drinks that are high in histamine or are known to trigger histamine release.
- Injuries such as cuts and bone fractures.
- Some pain medications such as aspirin, NSAIDs and narcotics.
- Strong scents including perfumes and chemicals.
- Friction, pressure, or vibration on the skin.
- Extremes of temperature.
- Exposure to sunlight.
- Exercise.
- Emotional and physical stress / excitement.

(Mastocytosis [& MCAS] Society Canada & 7/Patient.co.uk)

MCAS and a possible association with EDS/HSD

There seems to be a growing awareness in the medical and patient community that some patients with EDS/HSD also have signs and symptoms of mast cell activation (MCA). Indeed, results of a recent case control study by Dr Ingrid Cheung et al showed that two thirds of the patients, with a formal diagnosis of POTs and EDS, also had validated symptoms of a mast cell disorder suggestive of MCAS, based on diagnostic criteria and validated symptoms as reported by Akin et al (2010).

Writing in a recent publication (Fragile Links, spring 2015), Dr Brad Tinkle, clinical geneticist and expert in EDS, states that at the moment, he can't explain the connection between EDS and MCA, but the more he asks, the more (EDS) patients he finds who describe signs and symptoms of histamine excess (5/EDS Support UK).

It would seem this is a complicated intersection of two poorly understood illnesses for which further investigation is crucial, not only to validate patients symptoms, but also to improve the treatment approach for those affected.

In the meantime, we will consider a few areas of research which could provide some clues as to why people with EDS/HSD may also experience symptoms of mast cell activation:

The first clue relates to the high prevalence of food allergies found in those with EDS. In 2010, Dr Clair Francomano, a geneticist with a special interest in disorders of connective tissue, formed part of a team whose findings confirmed a high prevalence of food allergies in those with EDS when compared to the general population, and showed a significantly higher incidence of gastrointestinal signs and symptoms such as constipation, irritable bowel syndrome, gastroesophageal reflux disease, and chronic abdominal pain. The team's observations led them to postulate that a correlation exists between food allergies and gastrointestinal disfunction in some EDS patients, which they believe could be caused by collagen abnormalities. The team think that collagen abnormalities may allow lesions to form in the tissue of the mucosal membrane barrier. In 'normal' patients, this barrier prevents most large molecules passing from inside the bowel into the bloodstream, but the team hypothesize that altered tissue integrity in those with EDS/HSD increases the chance of larger proteins (such as undigested food particles or antigens found on the surface of cells), crossing the mucosal barrier and triggering an immunogenic response that would include mast cell activation (Zhang H. & Francomano C.A. 2010).

Further clues to mechanisms that may link EDS with mast cell activation can be found in a common comorbidity of both disorders; a subset of autonomic dysfunction called postural orthostatic tachycardia syndrome (POTs).

POTs is a disorder characterised by orthostatic intolerance and manifestations such as tachycardia, nausea, intolerances to heat and cold, flushing, brain fog, lightheadedness, fainting, breathlessness, fatigue, IBS-like symptoms and more which are, in fact, not dissimilar to symptoms seen in MCA.

In 2005, Shibao et al evaluated patients diagnosed with chronic disabling orthostatic tachycardia associated with episodes of systemic MCA. The number of patients involved was small, so the team did not attempt to perform a controlled study, but the observations they made led them to propose that, in *some* cases of POTs, particularly where patients present with flushing, there may be an underlying association with mast cell activation. They hypothesized that in these cases, activation of mast cell mediators, which are capable of causing constriction or widening of blood vessels, may trigger a 'feedback loop' which results in reflex sympathetic activation; a decrease in volume of blood plasma; norepinephrine release; and thus, orthostatic intolerance.

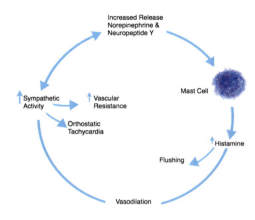

Recently confirmed evidence of *autoimmunity* in some forms of POTs could also potentially be associated with mast cell activation (Hongliang L. et al 2014). Two types of mast cells are recognised; those from connective tissue, and a distinct set that reside in mucosal tissue. The activities of the latter are dependent on T-cells (De S. 2015) a type of white blood cell best known for their role in autoimmune disorders. Mast cells and T-cells derive along different pathways from a single progenitor cell and may express complementary or overlapping functions (Wedemeyer J. & Galli S.J. 2000 / Seneviratne S. 2016 personal correspondence). A growing body of evidence indicates that mast cells and their mediator release are involved in the exacerbation of many autoimmune disorders (Walker M.E. et al 2012) including multiple sclerosis, rheumatoid arthritis and Sjögren's syndrome (Rozniecki J.J. 1995 / Hueber A.J. et al 2010), with some features of the immune response in autoimmune disorders very much like those of traditional allergic responses (Walker M.E. et al 2012).

The area of autoimmunity in POTs can be a difficult concept. After all, in most patients with EDS/HSD, it is generally attributed to abnormal connective tissue in the blood vessels, which permits veins to swell excessively in response to ordinary hydrostatic pressure, and allows excessive amounts of blood to pool in the patient's abdomen and/or lower limbs when they stand, triggering symptoms [Rowe P.C. 1999 / Bohora S. 2010 / Benarroch E.E. 2012 / Mathias C.J. 2012 / Eccles J. 2015). But POTs can be caused by many different factors, with different underlying causes in different people. It is, therefore, entirely possible for people with hEDS or HSD to acquire POTs through mechanisms unrelated to their connective tissue abnormalities, in the same way as any member of the general public. In some people, for example, symptoms of POTs start abruptly following trauma, surgery, pregnancy, and also as a secondary condition to viral infection (Soliman K. et al 2010). When POTs is acquired in this way, it is presently felt that is an autoimmune disorder (Vernino S et al 2000 / Grubb B.P. 2008), for which tell-tale serum auto-antibodies have been detected in blood samples (Conner R. 2012).

MCAS, EDS/HSD and POTs are three very complex areas of medicine. Research into any association is likely to be extremely difficult because a person's symptoms can cross so many areas of healthcare and lead to so many complications. However, these apparently unrelated symptoms might, in fact, fit together and they can and should be treated (Hakim A.J. 2016 in person).

Below we will look at the diagnosis of MCAS and its treatment.

Diagnosis of MCAS

MCAS is a diagnosis of exclusion, with primary and secondary mast cell activation disorders (see **Box 2**) as well as idiopathic anaphylaxis usually being ruled out before a diagnosis of MCAS is made (Picard M. et al 2013). It is, therefore, quite common for patients to have undergone multiple extensive medical evaluations to rule out all other causes before finally being given a diagnosis (Akin C. et al 2010).

Unlike rarer, but perhaps better known MCADs such as SM, tests carried out on those with MCAS do not show classic tell tale signs of mast cell proliferation and rarely show the '*significantly*' elevated tryptase levels that would traditionally alert most practitioners that they might be dealing with a more widely recognised mast cell activation disorder. Instead, tests are likely to show a normal number of mast cells and only a transient rise (or in some cases, normal levels) of tryptase despite all the physical symptoms of mast cell activation being very much apparent (Afrin L. 2014 / Seneviratne S. et al 2017).

According to Dr Andrew White, in these patients we need to look for other clues that their mast cells are not functioning normally. He says: '*There are many different chemicals that come out of mast cells which can be measured. Substances like histamine, prostaglandins and leukotrienes are usually measured in a 24 hour urine sample.'* If the symptoms fit, the patient has evidence of making too much mast cell mediator, and treatment with medications that block or treat the substances are effective, then many physicians are then willing to diagnose MCAS.

New proposed criteria for the diagnosis of MCAS was put forward by Dr Chem Akin et al in 2010 and, although MCAS is not yet internationally recognised, it is hoped this will be formally adopted over the coming years, resulting in better understanding and treatment for patients.

In the meantime, Dr Lawrence Afrin, a hematologist specialising in mast cell disorders, and Dr Suranjith Seneviratne, Consultant in Clinical Immunology and Allergy at the Royal Free Hospital and University College London, and Director of the Centre for Mast Cell Disorder, recommend doctors look for:

- symptoms indicating chronic/recurrent abnormal mast cell mediator release,
- and, at least partial response to therapy targeted against mast cells or their mediators,
- laboratory evidence of such release (or of mast cell proliferation not meeting World Health Organisation criteria for systemic mastocytosis),
- absence of any other evident disease which could better explain the full range of findings in the patient.

Treatment
Prof Seneviratne and his team in London are at the cutting edge of research and treatment of mast cell disorders, seeing what he believes to be the highest number of MCAS patients in any country in the world (close to 1000 as of Sept 2016). He hopes that their work will enable many more questions to be answered over the next few years.

In the meantime, however, there is no cure for MCAS, so treatment is primarily aimed at controlling and relieving symptoms. All or some of the same mediator-blocking medications used to treat SM may be used e.g. mast cell stabilisers and H1 and H2 antihistamines (Gerhard J. 2011). If patients are able to identify potential triggers for their symptoms (e.g. dietary, chemicals, medications, allergens), desensitisation therapy can be considered. Patients may be advised to follow a low histamine diet in general and, where required/possible, to make environmental modifications in order to reduce exposure to known triggers. Proton pump inhibitors may also be prescribed; if needed for stomach hyperacidity and, where tolerated, nonsteroidal anti-inflammatory medications. Like those with mastocytosis, some patients with mast cell activation syndrome may require higher then normal dosages to control their symptoms (Ref: The Mastocytosis Society Canada 2015). Further information on medications for MCAS can be found in the 2017 paper by Prof Seneviratne et al, entitled Mast Cell Disorders in Ehlers-Danlos Syndrome (see bibliography).

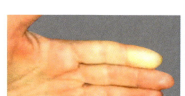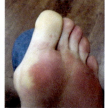

Raynaud's phenomenon & chilblains

In Raynaud's phenomenon, the blood vessels go into a temporary spasm, blocking the flow of blood to the extremities. The fingers and toes are most commonly affected, but the condition can also affect other areas of the body, such as the nose, lips and ears, causing them to feel cold and to loose colour. In the general population, Primary Raynaud's is usually triggered in cold temperatures, or by anxiety or stress. Secondary Raynaud's can be caused by various conditions of the blood vessels, joints, muscles, nerves or skin - for example, scleroderma, rheumatoid arthritis, multiple sclerosis, systemic lupus erythematosus (8/Patient.co.uk). Raynaud's sufferers are also prone to chilblains, which develop on the fingers and toes. These are seen as small, itchy and painful reddish-blue swellings which develop when the skin gets cold, causing the tiny blood vessels to constrict severely (Raynaud's Assoc.).

Raynauds-like symptoms and hEDS/HSD
Although chilblains are cited as a less common skin manifestation of hEDS/HSD, 'Raynaud's-like' symptoms are considered to be common co-morbidities. The type of Raynaud's that occurs in hEDS and HSD may be a secondary form, caused by over-reactivity of the sympathetic nervous system relating to the dysautonomia / postural orthostatic tachycardia commonly experienced by those with hEDS and HSD (Levy H.P 2004 / Castori M. 2010).

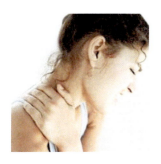

Fibromyalgia

Fibromyalgia is a long-term condition which causes widespread pain and tenderness in many areas of the body, often with accompanying pins and needles and numbness (6/Patient.co.uk). Other symptoms include feeling dizzy and faint, decreased concentration and memory ('brain fog'), being very sensitive to bright lights and crowds (this can feel unbearably amplified, especially during 'flare-ups'), difficulty sleeping, irritable bladder, muscle stiffness, headaches, extreme tiredness and feeling as if your hands or feet are swollen (although they are not) (2/NHS.uk). Symptoms tend to vary from person to person, and from day to day.

Fibromyalgia affects more women than men. It can develop at any age, but those between the ages of 30 and 50 are most likely to be affected (2/NHS.uk). The exact causes are not known and for many years there has been debate as to whether fibromyalgia is a physical disease affecting the muscles, or whether it is an emotional disorder. According to Professor Rodney Grahame, *'the prevailing view is that it is probably some form of distress signal that can arise in people with a number of different and unrelated conditions'*.

According to a study carried out by Tobias Schmidt-Wilcke et al (2007 & 2014), scans of patients with fibromyalgia showed that their brains process non painful stimuli, such as touch and sound, differently from the brains of people without the disorder. The data, obtained using MR-imaging and voxel-based morphometry VBM, revealed what was described as 'a conspicuous pattern of altered brain morphology', with a visible decrease in grey matter in both the right superior temporal gyrus and left posterior thalamus, and an increase in grey matter in the left orbitofrontal cortex, the left cerebellum and in the striatum bilaterally. This suggests that fibromyalgia is associated with structural changes in the central nervous system of patients suffering from this chronic pain disorder.

Writing for Arthritis Care, Jennifer Glass, Faculty Associate at the Research Centre for Group Dynamics at the university of Michigan, cites the study as *'adding more weight to the fact that there is some kind of very real disorder in people with fibromyalgia - one that is more of a central nervous system problem, rather than something out in the periphery causing pain.'* Changes in the way the body functions have also been noticed in people with fibromyalgia, including disturbed pain messages, low levels of hormones and sleep problems. However, it is not yet clear what causes these changes in the first place, and how they lead to fibromyalgia.

Fibromyalgia and hEDS/HSD

Several studies suggest a strong association between joint hypermobility and fibromyalgia (Ofluoglu D. 2006 / Sendur O.F. et al 2007), with symptoms such as multiple pain sensations, fatigue and proprioceptive disorders being common to both (also see **Box 1**, page 83). Findings by Dr Trinh Hermanns-Le show that some patients suffering from fibromyalgia present with clinical signs and alterations in the tissue, and ultrastructure of the skin similar to the hypermobile type of Ehlers-Danlos syndrome (hEDS) and, together with other experts such as Dr Faber from the Milwaukee Pain Clinic, she hypothesizes that some types of fibromyalgia possibly represent undiagnosed hEDS.

In one study conducted in fibromyalgia patients, 46.6% of patients were found to have joint hypermobility, against 22% in the control group. In another, 64.2% were affected versus 28.8% in the control group. Researchers are trying to establish whether joint hypermobility may play a part in the mechanism that causes pain in certain forms of fibromyalgia (Hermanns-Le T. et al 2012b / Cassisi G. 2014).

Dr. Faber, of the Milwaukee Pain Clinic states:

'In my professional experience often the greatest symptom (of Fibromyalgia) *is lack of endurance and the need to change positions. The pain discomfort is often described as a pulling or aching which worsens with time to a rather severe pain. It lessens with changing from standing to sitting or from these positions to lying. This cycle, of course, repeats as a chronic complaint. Often times the joints will be noted to crack and*

Box 1.

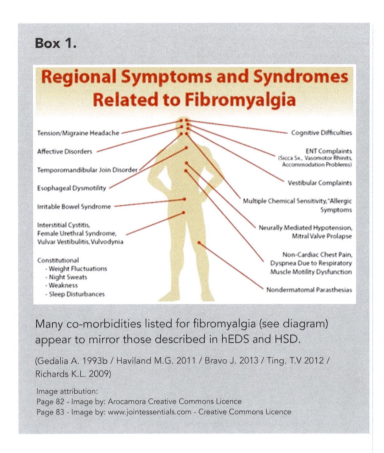

Many co-morbidities listed for fibromyalgia (see diagram) appear to mirror those described in hEDS and HSD.

(Gedalia A. 1993b / Haviland M.G. 2011 / Bravo J. 2013 / Ting. T.V 2012 / Richards K.L. 2009)

Image attribution:
Page 82 - Image by: Arocamora Creative Commons Licence
Page 83 - Image by: www.jointessentials.com - Creative Commons Licence

pop. My examinations have almost always revealed an undiagnosed hyper-mobility syndrome of the congenital or benign types.'

Dr Jamie Bravo MD (2008) also views Fibromyalgia as a co-morbidity of or, in some cases, possibly a misdiagnosis of, what is actually undiagnosed hypermobility spectrum disorder, stating:

'..all patients with fibromyalgia that I see fulfill the Brighton criteria that is diagnostic for joint hypermobility syndrome [now known as hypermobility spectrum disorder]. We'd call these pains "fibromyalgic pains of Joint Hypermobility syndrome [HSD]'.

Karen Lee Richards, author of Health Guide Fibromyalgia, agrees, stating: *'Fibromyalgia is rarely the only diagnosis a person has. Usually someone with fibromyalgia also has one or more comorbid or overlapping conditions, such as Chronic Fatigue syndrome, irritable bowel syndrome, restless legs syndrome, Migraines, allergies, etc [see* **Box 1***]. One possible comorbid condition we don't talk about frequently is joint hypermobility syndrome [now know as HSD]. ...Although we don't really know why, hypermobility and fibromyalgia seem to occur together more often than would be expected by chance.'*

A study by Gedalia et al (1993b) tested the hypothesis that joint hypermobility may play a part in the pathogenesis of pain in fibromyalgia. Researchers studied 338 children between the ages of nine and 15. They found that:

- 13% had joint hypermobility
- 6% had fibromyalgia
- 81% of those with fibromyalgia had joint hypermobility
- 40% of those with joint hypermobility had fibromyalgia

The investigators concluded, "This study suggests that there is a strong association between joint hypermobility and fibromyalgia in schoolchildren. It is possible that joint hypermobility may play a part in the pathogenesis of pain in fibromyalgia. More studies are needed to establish the clinical significance of this observation."

Treatment of fibromyalgia tends to be based around a combination of medicines such as antidepressants and painkillers, and self-help management strategies including exercise, physiotherapy, tens machine usage, myofascial release therapy, heated pool treatment (hydrotherapy), and cognitive behavioural therapy (6/Patient.co.uk).

Symptoms & Comorbidities

Part 2 - Area specific symptoms & comorbidities

Area specific symptoms & comorbidities

The remainder of the chapter is dedicated to a list of 'area specific' symptoms and comorbidities such as dental problems or disorders of the knee, working down from the head to the feet. Symptoms such as pain, which can be both area specific or body-wide have been placed at the beginning of the chapter. The following list should not be considered exhaustive.

Area Specific Symptoms

Headaches

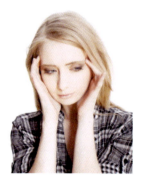

In a paper dedicated to his hypermobile patients (Pocinki A. 2010), Dr Alan Pocinki explains that people with hypermobile joints are predisposed to many different kinds of headaches, which often turn into migraines. He states that primary causes include chronic neck strain, temporomandibular joint problems, and severe autonomic dysfunction, and that dehydration or 'hangover-like' headaches may be related to inadequate blood flow. Cervical spine joint hypermobility is described as a causation factor for headaches (including persistent daily headaches), by Rozen T. D. et al. (NB/ headaches relating to Chiari malformation are discussed in 'The spine', page 91). Headache pain can be disabling in EDS (Jacome D.E. 1999), with migraine being the most common form in hEDS/HSD (Bendik E.M. and Tinkle B. 2011).

Photo attribution (above): marcolm - FreeDigitalPhotos.net

Ocular features

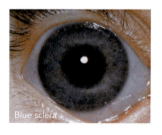

Overall, ocular complaints are usually mild to moderate in hEDS/HSD (Castori M. 2012). According to a study by Gharbiya et al, the most consistent association of eye anomalies in the hEDS/HSD group includes *'dry eyes, steeper corneas, pathologic myopia, and vitreous abnormalities, as well as a higher rate of minor lens opacities'*. Blue sclera is also commonly associated with hEDS (Castori M. 2012). All these eye conditions can be found in the general population, but are overrepresented in those with hEDS/HSD. Below, we look at some of these in a little more detail.

Keratitis sicca (dry eye syndrome): occurs when there is a problem with the tear film that normally keeps the eye moist and lubricated, resulting in decreased tear production or increased tear film evaporation. It can occur as a result of aging, as a side effect of some medications (such as antihistamines, antidepressants, diuretics, non-steroidal anti-inflammatories, and many others), and as a symptom of various medical conditions (9/Patient.co.uk). Symptoms include irritation in the eyes, which may feel gritty or like they are burning, or the sensation of a foreign body in the eye. Some people describe discomfort in their eyes when looking at bright lights and some experience temporarily blurred vision, which improves when they blink (1/NHS.uk & 9/Patient.co.uk). Dry eyes are common in those with hEDS/HSD, and may be associated with autonomic dysfunction and related dehydration (Castori M. 2012).

Keratoconus (steep corneas): occur when the normally round dome-shaped cornea progressively thins, causing a cone-shaped bulge to develop. The causes are not fully understood, but this disorder is more common in people who have atopic allergies such as eczema and asthma (Rahi A. et al 1977). Steep corneas are also associated with Down's syndrome and in some disorders of connective tissue such as EDS, Osteogenesis imperfecta and Marfan syndrome (Agarwal S. 2002). This disorder is usually first noticed in those in their teens and twenties, and symptoms include the distortion of images such as seeing 'starbursts' around the outside of lights, glare, halos and blurred vision (Allaboutvision.com).

Myopia (shortsightedness): Myopia causes distant objects to appear blurred, while close objects can be seen clearly; this is also known as short sightedness. Symptoms often start around puberty, and get gradually worse until the eye is fully grown. Myopia can range from mild to very severe (pathologic myopia). It is considered one of the less common features of eye problems in hEDS/HSD (Mishra B .P. et al 1996 / Castori M. 2012).

Blue sclera: The sclera (also known as the white of the eye), is the protective outer layer of the eye containing collagen and elastic fibres. The sclera should look opaque white but, in those with heritable disorders of connective tissue, blood vessels may be visible through the thinner sclerae, making the sclera appear faintly blueish (Bravo J. F. & Wolff C. 2006). Blue sclerae is seen in varying degrees in hEDS/HSD females, but is rare in males. Blue sclerae is normal in children up to 2 years of age (Bravo J. 2010).   Photo (blue sclera) by National Eye Institute

Less common features include: tilted optic disc, antimongoloid palpebral slant, unilateral ptosis, epicanthic folds and blepharochalasis (Castori M. 2012)

The nose and throat

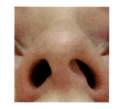

Deviated Nasal Septum
The septum is made of cartilage (composed of collagen) and divides the two nostrils of the nose. The term 'deviated septum' describes a septum that is off centre, making breathing difficult. The main symptom is nasal congestion, which is chronic and usually affects one side of the nose more than the other. People with a deviated septum may snore or suffer from sleep apnoea (see below). Other symptoms sometimes noted are sinus infections, headaches, postnasal drip and facial pain.

A deviated nasal septum may be caused by trauma to the nose, but for many it is present at birth, or occurs as a part of aging. It also has a significant appearance as a family trait, and in genetic conditions such as Ehlers-Danlos syndrome and Marfan syndrome (Fillingim R. B. 2009 / Child A.H. / Bravo J. 2011).

Obstructive sleep apnoea, and hypopnoea
Obstructive sleep apnoea (OSA) is a relatively common condition where the walls of the throat relax and narrow during sleep, or a partial blockage of the airway results in airflow reduction (known as hypopnoea), interrupting normal breathing that regularly interrupts sleep. OSA can have a big impact on quality of life and increases the risk of developing other health conditions.

Research by Dr Thomas Gaisl and his team (2017) showed that the prevalence of obstructive sleep apnoea (OSA) is higher in patients with Ehlers-Danlos syndrome than in a matched control group (in patients with EDS, OSA prevalence was 32% versus 6% in the matched control group). This is of clinical relevance as it is associated with fatigue, excessive daytime sleepiness and impaired quality of life'.

Dysphonia
Dysphonia is the name given to difficulty in speaking due to a physical disorder of the mouth, tongue, throat, or vocal cords. Chronic or recurrent dysphonia was found to be relatively common in hEDS during research by Marcos Castori et al, with 38.1% of patients displaying symptoms, with subsequent investigations demonstrating incoordination and/or low muscle tone/muscle weakness of the vocal cords. (Castori M. 2010a / Arulanandam S. et al 2016)

AREA SPECIFIC SYMPTOMS & COMORBIDITIES

Asthma-like symptoms

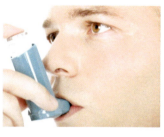

Some specialists think that certain forms of asthma, or asthma-like symptoms, may be caused by genetic connective tissue defects. In 2007, Morgan and Bird demonstrated an increased frequency of respiratory symptoms and reduced tolerance to exercise in subjects with HSD and EDS, compared with controls. Their findings confirmed:

- An increased prevalence of asthmatic symptoms.
- A genetic tendency to develop allergic diseases such as allergic rhinitis, asthma and eczema.
- Alterations in the mechanical properties of their lungs in many of the individuals, resulting in impaired gas exchange & increased lung volumes.
- An increased tendency of the airways to collapse.

In later work, Soyucen and Esen (2010), put forward the hypothesis that: *'Changes in the mechanical properties of the bronchial airways and lung parenchyma may underlie the increased tendency of the airways to collapse in asthmatic children'*. The paper agrees with the study carried out by Morgan et al, suggesting that HSD may lead to persistent childhood wheezing by causing airway collapse through a connective tissue defect that affects the structure of the airways.

'Asthma is not just a single disease, but a complex of several sub-types that should be genetically mapped and understood individually if we are to prevent and treat the disease properly in future' (Bønnelykke K. 2013)

FreeDigitalPhotos.net - Photo (Asthma) by marin.

Dental features

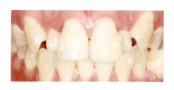

Features such as dental over crowding and a high narrow palate are found in most heritable disorders of connective tissue, including hEDS/HSD (Levy H.P. 2004).

© Understanding hEDS and HSD by C. Smith

Bleeding gums and gum disease, such as gingivitis, are often seen and may be caused by repeated damage to the fragile mucosa when brushing teeth (5/Patient.co.uk) and/or by ineffective oral hygiene due to restricted movement and pain in the hands and wrists (De Coster P. J. 2005a & 2005b).

Teeth may move more quickly than 'normal' when dental corrections, such as bracing or wearing a spring to expand the jaw, are carried out (7/EDNF.org / Porter S. 2016), and may tend to relapse after treatment is discontinued (Mitakides J. et al 2017). This may be due to the stretching, tearing and slow repair of the collagen fibres (7/EDNF.org). It is common to find that prolonged use of a retainer is required after treatment is finished. (Abel M.D. & Carrasco L.R. 2006 / Létourneau Y. 2001).

Fragility of the mucosa and increased susceptibility to dislocations of the temporomandibular joint means that orthodontic treatment should be carried out with great care in all those with EDS (Abel M.D. & Carrasco 2006 / Létourneau Y. 2001 / Pacak D.K. 2009).

Tooth enamel may show signs of minor pigmentation anomalies in the absence of 'normal' causes such as smoking, red wine, strong tea etc. (Castori M. 2012).

Resistance to local anaesthetics such as those used in dentistry have now been recognised in those with hEDS/HSD (also see page 25 and page 65).

Treatment and management of dental implications in hEDS, and HSD, can be found in Chapter 3, page 163)

Xerostomia (Dry mouth): Dry mouth results from reduced saliva production. As with 'dry eyes', dry mouth may be a reflection of the autonomic dysfunction often associated with hEDS/HSD. It can also be caused by dehydration, stress and medications (Castori M. 2012) such as antihistamines, antidepressants, diuretics, non-steroidal anti-inflammatories, and many others.

Temporomandibular joint dysfunction:
The temporomandibular joint (TMJ) is one of the most complicated joints in the body. Its muscles and ligaments enable it to move in multiple directions and to carry out tasks such as yawning and chewing food.

'Temporomandibular joint dysfunction (TMD)' is the term used to describe the many problems that can occur in the TMJ including difficulty in chewing

food; pain around the joint itself or around the ear, cheek and neck; grating, clicking noises when the jaw is moved; locking of the jaw, headaches, malalignment of the upper and lower jaw (Bupa.co.uk). The symptoms of TMD are reported in up to 70% of hEDS/HSD patients with an additional high incidence of myofascial pain, subluxation and dislocations (Castori M. 2012 / 7EDNF.org 1993), and is thought to be caused by hypermobility of the joint, combined with a dyspraxia of the muscles used for chewing food (Castori M. 2012).

> '[hEDS/HSD] *patients frequently report symptoms associated with TMJ and usually present in one of two ways. Pain in the area of the joint is reported in association with stiffness and reduced jaw opening due to muscle spasm, or at the other end of the scale patients report a feeling of 'looseness' in the joint, with clicking, subluxation or dislocation on wide opening of jaw'* (Keer R. & Grahame R. 2003).

Unfortunately, there are no specific interventions that have been *proven* to help TMJ laxity and dysfunction. Some may find intra-oral devices helpful (see page 164), but, usually, self-management techniques such as resting the jaw, taking smaller bites when chewing, making a conscious effort to open the mouth less widely when yawning etc., are recommended. In the case of acute flares of TMJ pain, local myofascial release and muscle relaxant medications may be beneficial. Dislocations which do not relocate spontaneously should be treated under medical supervision. '*Surgical intervention is often disappointing and should be considered only as a last resort*' (Castori M. 2012).

Information on dental management and TMD can be found on page 162.

Chronic neck strain

Nearly everyone with hEDS/HSD is affected by chronic neck strain, according to Dr Alan Pocinki MD. In his previously mentioned paper (page 85), he suggests that the two main reasons for this are:

• '*The ligaments that are supposed to support the head are too loose and*

© Understanding hEDS and HSD by C. Smith

therefore cannot do their job well. The muscles of the neck are forced to do more of the work of supporting the head than they are meant to do, so they become strained.

- *Second, most HMS [hEDS/HSD] patients have shoulders that are too loose, that is the "ball" of the upper arm is not held tightly in the "socket" of the shoulder. Because of the weakness of the shoulders, almost any activity that uses the arm, including reaching, pushing, pulling, and carrying, pulls not only on the shoulder but also on the neck.'*

These issues mean that the neck muscles are constantly under strain, and '…*what little healing may occur overnight is promptly undone the next day.*' He says he has found that this process occurs so gradually, that many people with hEDS/HSD do not even notice it and, when asked, they may say, "My neck is fine," when in fact their necks are a mass of knotted soft tissue; soft tissue that does not feel soft at all!

The shoulders

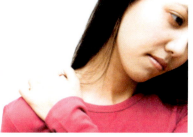

Multidirectional shoulder instability (MDI)
The humerus, glenoid, scapula, acromion, clavicle and surrounding musculature and ligaments make up the shoulder. There are three significant joints: the sternoclavicular joint, the acromioclavicular joint and the glenohumeral joint.

Multidirectional instability of the shoulder is defined as symptomatic-laxity of the glenohumeral joint. It is common in patients with EDS (Hawkins R.J. et al 1984 / Silliman J.F., 1993 / Johnson S.M. 2010) and can cause pain, nerve entrapment, stretched and torn ligaments and, of course, dislocations and subluxations (also see page 61).

Excessive laxity of the joint capsule in several, or all, directions (anterior, inferior, and posterior) is often experienced, which can lead to difficulty in maintaining the head of the humerus in a centered position within the joint.

AREA SPECIFIC SYMPTOMS & COMORBIDITIES

According to Johnson S.M. 2010, patients with hyperlaxity and instability are more likely to experience recurrent subluxation than dislocation, but dislocations are also common, with Ainsworth 1993 and Dolan 1997 citing shoulder dislocations as one of the two most commonly dislocated joints among those with EDS.

The term 'shoulder *laxity*' is used when excessive range of movement in one, or multiple, directions can be demonstrated, but the individual has no symptoms. In contrast, the term 'shoulder *instability*' is used when a patient presents shoulder laxity along with shoulder pain, weakness, fatigue, paresthesias, subluxation or dislocation (Anderson B.C. 2014).

Winging of the shoulder blade
A 'winged' scapula (shoulder blade) can suggest underlying problems within the shoulder and is often seen as a secondary symptom to instability. For example, winging of the scapula can often be seen in those who experience injuries, such as recurrent dislocations of the shoulder, and can lead to scapula dysrhythmia (muscles working out of time rather than all acting at the same time) and therefore, a dysfunction of the muscles that move and support the shoulder complex and scapula. Any painful condition of the shoulder can make a person more prone to problems with the scapula, because the pain often leads to abnormal movements of the shoulder as a whole.

Patients may complain of shoulder blade pain and may notice discomfort or pressure on the scapula when sitting in a chair. On examination, it may be clear that the scapula protrudes out on the back, rather than laying flat, or it may only become apparent when the shoulder is under increased load - for example, carrying a shopping bag or doing a press-up. Treating scapula dysrhythmia is an essential part of treating shoulder recurrent subluxations and dislocations.

Not all shoulder symptoms in hypermobile patients are caused by instability, and other causes such as rotator cuff tendonitis, rotator cuff impingement syndrome and rotator cuff tears should be considered during clinical assessment (Shirley E.D. et al 2012).

Photo attribution:
Photo (page 87) by: by marcolm - FreeDigitalPhotos.net
Photo (page 88) by: sixninepixels - FreeDigitalPhotos.net

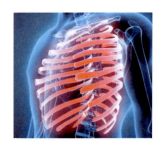

The chest and ribs

Less frequently described in medical literature, but problematic for many, are the joints where the ribs meet the breastbone, and where the ribs meet the vertebrae of the spine.

Slipping rib syndrome

Slipping rib syndrome is under-recognised and frequently misdiagnosed, which can lead to years of unresolved chest, abdominal and/or thoracic pain (Udermann B.E. 2005 / Tinkle B.T. 2010). When the sternocostal ligaments that hold the ribs to the sternum are weak, the ribs can intermittently slip out of place. This stretches the ligament even further, resulting in severe pain. For some, simply coughing or blowing one's nose can be enough to cause chronic chest pain from slipping rib syndrome.

Tests for investigating slipping rib syndrome include examining a patient for rib restriction by looking for a lack of symmetry of the posterior chest wall movements when a patient breaths deeply, and the Hook mnoeuvre, where the patient lies on their unaffected side while the therapist hooks their fingers under the lower costal margin and pulls forward. A positive test reproduces the patient's pain and causes a click.

Manual therapy, advice on avoiding poor posture and nerve blocks are all useful in treating this condition.

Rib subluxation / dislocation

Subluxated rib heads and rib dislocations are a problem commonly described in forums by people who have hEDS/HSD; seemingly occurring where the ribs connect to the spine or to the sternum. Unfortunately many find physicians are skeptical, as there is still scant scientific evidence supporting the existence of such a phenomenon. As mentioned on page 61, whilst ribs are not generally thought of as 'joints', they rely on the same problematic ligaments, tendons and cartilage that affect other areas of the body, so it may be feasible that they can be affected in the same way. Anecdotal descriptions from those who are hypermobile include rib subluxation and dislocation that can occur with normal movements such as coughing, laughing, sneezing, lifting, or throwing, and can be very painful. Often a sharp pain is described at the site, most often between the shoulder blades. Chest pain and muscle spasms may be induced by movement or breathing. If the nerves become pinched, symptoms such as numbness, and tingling may also be experienced. A lump at the dislocated site may be seen and swelling may occur.

Where muscle spasms and pain are fairly well controlled through pain relief, dislocations may resolve on their own, but otherwise injections of anaesthesia or muscle relaxants may be required (Tinkle B.T. 2010).

Costochondritis

In costochondritis, inflammation occurs at the junctions where the upper ribs join the cartilage that holds them to the breastbone (sternum), causing localised chest wall pain and tenderness that can be reproduced by pushing on the involved cartilage in the front of the rib cage (1/physiopedia.com). The cause of costochondritis is usually unknown. It may improve on its own after a few weeks, but it can last for several months or more. The condition doesn't lead to any permanent problems, but may sometimes relapse. Though painful, it often resolves without treatment (other than painkillers and anti-inflammatories), although corticosteroid injections may be recommended if pain is severe (15/NHS.uk).

> 'Many people with JHS [HSD] feel chest pain and tightness, and may even seek emergency care to rule out heart disease, when the source of their symptoms is the joints of the rib cage, a condition called costochondritis, or inflammation of the rib cartilage (Pocinki A.G. 2010).

Thoracic outlet syndrome (TOS)

If there is a narrowing of the passageway between the base of the neck and the armpit (the thoracic outlet), compression of the nerves and/or blood vessels that pass through this area can occur; this is known as thoracic outlet syndrome (Feinberg J H 2009). Symptoms can be constant or intermittent, and can vary in type depending on which structures are being compressed. Symptoms include pain/ discomfort along the top of the clavicle and shoulder, with pain sometimes spreading along the inside edge of the arm. Numbness and tingling, called paraesthesia, may also occur in the hand and fingers.

Symptoms tend to get worse when using the arms away from the body or overhead, for example when drying one's hair, folding washing, keeping arms in the 10 to 2 position when driving, lifting, carrying and writing. It may be difficult to hold and grip things, and the hand may feel clumsy. TOS can vary greatly in the range of symptoms it can cause. Some patients experience major symptoms, while others have only minimal discomfort or loss of function. Causes include: anatomical defects, pressure on the joints, repetitive activities, pregnancy, trauma, enlarged muscle/scar tissue, abnormal muscles in the neck, and a cervical rib (3/Mayo Clinic). The most common form of TOS is neurogenic (compression of the nerves), but two other forms of TOS also exist, which are related to compression of the vein or artery. These are far less common, accounting for only around 5% of cases, and are not discussed here.

Can hypermobility associated with TOS?
Hypermobility of the shoulder blade, and/or shoulder instability, can create tension or traction on the neurovascular structures in the thoracic outlet region and lead to 'thoracic outlet-type' symptoms (Feinberg J.H. 2009 / Chopra P. 2015).

The term 'disputed thoracic outlet syndrome' is sometimes used to describe features of pain, numbness, tingling and other subjective discomforts, when weakness/atrophy are not readily affirmable, and standard scans and imaging are inconclusive (Clinicalkey 2014). It is usually encountered in young or middle-aged, healthy, active adults (more women experience symptoms than men). Acceptance of this condition as a diagnostic entity is not universal; some doctors don't believe it exists, while others say it's a common disorder (3/mayoclinic.org).

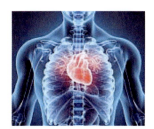

The heart

The supporting structures of the heart, including the valves and major blood vessels, involve connective tissue and therefore have the propensity to be affected by hEDS/HSD. Aortic root dilation and mitral valve prolapse are uncommon but can occur in hEDS (Pauker S.P. et al 2014). However, older estimates of the frequency of mitral valve prolapse (Grahame R. 1981 / Handler C.E. et al 1985) should be interpreted with caution, as the criteria defining MVP have evolved, and studies prior to 1989 may have overestimated its prevalence.

© Understanding hEDS and HSD by C. Smith

AREA SPECIFIC SYMPTOMS & COMORBIDITIES

In a cross-sectional and longitudinal study to outline the prevalence of cardiac findings in hypermobile and classical types of Ehlers-Danlos syndrome (and to provide longitudinal analysis of aortic root growth), aortic root dilatation was seen in twelve percent of patients with hypermobile EDS, and the frequency of mitral valve prolapse was reported as six percent in those with hypermobile EDS (Atzinger C.L. et al 2011).

The study concluded that, although aortic root size and mitral valve prolapse are increased in patients with both EDS hypermobile type and EDS classical type, in many cases they tend to be of little clinical consequence. Echocardiography may still be warranted as part of cardiovascular assessment, but decreased frequency of screening is recommended, especially in symptom-free adults.

Please note that cardiovascular dysfunction such as palpitations and tachycardia is discussed on page 69.

The elbow

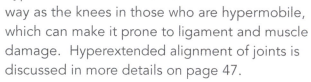

Hyperextension
The elbow joint is prone to hyperextension in the same way as the knees in those who are hypermobile, which can make it prone to ligament and muscle damage. Hyperextended alignment of joints is discussed in more details on page 47.

Pulled elbow
Pulled elbow is another name given to a dislocation or subluxation of the elbow joint (also see page 61). Variations in the anatomy of the radial head and surrounding structures, in combination with the degree of any violent injury that occurs, can cause a pulled/dislocated elbow. However, it should be noted that at least half of children who are seen for so called, 'pulled elbow' have no history of a 'pull' at all (Staheli L.T. 2008 / Tinkle B.T. 2010).

The association between pulled elbow and hypermobility indicates that pulled elbow can also be considered one of the effects of this condition (Amir D. et al 1990). Indeed, the results of the study by Amir et al, over a 2 year period, found that the prevalence of hypermobility among children with pulled elbow was 73%, which is 23% higher than in non-hypermobile children of similar age. In 48% of the cases of children with pulled elbow, at least one of the parents was also hypermobile, whereas only in 10% of the control group were parents hypermobile.

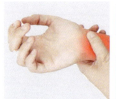 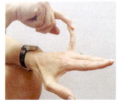 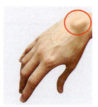

The wrist / hand / fingers

The hand

Hand dysfunction is commonly linked to ligamentous laxity (Murray K. 2006). In those who are hypermobile, the small joints of the hand are often affected, and finger and thumb instability, joint dislocations and hyperextension is commonly seen. The carpometacarpal joint of the thumb may be particularly susceptible to weakened ligamentous constraints in Ehlers-Danlos syndrome (Moore J.R. 1985). Carrying out normal day to day tasks, such as writing or chopping vegetables, can result in overuse injuries such as hand fatigue, aching, pain, cramp and dislocations. Assistive aids, accessed via occupational therapy, can be of great assistance. Such aids may include 'fat' pens with a wide nib to encourage a more stable grip and finger position when writing, and adapted cutlery to help with tasks such as chopping. Hand therapists may also suggest 'ring splints', to stabilise the finger joints when carrying out certain tasks.

The wrist

In the general population, the wrist is the most commonly injured joint in the body (You J.S. et al 2007)

> 'Over the last 20 years, significant advances have occurred in the understanding of wrist anatomy, pathophysiology, and carpal kinematics. Even so, some wrist injuries remain a diagnostic enigma, while others remain frustrating to treat either conservatively or with operative intervention.'
> (Morhart M. 2015)

Weakness of the wrist, nerve compression with carpal tunnel-type symptoms, and ulnar nerve entrapment/neuropathy are all described as affecting those with hEDS/HSD (Tinkle B. 2010 and Aktas I. 2008). Nerve compression can cause weakness in the muscles of the hand, making tendinosis more likely, and making small dextrose tasks, such as sewing or doing up buttons, difficult. Numbness and pins and needles in the fingers is described, along with chronic arm/hand pain. Carpal dislocations can lead to chronic pain and wrist instability. They are difficult to diagnose and often missed (3/ patient.co.uk).

Ganglion cysts

A ganglion cyst is created when there is a weakness in the connective tissue (fascia) over the tendon sheaths. This allows the sheath to bulge out and fill with synovial fluid, which may cause pain and/or problems with mobility in the joint (often found in the wrists). Baker's Cysts (behind the knee) are also associated with hypermobility, especially in childhood (Neubauer H. 2011).

Arachnodactyly

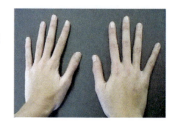

Arachnodactyly is condition in which the fingers are abnormally long and slender, in comparison to the palm of the hand and arch of the foot. Some individuals may also have thumbs which are pulled inwards towards their palms. This feature can occur on its own in the general population, but is also be associated with heritable disorders of connective tissue such as EDS and Marfan syndrome.

Other areas of this book, which deal with symptoms affecting the hand / wrist, include Raynaud's phenomenon (page 81) and complex regional pain syndrome (page 53) and dislocations (page 61).

The spine

When the ligaments that normally support the spine and pelvis, keeping them stable, are hypermobile, they are too loose and put muscles under extra strain in their effort to try and support the upper body.

When the hips are hypermobile, the lower back can be put under strain in an attempt to stabilise the pelvis. These imbalances often lead to lower back pain. The spine is particularly susceptible to problems such as disc prolapse (also known as a slipped disc or herniated disc), pars interarticularis defects and spondylolisthesis (Graham R. 1999) and spinal pain syndrome (Stodolna-Tukendorf J. 2011). Degenerative disc disease, facet arthrosis, dural ectasia and dural cysts are also seen in those with EDS (Francomano C.A. 2006). Photo attribution: yodiyim - FreeDigitalPhotos.net

Some of these are described in more detail below:

Spinal pain syndrome

The most common cause of spinal pain syndrome is overload of the spine. It damages the function of the spine and the morphology of the spine's tissues.

Literature suggests that a generalised insufficiency of connective tissue, which manifests itself as a hypermobility of joints, might be one of the causes of overload.

Joint hypermobility is recognised much more often in patients with spinal pain syndromes than in patients treated because of other diseases, and twice more often in females than in males. Amongst young people under 30 years of age, hypermobility occurs in 55% of the population with spinal pain syndrome. In the youngest patients, HSD may be the cause of overload spinal pain syndromes, and a predisposition factor towards spinal pain syndromes in older patients (Stodolna-Tukendorf J. 2011).

Lumbar disc prolapse (also known as a slipped disc or herniated disc)

Lumbar disc prolapse occurs when a tear in the outer ring of an intervertebral disc allows the soft, inner material to bulge out beyond the damaged outer rings. This can aggravate a nerve and trigger back and leg pain. Excessive lumbar spinal mobility and abnormal collagen alignment in the lumbar spinal discs of those with EDS/HSD can leave them vulnerable to lumbar disc prolapse (Aktas I. et al 2011). From their findings, Aktas et al concluded that *'there is a positive correlation between Lumbar Disc Prolapse and JHS/EDS-H* [HSD/hEDS].*'*

Pars interarticularis defects

The 'Pars interarticularis' is a small segment of bone that joins the facet joints in the back of the spine. A 'defect' would include a lumbar spondylolysis; a unilateral or bilateral stress fracture of the narrow bridge between the upper and lower pars interarticularis, leading to a condition called spondylolisthesis (3/spine-health.com). The pars interarticularis defect is generally believed to represent a fatigue fracture caused by repetitive loading and unloading of this region of the vertebrae from physical activity. It should be remembered that, for those with a connective tissue abnormality such as hEDS/HSD, the physical activity necessary to cause such symptoms may only be minor day to day activities.

Spondylolisthesis

This can occur through degeneration of the spine as a natural occurrence of aging, but it can also develop as a result of stress fractures (see Pars interarticularis defects above) caused by excessive hyperextension of the spine (commonly seen in gymnasts), physical trauma or as a congenital birth

---

AREA SPECIFIC SYMPTOMS & COMORBIDITIES

Imaging and radiological findings
Though CT scans and MRI remain the standard for most spinal practitioners, radiological findings do not always correlate well with clinical findings or surgical outcome in those with hEDS (Arnasson O. et al., 1987 / Tinkle B. et al 2017).

In those with hEDS, it should be borne in mind that dynamic instability is unlikely to be demonstrated in a resting supine subject, and pathological instability will often only be revealed when the ligaments are placed under stress. Though not yet validated, dynamic MRI in the upright position subjects the vertebral spine to physiological loading, and can be performed in the flexed and extended positions to demonstrate instability (Milhorat T.H. et al., 2010 / Klekamp J. 2012 / Tinkle B. et al 2017).

defect. In a healthy spinal column, each vertebrae is stacked above the other and separated by intervertebral discs. When spondylolisthesis affects an individual's spinal column, it means that the fibrous tissue connecting the solid central part of a vertebra to the vertebral arch has become weakened. This weakness allows the affected vertebra to slip backward or forward over the vertebra below it, causing spinal misalignment (this is not to be confused with a 'lumbar disc prolapse', when one of the spinal discs in between the vertebrae rupture - see above). The degree of slippage in spondylolisthesis can vary, and patients with slight spondylolisthesis may be unaware that they have the condition. For others, even minor vertebral slippage can lead to lower back pain, muscle spasms, tight hamstring muscles, stiffness and abnormal curvature of the spine. Spinal cord or nerve root compression symptoms include numbness, tingling, shooting pains in the legs, muscle weakness and even bladder and bowel dysfunction, the latter of which should be treated as a serious medical emergency. (laserspineinstitute.com 2014)

Postural Kyphosis

Postural Kyphosis commonly develops in those with hEDS (el-Shahaly H.A. 1991); the normal curve in the middle section of vertebral column (the thoracic vertebrae) is more curved than normal. It is thought that in hEDS, this is primarily due to the combination of loose ligamentous structure and poor posture (also see 'Considering postural alignment' in Chapter 3, page 140).

Scoliosis (Abnormal twisting or lateral curvature of the spine):

Idiopathic scoliosis (scoliosis of unknown cause) is the most common spinal abnormality in children in the general population, and joint hypermobility occurs more frequently in children with idiopathic scoliosis than in healthy sex and age matched controls (Czaprowski D. 2011). Sometimes however, scoliosis forms as a direct manifestation of a disorder of connective tissue, such as Marfan syndrome or Ehlers-Danlos syndrome. When this is suspected, it is known as 'syndromic scoliosis', which may progress faster than other types of scoliosis and may continue to progress even into adulthood (Tinkle B.T. 2010). In an evaluation of patients with hypermobile and classical EDS, 52% of 58 patients had scoliosis (Stanitski D.F. et al 2000). The same study found that substantial back or neck pain was present in 82% of patients with scoliosis, and in 71% of patients without spinal deformity.

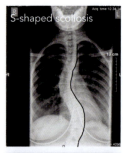
S-shaped scoliosis

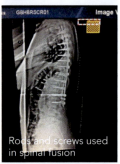
Rods and screws used in spinal fusion

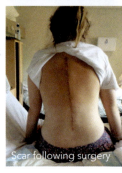
Scar following surgery

Dural ectasia
Often detected when reviewing spinal MRI's, dural ectasia is a widening or ballooning of the dural sac surrounding the spinal cord. It usually occurs in the lumbosacral region, as this is where the cerebrospinal fluid pressure is greatest, but any area of the spinal canal can be affected.

Dural ectasia can occur as part of several disorders including Ehlers-Danlos syndrome (Francomano C.A. 2006), but is perhaps best known as a manifestation of Marfan syndrome, occurring in 63–92% of people with the syndrome (Judge D.P. 2005).

In many people, dural ectasia causes no symptoms, but for those who do experience symptoms, the most common are headaches, weakness, numbness above and below the involved limb, and leg pain. Sometimes rectal and genital pain, bowel and bladder dysfunction, urinary retention or even incontinence may be experienced. Symptoms are usually, but not always, relieved when a person lies down.

Craniocervical instability (CCI)
The craniocervical junction (the interface between the skull and cervical spine comprise a joint(s) which seems to be susceptible to the same strain and injuries as seen in other joints in EDS (Tinkle B. et al 2017). The lack of structural stability at the craniocervical junction may lead to a deformation of the brainstem, upper spinal cord, and cerebellum. Studies about the prevalence as well as the symptoms, imaging, and management are scarce, but in some individuals it is thought CCI can result in one or more of the following:

Nerve dysfunction, compression of the brain stem (loose ligaments can misalign the proper angle of the odontoid bone causing it to push backwards, compressing the brainstem), cranial settling (the skull sinks downward onto the spine), and Chiari malformation - please see below.

Chiari Malformation (CMs)
There are four different types of Chiari malformation. The association with hypermobile Ehlers-Danlos syndrome concerns Chiari malformation type 1 (CM-1) (Milhorat T. et al 2007 / Henderson Sr. F.C. et al 2017), a type that can be acquired or congenital.

Chiari malformation occurs when the cerebellar tonsils (the lowest part of the back of the brain) extend into the spinal canal. This can put pressure on the brainstem and the top of the spinal cord, which can cause symptoms (18/ NHS.uk)

At the time of writing, insufficient research has been carried out to know whether Chiari Malformation is more common in people with EDS than in the general population. In the general population, CM-1 is usually congenital; due to structural defects. However, in hereditary disorders of connective tissue, such as EDS, it would seem that CM-1 may be caused by something else, such as:

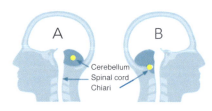
Diagram A above, shows the average position of the cerebellum. Diagram B shows a Chiari malformation

- sliding of tissues down from their normal resting position when in the upright position (Milhorat T.H et al 2007 / Hakim A.J. 2014c)

and or

- hypermobility at in the vertebral bones at the very top of the neck, leading to changes in the position / angle of these bones when upright (Milhorat T.H et al 2007 / Hakim A.J. 2014c)

CM-1 may also be associated with tethering of the spinal cord (Milhorat et al 2009); a condition where the cord has become abnormally attached within the spine and is less free to move with movement of the spine (Hakim A.J. 2014c). In this instance, the tethered cord exerts tension on the cerebellum tonsils, 'pulling' downward. However, the research team carrying out the study did not look at how often this specifically occurred in EDS cases. (More on tethered cord can be found in the section below).

Differences between patients with the combination of a hereditary disorder of connective tissue *and* CM-I, and those presenting solely with CM-I were found to be:

- an earlier onset of symptoms,
- a greater female prevalence,
- higher incidences of lower brainstem problems retroodontoid pannus formation,
- scoliosis,
- temporomandibular joint disorders,
- a flattened occiput,
- oropharyngeal hypoplasia,
- increased incidence of lower brainstem symptoms signs / dysautonomia.

(Milhorat T.H. et al 2007 / Ions G. - EDS Support UK).

CM-I symptoms include but are not limited to:

- headaches (usually at the back of the head – these are brought on, or made worse by, exercise, straining, laughing or bending over) (Hakim A.J. 2014c)
- fatigue,
- muscle weakness in the head and face,
- neck pain,
- swallowing issues,
- impaired gag reflex,
- brain fog and memory issues,
- dizziness,
- nausea,
- insomnia,
- impaired co-ordination,
- cranial cervical instability and pain,
- ringing in the ears,
- retro-orbital pain or pressure, and disordered sensation in the lower limbs are also noted.

(Milhorat T. H. et al 2007, Francomano C.A. 2006)

'The difficulty with many of these symptoms is that they might also come from a combination of other musculoskeletal problems, migraine, cardiovascular autonomic problems (e.g. POTS and hypotension, and gastric problems. A detailed assessment by a doctor is required to determine how all the symptoms might fit together' (Hakim A. 2014C).

Many doctors are still trained to look for CMs that are long and pointy in shape, but CMs can also be short, rounded or off-centre. The conventional definition of a

AREA SPECIFIC SYMPTOMS & COMORBIDITIES

Chiari malformation states that the cerebellum tonsils must protrude at least 5mm below the foramen magnum. However, patients with less extreme herniations can also experience significant neurological symptoms involving the brain stem and cerebellar functions (Oro J. 2010) (Also, see 'Tethered cord' below)

It has been found that in those with EDS, the position of the cerebellar tonsils may appear lower than expected if the patient is MRI scanned in an upright (vertical) position (Silva J.A. 2005), something that may be missed if MRI's are taken in a horizontal position (Freeman M.D. 2010), and that it is necessary to check for hypermobility at the craniocervical junction, which usually cannot be seen from X-rays.

Tethered cord syndrome (TCS)

In normal circumstances, the spinal cord hangs loose in the spinal canal. It is free to move up and down as we bend, stretch and grow. However, in some people the cord becomes tethered; meaning it is held taut either at the end, or at some point within the spinal canal (Hakim A.J. 2014c). In the case of a child, a tethered cord may force the spinal cord to have to stretch as their body grows. In adults, the spinal cord can stretch in the course of normal day to day activity.

Although an association between tethering of the spinal cord and type 1 Chiari malformation was found in research by Milhorat et al (2009) and it's occurrence is recognised by many experts as also being associated with EDS, unfortunately, insufficient research means that, as yet, no definite link can be proven (Hakim A. 2014C). It is, however, known that, when seen in individuals with EDS, tethered cord syndrome is most often associated with a structurally abnormal filum terminale (Henderson Sr. F.C. et al 2017).

'Tethered cord syndrome is usually characterised by low back pain, neurogenic bladder, lower extremity weakness and sensory loss, as well as musculoskeletal abnormalities' (Henderson Sr F.C. et al 2017). Where the filum (a flexible strand of connective tissue that attaches the bottom of the spinal cord to the lower end of the spine) is wrapped around the base of the spinal cord, pressure may be exerted on the nerves that go to the pelvis, bladder, bowel and legs, causing a range of symptoms including low back pain; lower extremity weakness, numbness and sensory loss;

severe constipation and urinary complaints (e.g. urgency, frequency, and incontinence) and bowel incontinence.

Traditionally, it has been presumed that a low-lying conus medullaris is the best indication that a spinal cord is under tension. However, Henderson et al (2017) state: *'Controversy exists over whether it is necessary to radiologically demonstrate a "low lying conus medullaris," that is, a conus ending at the lower L2 [vertebrae] level or below' '...A growing body of evidence supports the clinical diagnosis of tethered cord syndrome with or without the radiological demonstration of a low-lying conus medullaris, which justifies surgical intervention when the clinical criteria are met'* (Tu A. & Steinbok P. 2013 / Henderson Sr F.C. et al 2017).

When no imaging evidence of tethered cord is found on MRI (i.e. the conus medullaris appears to be in the "normal" position), but signs and symptoms are consistent with tethered cord and all other conditions have been excluded, a diagnosis of 'occult tethered cord' may be made (also known as 'suspected tight filum terminale syndrome').

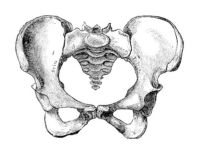

The bony pelvis

At the rear, the pelvic skeleton is formed of the sacrum (tailbone) and the coccyx. The sacrum creates a restricted joint with the pelvis, also known as the sacroiliac (SI) joint. At the front is the pubic symphysis (pubic bone) and, to either side, the ilia (hip bones). The hip bones connect the spine with the lower limbs. They are attached to the sacrum posteriorly, connected to each other anteriorly, and joined with the two femurs at the hip joints.

The gap enclosed by the bony pelvis, called the pelvic cavity, is the section of the body underneath the abdomen and mainly consists of the reproductive organs and the rectum, which are discussed separately in later sections of this chapter (page 101).

A combination of factors are often responsible for the instability in joints that cause pain / dysfunction in the bony pelvis. Uneven movement of the pelvic joints such as standing on one leg to pull on trousers, stretching the legs apart during sporting activities or getting out of the car, postural changes such as bad sitting postures, or changes in the muscles and ligaments due to pregnancy, can make the joints less stable, resulting in pain. External support, such as a pelvic belt, is often necessary in order to obtain relief of symptoms (Keer R. & Grahame R. 2003).

Sacroiliac joint dysfunction

The sacroiliac joints (SI joints) are located on either side of the area where the sacrum bone interconnects with the pelvis at the bottom of the spine.

When problems occur, they can often be due to one, or both, of the joints being too loose (hypermobility), or being *jammed* or *stuck* (hypo-mobility). In hEDS/HSD, the SI joint(s) can remain loose and cause pain or discomfort with spinal motion such as bending forward, backward, or side-to-side, as well as spinal pressure from sitting (Tinkle B.T. 2010). Alternatively, tightness can form in the surrounding tissues and the ligaments then shorten in an effort to stabilise the area, but instead create restriction. It is not uncommon for one SI joint to be too loose whilst the other is too tight, and it is possible that this difference in mobility between the two joints is a primary producer of pain (Pool-Goudzwaard A.L. 1998).

The pregnancy hormone, relaxin, can also loosen the SI joints and cause pain during the latter part of pregnancy, triggering pain in the buttock or lower back (Tinkle B.T. 2010). The position of the baby in the womb can also be a factor. In severe cases, crutches may be needed by those with SI joint instability (Keer R. & Grahame R. 2003).

Pelvic Girdle Pain (PGP)

PGP describes a set of painful symptoms caused by a misalignment or stiffness of the pelvic joints at either the back or front of the pelvis. Pain can also radiate to the thighs and/or lower back, and some women feel or hear a clicking or grinding in the pelvic area. There can also be pain in the perineum; the area between the vagina and anus.

In the general population, pelvic girdle pain is most commonly experienced as a result of pregnancy or childbirth, when hormones such as relaxin remodel this ligamentous capsule, allowing the pelvic bones to be more flexible for delivery. In hEDS/HSD, however, PGP can also occur without being related to pregnancy or childbirth; the ligaments may fail to provide sufficient reinforcement of the fibrocartilage between the pubic bones when the legs are stretched far apart, for example when taking part in activities such as ballet or gymnastics (Hakim A. 2013h).

In addition to symptoms in the thighs, back and pelvic area, the pelvis can feel very unstable making walking / weight-bearing potentially very painful.

The pain can be most noticeable when in an unbalanced position, such as when:

- standing on one leg (e.g. when getting dressed),
- walking,
- going up stairs,
- turning over in bed,
- moving your legs apart (e.g. when getting out of a car).

With the right advice, PGP can usually be managed, and the symptoms minimised. A physiotherapist can advise on treatment and techniques to manage the pain and discomfort (Hakim A.J & Keer R. 2013h), and occasionally the symptoms even clear up completely (10/NHS.UK). During pregnancy, low back and pelvic pain can often be eased by the use of a maternity or sacroiliac support in conjunction with exercise and pacing of activities (Hakim A.J & Keer R. 2013h).

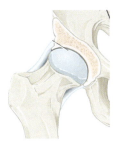

The Hip

The hip joint is a ball-and-socket synovial joint. It is the junction which allows motion between the pelvis and the femur and which connects the axial skeleton with the lower extremities. The hypermobile hip joint is frequently a cause of symptoms in the hEDS/HSD patient, with an increased range of motion and ligamentous laxity causing symptoms similar to those seen in developmental hip dysplasia, but without the developmental changes of the socket (Keer R & Grahame R 2003). There may be pain in the hip, and the inner thigh muscles and adductors may be extremely painful when pressed. Pain may be described as radiating towards the knee. Walking may cause pain on the side of the hip or in the groin area. Other common hip problems include hyperextension, clicking (snapping hip syndrome) or subluxation (Keer R & Grahame R 2003).

AREA SPECIFIC SYMPTOMS & COMORBIDITIES

Snapping hip syndrome

This is a condition characterised by a snapping sensation which is felt when the hip is flexed and extended. It may also be accompanied by discomfort or pain. If it is painless, there is little cause for concern. Rombaut et al (2010) reported that snapping hip was a frequent complaint in hEDS. Those affected by pain find it often lessens to some extent with rest and a combination of ice, compression, elevation, hydration and Ibuprofen. In some cases, the condition is curable with appropriate treatment, or sometimes it heals spontaneously. MRI can sometimes identify intra-articular causes of snapping hip syndrome.

Hip dislocation

At birth, hip dislocation is not typically seen in hEDS/HSD. However, once outside the infantile period, hip dislocations are common and those with hEDS/HSD are more likely to dislocate a hip with smaller amounts of traumatic force than you would expect in a non-hypermobile individual (Tinkle B.T. 2010 / Davenport M. 2014).

Femoro acetabular impingement

Femoro acetabular impingement (FAI) refers to a condition of the hip, where the shape of the ball and the shape of the socket do not correspond as they should, and there is abnormal contact, causing pinching between the ball of the hip and the edge of the socket . This results in damage to the tissues which can then cause pain and lead to some restriction of hip movement.

Occasionally, FAI can occur in individuals with normally shaped balls or sockets. These individuals have hypermobile joints and impingement occurs when the joint is at an extreme of its range of movement (Park Clinic Orthopaedics.com).

Bursitis

There are two major bursae in the hip that are prone to becoming inflamed or irritated. The most commonly affected covers the bony point of the hip bone, called the greater trochanter. The less commonly affected of the two, is the iliopsoas bursa, located on the inside of the hip near the groin.

Bursitis is discussed in more detail under 'Recurrent Musculoskeletal Disorders' on page 45.

Above Image by: Henry Gray - Anatomy of the Human Body 1918.
Image (page 96) by: cnx.org/contents/FPtK1zmh@8.25:fEl3C8Ot@10/
Prefacecreativecommons.org/licences/by-sa/3.0/

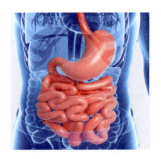

Gastrointestinal Dysfunction

Only in recent years has the significant association between hEDS/HSD and functional gastrointestinal and motility disorders been recognised, despite scholarly articles having described the association as far back as 1969 (see Beighton P.H. et al 1969). Research carried out by leading specialists such as Professor Qasim Aziz, Doctor Natalia Zarate, Professor Rodney Grahame and Dr Alan Hakim has led to a better understanding of the symptoms and possible causes. Experts now recognise gastrointestinal (GI) symptoms as common in those with hEDS/HSD (Zarate N.et al 2010), and the revised International EDS nosology 2017, states evidence is now in existence demonstrating involvement of the entire GI tract in EDS (Fikree A. et al 2017).

For many hEDS/HSD patients seen in gastroenterology clinics, no underlying cause for their symptoms can be identified resulting in a diagnosis of 'functional gastrointestinal disorder' (See **Box 1**, A). Research carried out by Zarate et al (2010), and Fikree et al (2013) suggests possible structural connective tissue abnormalities as a major cause (see **Box 1**, B) although conclusive evidence is yet to be established. Other causes include use of medications affecting the gut (see **Box 1**, C), EDS associated autonomic dysfunction (see **Box 1**, D), and bacterial overgrowth in the bowel (see **Box 1**, E) (Collins H. 2013). Lack of connective tissue integrity, altered absorption and lesions in mucosa leading to mast cell disorders in EDS are all avenues which should be explored in coming years (Collins H. 2013).

What is the gastrointestinal tract?

The gastrointestinal (GI) tract is a connective tissue-rich system of the body, made up of a long muscular hollow tube that extends from the oral cavity where food enters the body, through the oesophagus, stomach, small intestine, large intestine, rectum, and finally the anus. It is involved in processes such as mechanical and chemical digestion; breaking down food to be absorbed, absorbing nutrients from that food, and metabolising carbohydrates, fats and water. The mucosal layer of the gut is also a major contributor to basic immune function; acting as a physical and immunological boundary that senses and eliminates pathogens such as viruses, bacterium, funguses and parasites (Nochi T. 2006). There is also increasing evidence that the gut mucosa plays a central role in mediating intestinal allergic reactions (see mast cell activation disorder, page 77) (Bischoff S.C. 1996). Image attribution: yodiyim - FreeDigitalPhotos.net

How do hEDS/HSD manifest themselves?

HEDS/HSD may manifest in any segment of the GI tract (Farmer A.D 2009) and have wide-ranging effects on these complex processes and, in turn, on our health and wellbeing. However, few are aware of the role of non-inflammatory connective tissue abnormalities such as these, in causing gastrointestinal symptoms and dysfunction (bowelcancerresearch.org).

What are some of the gastrointestinal issues that hEDS/HSD patients may experience?

i)
- Generalised abdominal pain
- Bloating
- Nausea
- Heartburn (acid reflux from the stomach in to the gullet)
- Vomiting
- Constipation (having to strain to pass faeces, or being unable to pass faeces as often as 'normal'.
- Diarrhoea

ii)
- Dysmotility - sluggish or spasming movements of the gut
- Gastroparesis - a severe delay in emptying of the stomach into the small bowel, which can cause nausea, vomiting and bloating (NB/ so far, a definitive link between hEDS and gastroparesis has not been established) (Hakim A. 2016b).

iii)
- Hernia (where the bowel pushes through the abdominal wall e.g. around the belly button, or at the groin)
- Hiatus hernia (where part of the stomach squeezes into the chest through an opening in the diaphragm)

iv)
Up to 10-15% of individuals with EDS, including those with hEDS, also describe:
- A sense of urgency when needing to pass faeces

A note from the author:

Hello,

Thank you for ordering 'Understanding Hypermobile Ehlers-Danlos Syndrome and Hypermobility Spectrum Disorder.' I have been truly overwhelmed by the encouragement I've received whilst writing this book and would like to thank all those who showed faith in me by pre-ordering.

Hypermobile Ehlers-Danlos syndrome and hypermobility spectrum disorder are extremely complex subjects, but I have done my absolute utmost to explain them in a clear and concise way, and have been fortunate enough to have several professional and patient experts in these disorders review my work for me along the way.

As is the case with my own family, many of you will have struggled for years to obtain diagnosis, and may have received only fragmented, single-body-system, rather than holistic, care; something that urgently needs to change. You will, likely, have a huge number of questions, which I very much hope this book will help answer. The content of this book cannot and should not, however, replace advice from your own healthcare professional(s). Any person who experiences symptoms or feels that something may be wrong should seek individual, professional help for evaluation and/or treatment. This book is for information only and is not intended to provide individual medical advice.

Although social media is a convenient communication tool, if you have any queries or comments relating to your purchase, I would be really grateful if you could contact Redcliff-House Publications (editor@redcliffhousepublications.com), directly, in the first instance. Redcliff-House Publications is a new, small business, who very much care about the EDS/HSD community and will do their very best to help.

Many thanks

Claire Smith
Author

Redcliff-House Publications, Unit 1, Westside,
Warne Road, Weston-super-Mare, Somerset, BS23 3TS
Email: editor@redcliffhousepublications.com

- Haemorrhoids (piles)
- Skin tears with bleeding
- Faecal incontinence (soiling themselves due to the inability to control when they pass faeces)
- Prolapse of the rectum (very rare)

(Above list of symptoms - Dr Alan Hakim, HMSA website 2014 www.hypermobility.org, together with articles by Levy H.P et al 1999 / Zarate N. et al 2010, Fikree A. et al 2013 and 5/NHS.uk).

Box 1

A/ Functional Gastrointestinal Disorders (FGID):

For many with EDS/HSD, the type of symptoms shown in List **i** (above) are investigated, but no underlying cause is found. Such lack of findings frequently results in their symptoms being diagnosed as 'functional gastrointestinal disorders.' FGIDs are unexplained disorders of function (how the GI tract *works*), rather than structural or biochemical abnormalities, and are also commonly diagnosed in the general population.

More than twenty FGIDs have been identified (Centre for FGI and Motility Disorders 2015). They can affect any part of the GI tract, including the oesophagus, stomach, bile duct and/or intestines. The most common and best researched FGID is irritable bowel syndrome - a disorder causing abdominal pain associated with altered bowel habits of diarrhoea, constipation or alternating between both. Other common FGIDs include functional dyspepsia (pain or discomfort in the upper abdominal area, feeling of fullness, bloating or nausea), functional vomiting, functional abdominal pain, and functional constipation or diarrhoea.

In 2009, Farmer et al decided to evaluate the incidence of hEDS in a cohort of 115 patients who had been referred to their tertiary referral neurogastroenterology clinic. 72 of these patients were attending the clinic without previous doctors having been able to find a cause for their symptoms and many of them had been labelled, in secondary care, as having irritable bowel syndrome. Upon clinical assessment, it was evident that 42 of these patients had evidence of joint hypermobility and, of these 42, 26 were diagnosed as having hEDS.

> '...an intriguing possibility is that patients with EDS may present with a disorder with a clinical phenotype similar to that which is currently termed and understood as irritable bowel syndrome' (Farmer A. D & Aziz Q, writing for EDS Support UK)

More recent research by Fikree et al (2014) specifically investigated the importance of connective tissue and its relationship to FGID. They set up a large epidemiology

AREA SPECIFIC SYMPTOMS & COMORBIDITIES

case-control study, in which scientists compared the prevalence of hypermobility in patients with and without gut disorders, to discover whether hypermobility and gut disorders were linked and, if so, how. A total of 708 patients were split into those with functional gastrointestinal disorders, those with no gastrointestinal disorders, those with organic diagnoses (disorders with a known a structural/biochemical cause), and those with a reflux disorder (e.g. heartburn, acid reflux). The prevalence of hypermobility was found to be highest in those with functional gastrointestinal disorders (38%) and reflux disease (40%), as compared to those with organic GI disease (26%) and patients without GI disorders (26%).

B/ Structural abnormalities:

It is hypothesized that, in some cases, fragility and extensibility of the connective tissue in the gastrointestinal tract may lead to structural abnormalities (8/EDNF.org). Some leading experts believe that abnormalities in the collagen structure of the extracellular matrix surrounding the gastrointestinal tract may influence gut biomechanics, leading to disordered sensory/motor function and contributing to the development of many of the gastrointestinal symptoms, such as sluggishness and pain, which are seen in hEDS/HSD(Farmer A. D & Aziz Q, writing for EDS Support UK).

The previously described research by Aziz et al has certainly demonstrated that a sluggish gastrointestinal tract is present in a significant proportion of patients with hEDS/HSD and, in an article for the Hypermobility Syndromes Association, Aziz explains: '*this sluggishness is likely to be due to the increased elasticity of the gut due to abnormal connective tissue, in the same manner the abnormal connective tissue in the muscles and joints make them more flexible. The increased elasticity of the gut would make it more compliant (floppy) and hence the peristalsis (sequential movements that push the food through the gut) would be less effective.*'

> '*Things have to move along the conveyor belt at a rate expected, otherwise dysmotility occurs and with problems such as reflux, delayed gastric emptying etc*' (Collins H. 2013).

Previous work, carried out by Al-Rawi et al in 2004, also found a positive correlation between the presence of joint mobility and structural defects such as hiatus hernia. Ligamentous laxity and weakness of supporting structures, such as the phrenico-oesophage ligament, were cited as possible aetiological factors for their development (Al-Rawi Z.S. 2004). Even in the last century, research such as that by Levy & Francomano et al, concluded that EDS (including both the hypermobile and classical forms) may cause reduced lower esophageal sphincter tone, increased distensibility, and/or decreased GI motility, resulting in gastroesophageal reflux disease and irritable bowel-like symptoms (Levy H.P et al 1999).

Some experts hypothesize that structural abnormalities such as lesions in the gut, caused by poor collagen integrity, may allow undigested foods, bacteria, yeast, and other pathogens into the bloodstream (Collins H. 2013). They believe that this can 'drive the immune system wild', triggering disorders such as gluten intolerance, celiac disease, immune disorders and mast cell disorders (see page 77) but so far, this theory remains unproven (Collins H. 2013).

C/ The effects of pain medications:

Patients with EDS often experience chronic pain, which is commonly treated with non steroidal anti-inflammatories (NSAID), or drugs such as Codeine or Tramadol. Unfortunately, side effects of such medications include NSAID-induced gastritis, which mimics gastroesophageal reflux disease, and narcotic-induced symptoms, which can mimic the symptoms of irritable bowel syndrome (Levy H.P. et al 1999).

The most common side effects are:
• Heartburn and nausea (e.g. from NSAIDs)
• Ulcers and bleeding (e.g. from NSAIDs)
• Constipation (e.g. from Codeine or Tramadol)

(Ref: Hakim A.J. 2013d - HMSA website)

D/ Autonomic dysfunction and GI disorders:

There is increasing agreement that autonomic abnormalities can often be associated with functional disorders of the gut (Tougas G. 2000), with a growing number of reports demonstrating disordered autonomic function in subgroups of functional bowel patients (Spaziani R.M. et al 1996). In an article for EDS Support UK, Dr Alan Hakim and Professor Rodney Grahame write: 'It has been suggested that some individuals may have autonomic dysfunction of the bowel as a consequence of imbalance or over-sensitivity to the same chemicals that are associated with pain and autonomic dysfunction in the brain and the heart. Changing the effect of these chemicals in the bowel may be one way in which classes of drugs like the anti-depressants help reduce the symptoms of

irritable bowel' (3/EDSUK.org).

Dysfunctions of the autonomic nervous system (such as postural orthostatic tachycardia), are commonly associated with those with hEDS/HSD (see page 69) and may also be involved in gastrointestinal conditions such as gastro-oesophageal reflux disease and neuropathic upper gastrointestinal motility disorders (Chakraborty T.K. 1989 & Ogilive A.L 1985). Indeed, research carried out by Levy, Francomano et al showed that 9 out of 10 of their patients with EDS and suspected or confirmed cardiovascular autonomic dysfunction also had gastrointestinal complications (Levy H.P. et al 1999).

'[From the studies available], it would appear that hEDS and, autonomic symptoms, and GI symptoms are indeed linked, though the exact mechanism for the association is unknown' (Fikree A. et al 2017 / Castori M. et al 2017).

A better understanding of the mechanisms responsible in the pathogenesis of functional disorders of the GI system, including altered autonomic function, is urgently needed, with studies that focus on the mechanisms of disease rather than its clinical manifestation, and on pathophysiology rather than just symptoms (Tougas G. 2000).

E/ Bacterial overgrowth in the gut:

100 trillion microbial cells live in our gut, primarily bacteria. For a long time, scientists assumed that these bacteria, despite their numbers, did very little. But in the past decade or so, researchers have come to realise that gut bacteria influence the way our bodies work, including the way we metabolise the food we eat, the nutrition we receive from that food, and our immune function. For example, factors such as having an unbalanced diet, stress and taking antibiotics can all deplete the good bacteria in our gut and allow an overgrowth of 'bad' bacteria to form.

Disruption to the gut bacteria has been linked with gastrointestinal conditions such as diarrhea, bloating and cramps, inflammatory bowel disease and obesity (Guinane C.M. 2013), immune disorders (Bischoff S.C. 1996 / Collins H. 2013) including mast cell intolerances and skin conditions such as eczema and psoriasis, and with low mood, negative thoughts and depression (Steenbergen L. et al 2015).

Good bacteria in our gut also support the contraction and relaxation of the intestinal walls, which moves food along says Cassandra Barns, nutritionist at the

NutriCentre (Burns C. 2015). An overgrowth of bad bacteria may, therefore, contribute to sluggish motility. According to Dr Heidi Collins, Chair at the Ehlers Danlos National Foundation, in those with EDS/HSD, enlargement and dilation of the small bowel may provide the conditions needed for high bacteria overgrowth to form (Collins H. 2013).

AREA SPECIFIC SYMPTOMS & COMORBIDITIES

In an article for EDS Support UK, Marianne Williams, NHS & Private Specialist IBS & Allergy Dietitian, writes that EDS patients are starting to experiment with different dietary interventions to help their GI symptoms, and some are reporting success with exclusion diets, such as the new Low FODMAP Diet.

In a healthy GI system, FODMAPs (a group of fermentable short-chain carbohydrates) are very beneficial; they contain prebiotics which feed the good bacteria that we need to function properly (Bouhnik Y. 1996 / Davis L.M.G. 2010). However, if a person whose gut bacteria is out of balance consumes FODMAPs, the resulting fermentation can cause symptoms such as bloating, wind, constipation, diarrhea, stomach cramps and pain.

It would seem that, in many cases, a low-FODMAP diet can help people with hEDS/HSD suffering from IBS-like symptoms find a way to control them (Halmos E.P. - 2014 / Fikree A. et al 2017). By removing foods on which bacteria thrive, the diet is effective at keeping symptoms in check. But it is important to realise that avoiding 'trigger foods' only removes the *symptoms*; it does not address the underlying problem (the unbalanced overgrowth of bad gut bacteria) and means having to avoid a long list of otherwise beneficial foods.

For this reason, many dietitians consider the Low-FODMAP diet should be used only as a temporary measure, until symptoms and inflammation have calmed. According to the International Foundation for Gastrointestinal Disorders, the diet should be undertaken under expert guidance from a dietician trained in the area. They suggest that a typical approach would involve restricting problematic FODMAPs for 6–8 weeks, or until good symptomatic control is achieved. Once the symptoms have been alleviated, patients work to rebuild the balance of their gut flora (the complex community of microorganism species, including bacteria, which live in the digestive tract). A combination of strategies can be implemented such as taking probiotic (good bacteria) supplements or eating foods such as 'live' probiotic yoghurt, before very slowly (and in small quantities) re-introducing restricted foods. Having a healthy, diversified gut flora should allow many individuals to tolerate most beneficial FODMAP foods again.

Embarking on any such changes to diet should be carried out under the supervision of a patient's GP, nutritionalist or gastroenerologist.

Treatment of GI disorders seen in hEDS/HSD

In his 2004 paper describing hEDS, Howard P Levy, MD, PhD, suggests the following action for patients presenting with gastritis, reflux, motility issues and pain:

- Gastritis and reflux symptoms may require intensive therapy. Other treatable causes, such as H. pylori infection, should be investigated.
- Upper endoscopy is indicated for resistant symptoms, but frequently is normal other than chronic gastritis.
- Delayed gastric emptying should be identified if present, and treated as usual with promotility agents.
- A motility enhancer may be helpful for those with constipation only.
- Tricyclic antidepressants may be especially helpful for persons with both neuropathic pain and diarrhea.
- Irritable bowel syndrome is treated with antispasmodics, antidiarrheals and laxatives as needed.

With regard to FGID, Alan Hakim, Chief Medical Advisor for the HMSA writes:

'For the majority of individuals the self-management & medical treatments used to manage Irritable Bowel syndrome in the general population will work.

Types of treatments used in IBS for which there is evidence of effectiveness include:

- *exercise,*
- *pelvic floor biofeedback,*
- *CBT and hypnotherapy,*
- *herbal remedies (peppermint oil, STW5 (Iberogort), Padma Lax),*
- *medications [serotonin antagonists (e.g. Ondansteron), 5HT4 agonists (e.g. Prucalopride), & Guanylate Cyclase C agonists (Linaclotide),*

and also:

- *probiotics,*
- *exclusion diets.'*

© Understanding hEDS and HSD by C. Smith

100

Rectal Prolapse

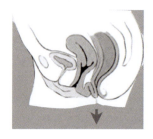

Although rare, rectal prolapse is a complication seen in hEDS/HSD. Rectal prolapse is the protrusion of either the rectal mucosa or the entire wall of the rectum, that occur either with bowel movements or independently. Ligaments and muscles should securely attach the rectum to the pelvis, but sometimes the supporting structures stretch or detach from the rectal wall. A complete prolapse is diagnosed when the entire rectum extends out of the anus, whereas a partial prolapse involves only a few centimetres of rectal lining (mucosa). In some cases, the rectum begins to drop down but does not actually extend outside the anal opening. Instead, it forms an internal prolapse.

Gastrointestinal disorders such as long term constipation and long term diarrhea can increase the risk of rectal prolapse, as can aging, pelvic floor dysfunction (see page 106) and having a long term cough and the stresses of pregnancy/childbirth.

Signs of a rectal prolapse may include the noticing of a soft, red tissue protruding from the anus after a bowel movement, which may initially be confused with a large hemorrhoid. There may also be pain, constipation, faecal incontinence, discharge of mucus or rectal bleeding.

Fecal incontinence

Fecal incontinence is an inability to control bowel movements, resulting in involuntary soiling, also sometimes known as bowel incontinence. The experience of fecal incontinence varies from person to person. Some people may experience an urgent need to go to the toilet but are unable to make it to a toilet in time. This is known as urge bowel incontinence. Others experience no sensation before soiling themselves (known as passive incontinence or passive soiling) or experience slight soiling when passing wind. Incontinence may occur on a daily or infrequent basis.

A survey by Arunkalaivanan et al (2009), found the prevalence of fecal incontinence to be significantly higher in women with JHS (HSD) when compared with women without this condition (14.9% in those with JHS (HSD) compared with 2.2% in the general adult population). A later survey of 89 children, aged 5 to 12 years and diagnosed with generalised joint hypermobility, also found an increase in fecal soiling in comparison to controls (De Kort L.M et al 2003)

Contraception, pregnancy & childbirth

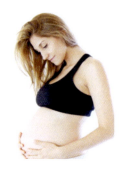

Considering hormonal contraception

As discussed on page 35, it is thought that changes in female hormones during the monthly cycle can lead to increases in pain, dislocations and clumsiness in the days leading up to menstruation in those affected by hEDS/HSD. Perhaps unsurprisingly then, some female hormonal contraceptives also appear to lead to an increase in hypermobility of the joints (4/HMSA 2014 - Bird H / McIver H 2014).

Dr Howard Bird states that: *'when careful gynaecological and rheumatological histories are taken together, it is surprising how frequently hypermobility, which was only slightly worse at the time of normal unmodified menstruation, becomes significantly worse with certain contraceptive pills, especially those containing progesterone alone or with progesterone depo contraception preparations or with mechanical devices impregnated with progesterone.'* (4/HMSA 2014)

For this reason, female patients may wish to discuss the possibility of using a combined oestrogen/progestogen contraceptive product with their general practitioner. In recent years, research in the general population has highlighted potential side effects associated with oestrogen-based contraception (e.g. slightly increased risk of blood clots), making it more likely that GPs prescribe progesterone-only preparations instead of combined products. For this reason, it may be helpful to take printed information about hypermobility and hormones (available from the Hypermobility Syndromes Association or Ehlers-Danlos Support UK websites) along to the appointment, in order to explain concerns. Professor Bird states: *'whether any slight risk in using such a (combined) preparation is worth taking for the significant improvement in the joints might ultimately be a decision for the patient, though it should be taken in conjunction with the* general practitioner, if necessary with expert gynaecological advice. (Links to further information on 'hormonal contraception and hypermobility' can be found in the resources section of this book).

What are the different types of hormonal contraceptive?

- The combined pill (containing both oestrogens and progestogens).
- The progestogen only pill (contains only progestogens).
- The contraceptive injection (progestogen only).
- The contraceptive implant (inserted under the skin of your upper arm).
- Hormone containing intra-uterine devices (placed directly in the womb, deliver small amounts of progestogen locally into the uterus).

Pregnancy and childbirth - introduction

HSD, and hEDS, are quite a broad diagnoses with varied severity and complexities seen between individuals. It is not surprising then, that the experience of childbirth within this group is also varied. Some pregnant women with hEDS/HSD experience more severe forms of the problems that many women (hypermobile or not) do during pregnancy; some experience these problems earlier in the pregnancy than would be expected in non-hypermobile women; some find the impact of any problems that occur may have a lasting or greater affect. Others, however, experience few problems (if any). In some cases, the effects of childbirth on the body remain unclear until average recovery periods have passed. Women's experiences are also affected by local standards of general, maternal and postnatal healthcare, personal circumstances and so on.

In 2016, an important paper was published from Sweden (Sundelin H.E. et al), which has helped to clarify concerns raised in the past. Dr Alan Hakim explains: 'The researchers identified 314 cases of pregnancy in women with either EDS or JHS [HSD] through the Swedish Patient Register and Medical Birth Register. The cases were compared with 1,247,864 controls (pregnant women without a diagnosis of EDS/HSD). The risk of complications in EDS/JHS [EDS/HSD] was assessed after adjusting for maternal age, smoking, number of pregnancies, and year of birth. Reassuringly, EDS/JHS [EDS/HSD] was not associated with any increased risk of preterm birth, the need for a caesarean section, stillbirth, complications in the infant at delivery (a low Apgar score), or the infant being small for gestational age or large for gestational age.

At the same time similar observations have been published by Hugon-Rodin et al (2016). The obstetric outcomes in those participants with EDS-H/JHS [hEDS/HSD] were similar to those of the general French population for deliveries by caesarean section and premature births. However, they did find that the risks of spontaneous abortion (28%) and multiple spontaneous abortion (13%) in females with EDS-H/JHS [hEDS/HSD] were somewhat higher than is seen in the general population. General population studies show spontaneous abortion (loss of the fetus before 20 weeks gestation) occurs in 10-20% of women (Tulandi T. et al 2016).'

Thankfully, awareness and understanding of hEDS/HSD among medical staff in the UK is on the rise and the age at which people are diagnosed has fallen dramatically over the last ten years alone. Naturally this improves the incidence of uneventful pregnancies (McLuckie F. 2015 HMSA).

Medication check

Very few medications have been found to be completely safe during pregnancy, so it is a good idea for all medicines to be reviewed with the pharmacist and/or primary care doctor, for advice on whether or not they can be discontinued altogether. Depending on the type of medications, it may be possible to stop some straight away, while others need to be weaned gradually. Where possible, medicines should be completely out of the system before the woman attempts to become pregnant.

Pregnancy

During pregnancy, there are changes in the blood level concentration of various hormones such as oestrogen and progesterone, necessary to enable the fetus to grow in a proper well-balanced environment and to prepare the mother for the birth. Along with weight gain, a female's body is out of balance with their shape taking a different form. Significant musculoskeletal strain can occur as a result of the increase in weight, borne primarily by the lower back and pelvis (Taylor D. et al 1981). At the same time, female hormones and relaxin work to increase joint laxity (Ainsworth S.R. & Aulincino P. 1993). For some females, this may cause pre-existing problems to worsen and may trigger new joint pains and instability. Commonly described symptoms include pelvic girdle pain and sacroiliac joint dysfunction (see page 95 for more information on both) caused by increased instability of the joints, and low back pain caused by increased laxity in the spinal joints and weight gain. Everyone's experience is different however; some find pregnancy debilitating, experiencing symptoms that make walking or weight-bearing difficult or impossible; others report feeling much better during pregnancy, even experiencing a reduction in symptoms (Molloholli M. 2011 / Tinkle B. 2010/ & Hakim A.J. 2013h). The reason for this improvement in some women may be due to hormonal changes that cause positive psychological mood changes and decreased sensitivity of the muscle pain receptors.

Management

Pacing of activities and getting proper rest to reduce the chance of symptom flare-ups are recommended (Hakim A. J. 2013h). Activities that cause pain should be limited or avoided, but overall, it's important to remain as active as possible. If able, exercise such as walking, swimming or exercise in water is usually recommended (Hakim A. J. 2013h).

Dr Brad Tinkle recommends hypermobile women begin pelvic floor exercises while they are pregnant (Tinkle B. 2010). Physical rehabilitation with support from a therapist may also be required; early and throughout pregnancy. (Hakim A. J. 2013h). If lower back pain or pelvic instability occur, use of a pelvic belt / sacroiliac support may be beneficial.

Informing appropriate medical staff

The midwife allocated will go through the mother-to-be's medical history and concerns at the first meeting. Ensuring the healthcare team are aware of potential problems from the start can help to reduce the risk of them arising, and speed up any necessary interventions (should they occur) so that complications or difficulties for both mother and child may be minimised (Hakim A. J. 2013h). It is advisable to take some information on hEDS/HSD along for reference (see www.hypermobility.org), as midwives don't know every medical condition. In some cases, referral may be made to an obstetrician who can asses the level of medicalised care needed, and will discuss any concerns there may be regarding birth positioning, anaesthesia, natural delivery versus caesarean etc.

At the time of writing, there are no formal obstetric management guidelines for patients with hEDS/HSD. Instead, management and birth plans should be made on a case-by-case basis, taking into account the diagnosis and severity of EDS, to optimise maternal and neonatal outcomes. 'Careful, collaborative antenatal planning should help reduce risks. Clear documentation of risks, together with birth and care plans, should be used to alert staff on duty when a woman with EDS-H/JHS [hEDS/HSD]

presents in labour, thus reducing the incidence of complications' (Molloholli M., Specialty Registrar in Obstetrics and Gynaecology,Horton General Hospital, Oxford Radcliffe Hospitals NHS Trust).

Childbirth complications

Studies to determine how often women with EDS experience obstetric and gynecologic issues compared with the general population are scarce, with those that are available concentrating mainly on the vascular type. In EDS hypermobile type, maternal and fetal outcomes are generally good, but maternal complications related to the abnormal connective tissue occur more often than in the general population. Reported complications include increased rate of wound ruptures along surgical incisions and delayed wound healing, the uterus failing to contract after the delivery of the baby, hemorrhage, pelvic prolapse, deep venous thrombosis and coccyx dislocation (Hermanns-Lê T. et al 2014). Ehlers-Danlos National Foundation state: 'In connection with natural delivery, women with EDS have experienced incontinence, weak pelvic floor, prolapse of the uterus, sprained joints of the pelvis, separation of the symphysis pubis (the joint between the two pubic bones in the frontal lower part of the pelvis) and rupture of the rectal musculature' (12/EDNF.org). In medical terms, these disorders may be considered less severe complications of birth than those seen in other forms of EDS (e.g. vascular type), but they can have a profound effect on life and confidence.

Also see pages 95, 101, and 105-109).

Other considerations

Deciding whether to opt for a vaginal delivery or a caesarean section can be difficult. There is no absolute indication for caesarean section and, indeed, possible delays in wound healing with such a procedure may need to be taken into account (Kochharn P.K. 2011). The benefits and risks are decided through clinical judgement (Hakim A. J. 2013h & 12/EDNF.org). In general, the additional risks that should be taken into account when considering vaginal delivery include:

- A higher risk of unusually rapid delivery (Charvet P.Y. et al 1991, Lind J. & Wallenburg H.C. 2002 / Sorokin Y. et al 1994 / Castori M.2012).
- The chance of perineal trauma either by spontaneous delivery or instrumental delivery (Molloholli M. 2011).
- Any perineal trauma caused by tearing or episiotomy may heal more slowly than 'normal' or healing may be impaired (Hakim A. J. 2013h HMSA).

AREA SPECIFIC SYMPTOMS & COMORBIDITIES

- In order to minimise the risk of pelvic prolapses, caesarean section should be considered the first choice when a vaginal delivery without episiotomy cannot be anticipated (Castori M. 2012 / 2012b).
- Large tears and tissue disruption leading to fistulas and sphincter dysfunction have been described (Molloholli M.2011).
- Any other surgery required will need to take the possible effect on healing into account. (Molloholli M.2011.)
- According to Bird H. 2007 and Kochharn P.K. 2011, there is an increased risk of postpartum haemorrhage, and any factors likely to cause obstetric haemorrhage (placental abruption or placenta praevia) may be exacerbated by the laxity of the connective tissues.

Positioning

Hypermobile women with unstable hip/pelvic, knee or spinal joints are vulnerable to injury if placed in inappropriate positions during labour or operative delivery (Molloholli M. 2011). When regional or general anaesthesia is effective in eliminating pain, great attention to positioning is required in order to avoid inadvertent joint dislocations or subluxations (Molloholli M.2011 / Kochharn P.K. 2011).

'Positioning during delivery should be carefully thought through to make this as comfortable and physically safe as possible. It is worth discussing this with the midwife and trying out positioning for a normal delivery, noting what works. Try to ensure the hips/legs are supported and those with pelvic girdle pain will benefit from delivery positions that do not involve lying on their backs.'
(Hakim A. HMSA Website - Jan 2016)

Anaesthesia

Due to what is hypothesized to be a *resistance* to anaesthesia or a *faster rate of anesthesia absorption* through the extracellular matrix of the connective tissue, in some cases those with hEDS/HSD may gain little or no benefit from epidural anaesthesia or from other local painkillers given before the repair of an episiotomy or tear (Hakim A.J. 2013h / Tinkle B. T.2010 / Hakim A. et al 2005 / Kochharn P.K. 2011). The subject of anesthesia is also discussed in Chapter 1 (page 25), Chapter 2 (page 65), and Chapter 3 (page 165).

Dysautonomia and childbirth

Although not specific to hEDS/HSD, a study of women with dysautonomia by Dr. Blair Grubb & Dr Kanjwal et al, found that about 30% of women felt their symptoms worsened after giving birth, while 70% of women reported that their symptoms remained stable (Kanjwal K.K. et al 2009). A later study by the Mayo Clinic found no differences in the autonomic function tests scores in women with a form of dysautonomia called postural orthostatic tachycardia (POTs) who had children, compared to women with POTs who did not (Kempinski K. 2010). For more information on dysautonomia and POTs in relation to hEDS/HSD, see page 69.

As previously discussed, the effects of taking most medicines, including those for dysautonomia, on the unborn baby, are often unknown and should be discussed with the GP, ideally before conception. Existing dysautonomia should also be discussed with the anaesthetist prior to the birth, as it may trigger exaggerated hypotension during regional or general anaesthesia (Kochharn P.K. 2011 / Jones T.L 2008).

Postpartum and beyond

For those experiencing pain, muscle weakness or subluxations/dislocations etc., the work involved in nursing, lifting, carrying and general handling of an infant can prove difficult, and it may be necessary to enlist some help in the weeks postpartum (Molloholli M. 2011 / Hakim A. J. 2013h). Sleep deprivation and physical and emotional stress can cause flare-ups of pain, fatigue and anxiety. These can be hard to manage, especially as women who usually take pain or anxiety mediations may not be able to do so. Women should be encouraged to raise any concerns with their healthcare team. Implementing self management techniques such as; pacing and resting, considering posture when lifting, carrying, pushing prams or buggies, and changing nappies can all reduce fatigue and strain on muscles and joints.

The infant

New mothers, who are themselves affected by hEDS/HSD, are often, understandably, watchful for signs that their child may have inherited the same disorder. According to Dr Alan Hakim, even though hypermobility has a high inheritance, it does not mean the child will necessarily develop any symptoms, either in childhood or later on in life. It is important to note that infants and children are generally more hypermobile and may lose this to some degree as they grow. Even if they remain hypermobile, it does not necessarily mean that they will develop symptoms. The important thing is that, if they do develop any problems, their doctor appreciates that hEDS/HSD is present in the family and recognises that this may explain their symptoms (Also see page 22 and page 125).

Image attribution (Page 101 column 2) : nenetus FreeDigitalPhotos.net

© Understanding hEDS and HSD by C. Smith

Urogynaecological symptoms

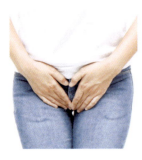

Urogynaecology is the area of medicine that deals with symptoms relating to female incontinence and pelvic floor disorders. As with the general female population, those with hEDS/HSD most commonly develop incontinence and pelvic floor disorders after childbirth; however, those with hEDS/HSD often develop them earlier or after fewer births (Tinkle B.T. 2010). In the hEDS/HSD community, urinary incontinence has also been found at increased frequency in females who have never given birth (the nulliparous female) (Castori M. 2010a / Smith M.D. et al 2012). In the general population, urinary stress incontinence is invariably the consequence of pelvic floor trauma following childbirth, so it is exceedingly unusual in the woman who has not given birth, and should be regarded as a clue that may suggest a diagnosis of hEDS/HSD. (Dickson M.J & Davis S. 2011). According to Mastoroudes et al (2013), doctors spend an insignificant amount of time asking those with hEDS/HSD about (uro)gynaecological issues. They state that '*under-diagnosis of these issues may be, in part, due to patient-underreporting of their symptoms to their physicians and, in part, to a failure by general practitioners and rheumatologists to routinely screen for these symptoms.*' Careful attention should be paid to this subject and women should be (routinely) questioned regarding incontinence and other issues such as genital prolapse, endometriosis, and dyspareunia (McIntosh L.J. 1995).

Malcolm John Dickson, Consultant Obstetrician & Gynaecologist, from Rochdale Infirmary agrees, stating: '*In recent years we have encountered several nulliparous women with urinary stress incontinence. They were referred for a geneticist's opinion, and all of these nulliparous women with urinary stress incontinence were found to have Joint Hypermobility syndrome* [now known as HSD] *or Ehlers-Danlos syndrome. These women were all young when they presented to the uro-gynaecology clinic. We hope that by early identification of their joint hypermobility syndrome* [now known as HSD], *appropriate advice and physiotherapy may delay, or possibly prevent, the development of pain and disability that can develop in people with Joint Hypermobility syndrome* [now known as HSD].' If a nulliparous female is found to have stress incontinence, the physician should inquire about collagen function and joint flexibility; questions such as these may reveal signs that can lead to expedited management for patients with previously unrecognised joint problems (Smith M.D. et al 2012).

Urinary tract dysfunction

The lower urinary tract includes the bladder and urethra, and allows for storage and timely expulsion of urine. Hakim (2013f) states: 'In both male urology and female urology, it is currently unclear whether bladder symptoms are more common in those with hypermobility than in the general population'. However, loosely knit collagen fibres can mean that the pelvic floor is far less able to adequately support the internal organs, and this lack of strength may play a role in incontinence. Stretchy collagen in the bladder-wall can also allow the bladder to stretch far more than that of a non-hypermobile person, meaning a patient often 'holds on' far longer than they should before urinating; causing urination problems, infection, or leaking. '*The causes of urinary tract dysfunction in the hypermobility syndromes may be related to changes in the anatomy of the bladder and pelvis, or may be neurological and affecting the sympathetic nerve autonomic control of the bladder, psychogenic* [influenced by things like anxiety and pain], *or as a consequence of infection and inflammation of the urinary tract. It is also important to consider the presence of bowel problems too in the hypermobility syndromes as things like chronic constipation may affect bladder function.*'
(Hakim A.J. & Grahame R. 2004, Bravo J. and Wolff C. 2006, Mathias C.J. et al 2011, Hakim A.J. 2013f)

Dysfunction of the urinary tract covers disorders such as:

- **Frequency** - the need to urinate frequently.
- **Urgency** - the need to urinate urgently; sometimes urine leaks before you have time to get to the toilet. It is usually due to an overactive bladder.
- **Dysuria -** painful or difficult urination.

- **Nocturia -** the need to wake and pass urine at night.
- **Urinary incontinence** - the involuntary loss of urine as a result of more pressure in the bladder than in the sphincter.
- **Stress incontinence** - a condition (found chiefly in women) in which there is involuntary emission of urine when pressure within the abdomen increases suddenly, such as in coughing or jumping. Commonly found in women who have given birth, urinary stress incontinence is found at increased frequency in females who have never given birth within the hEDS/HSD community (Castori M. 2010a).
- **Urinary tract infections** - reported more frequently in girls with hypermobility compared to controls (De Kort L.M. et al 2003 / Adib N. et al 2005 / Tinkle B.T. 2010).
- **Voiding symptoms** - this can be due to nerve dysfunction, non-relaxing pelvic floor muscles or both. Voiding dysfunction is also classified as being caused by under-activity of the bladder. Symptoms include difficulty emptying the bladder such as slow or weak urine stream, urinary hesitancy, dribbling of urine, and overflow incontinence (due to chronic urinary retention).

Doctors treating those with hEDS/HSD who have symptoms of urinary tract dysfunction may need to modify the standard advice they would usually give to non-hypermobile females, paying greater attention to considerations such as fluid intake and surgical implications (see page 165), to take into account problems that tend to arise in the hypermobility syndromes. (Hakim A 2013f / Cuckow P. EDS Support UK).

Gynaecological aspects

The pelvic floor:
The pelvic area is a bowl-shaped grouping of bones, muscles, and ligaments that provide protection for the bladder, urethra, uterus, and rectum. The pelvic floor of this bony structure consists of tissues that span the opening. In basic terms, it is a broad sling of muscles, ligaments and overlapping sheets of fibrous connective tissue (fasciae) stretching from the pubic bone at the front of the body, to the base of the spine at the back. These bear the load of the visceral organs, as well as controlling the openings for the vagina, urethra and rectum (Hakim A.J. 2013h).

Examples of research illustrating an increased risk of urogynaecological symptoms in those who are hypermobile than in the general population.

In a research questionnaire by de Kort *et al* (2003), the relationship between generalised joint hypermobility (GJH) and lower urinary tract symptoms; presenting as nonneurogenic bladder / sphincter dysfunction in children, was researched. It concluded that, in children with GJH of the joints, symptoms of nonneurogenic bladder/ sphincter dysfunction are more prevalent. In girls, symptoms manifest as urinary incontinence and possibly urinary tract infections. In boys, this condition manifests as constipation and possibly fecal soiling (de Kort et al 2003).,

A cohort study by Jha *et al* (2007) found the prevalence of urinary incontinence to be significantly higher in women with JHS [HSD] when compared with women without this condition (Jha S. et al 2007).

In 2009, a survey of members of the hypermobility syndromes association (all with hospital specialist diagnoses of JHS [HSD]) was carried out by Arunkalaivanan et al (2009). Overall prevalence of urinary incontinence in this group was 68.9%. The estimated prevalence of incontinence in a similar population without JHS [HSD] was 30%. (Arunkalaivanan A.S. et al in 2009).

'*Such a high prevalence of incontinence* (in hEDS/HSD) *may justify the need for an integrated continence pathway in the larger specialised hypermobility units in the country.*' (Mastoroudes H. et al 2013).

Pelvic floor weakness:
Some degree of pelvic floor weakness is experienced by many women in the general population who have given birth. When the muscles of the pelvic floor are weak or have been damaged, the ligaments and fasciae have to provide support for the pelvic organs. In those with inherent connective tissue fragility however, the strength of these ligaments and fasciae may already be compromised, increasing the likelihood that pelvic organs may prolapse at a younger age or after fewer births (Tinkle B. T. 2010, 9/NHS.uk, McIntosh L.J. 1996). They are most often facilitated by episiotomy and vaginal tears following childbirth (Castori M. 2012 / Castori M. et al 2010).

What is pelvic organ prolapse?

A prolapse occurs when the pelvic muscles and tissues become weak and can no longer hold the organs in place correctly. According to Marco Castori (2012b), pelvic organ prolapse (the bulging of one or more of the pelvic organs into the vagina) is the most debilitating gynecological feature of hEDS/HSD, and, accordingly, it was recognised in the revised 2017 International classification.

The risk of developing pelvic organ prolapse can be increased by:

- Heritable disorders of connective tissue.
- Age – prolapse is more common as women get older.
- Childbirth, particularly if it is long or difficult.
- Repeated heavy lifting and manual work.
- Long-term coughing or sneezing (for example, if the individual smokes, has a lung condition or allergy).
- Excessive straining when going to the toilet. because of long-term constipation.
- Hysterectomy or bladder repair.
- Changes caused by the menopause such as reduced oestrogen levels and weakening of tissue.
- Being overweight.
- Fibroids (non-cancerous tumors in or around the womb) or pelvic cysts (which create extra pressure in the pelvic area).
- Weakening of the muscles of the pelvic floor can develop due to, or be worsened by, many factors including: carrying excessive weight, a long term cough, chronic constipation, pregnancy and childbirth.

(Rinne K.M. & Kirkinen PP. P. 1999, 9/NHS.uk, Hakim A. J. 2013h)

Symptoms:

Some women with a pelvic organ prolapse don't have any symptoms and may not discover that they have the condition until they undergo an internal examination, such as a cervical screening.

Others may experience:

- A sensation of dragging, aching or pulling, heaviness or bulging in the pelvic region (as if something needs to be pushed back into the vagina). In severe cases, the pelvic organs may protrude through the vaginal opening.
- Difficulties in using a tampon.
- Problems passing urine such as slow stream or a feeling of not emptying the bladder fully.
- Difficulty starting to urinate, or a spraying or weak stream of urine.

'Certain conditions can cause the tissues in your body to become weak, making a prolapse more likely, including:

- *Joint hypermobility syndrome [now known as HSD] – where your joints are very loose*
- *Ehlers-Danlos syndrome – a group of inherited conditions that affect collagen proteins in the body.*
- *Marfan syndrome – an inherited condition that affects the blood vessels, eyes and skeleton.'*

(Quote: 9/NHS.uk)

- The need to urinate more often and/or the sensation that you are unable to empty the bladder well.
- Urinary incontinence, including leaking urine when you cough, sneeze or exercise.
- Urinary tract infections.
- Difficult bowel movements - the need to strain or push on the vagina to have a bowel movement.
- Fecal incontinence.
- Needing to push the stool out of the rectum by placing fingers into or around the vagina during a bowel movement.
- Lower back discomfort.
- Vaginal dryness or irritation.
- Pain or discomfort during intercourse.

Types of pelvic organ prolapse:

Pelvic organ prolapse can affect the front, top or back of the vagina. It should be noted that it is possible to have more than one of these types of prolapse at the same time. (9/ NHS.uk)

The main types of prolapse are:

Anterior prolapses:

Cystocoele (bladder prolapse) - These forms of prolapse occur where the bladder's supportive tissues (called fascia) stretch or detach from the attachments securing it to the pelvic bones, allowing it to move from its normal position, and press against the wall of the vagina, forming a bulge (Pocinki A. G. 2010).

Urethrocele (urethral prolapse) - occurs when the tissues surrounding the urethra sag downward into the vagina. (9/NHS / Pocinki A. G.2010 / Palm S. / WebMD 2014)

In some severe cases, the prolapsed pelvic organs may bulge outside the opening of the vagina.

Symptoms include:

© Understanding hEDS and HSD by C. Smith

107

- A feeling of pressure or fullness in the pelvis and vagina which may increase when lifting, coughing or straining.
- A feeling of incomplete emptying of the bladder
- Repeated bladder infections
- Pain or urinary leakage during intercourse

Posterior wall prolapse:

Rectocele - occurs when the support tissue or fascia stretches or detaches from its attachment to the pelvic bones, and allows the end of the large intestine to fall, bulging forward and pushing into the vaginal wall (Pocinki A. 2010).

Symptoms typically include:

- A bulge sensation.
- Chronic constipation or incomplete bowel movements requiring the woman to insert a finger in or around the vagina or rectum to help empty bowels (Mohammed et al 2010).
- Intercourse may be uncomfortable or painful because of the pressure of a full bowel.

Enterocele - occurs when the intestines (or small bowel) protrude through a fascial defect or weak tissues, pressing against and moving the upper wall of the vagina. Enterocele are most commonly caused by prolonged delivery or forceps deliveries in childbirth.

Symptoms may include:
- a sensation of mass bulging into the vagina or pushing against the perineum or pain with intercourse. Other symptoms include a pulling sensation in the pelvis or low back pain that eases up when you lie down, or a feeling of pelvic fullness, pain or pressure.

The 'degree of drop' of enteroceles varies, from halfway down the length of the vagina, down to the perineum, or may even protrude out of the anal canal to form rectal prolapse. (9/NHS.uk / Pocinki A.G. 2010/ Palm S.)

NB/ Despite their impact on deification, both rectocele and enterocele are defects of the pelvic supporting tissue and not the bowel wall, hence their inclusion in this section.

In a study by Mohammed et al, 56 of JHM patients (86%) were found to have significant morphological abnormalities, such as rectocele, compared with 64% of the non-JHM group. 'The greater prevalence of joint hypermobility in patients with symptoms of rectal evacuatory dysfunction, and the

AREA SPECIFIC SYMPTOMS & COMORBIDITIES

A study of women with Marfan syndrome, and Ehlers-Danlos syndrome, by Carley and Schaffer (2000), from the Department of Obstetrics and Gynecology at the University of Texas, concluded that women with these HDCTs suffer high rates of urinary incontinence and pelvic organ prolapse. Their findings supports the hypothesized causative role of connective tissue disorders as a factor in the mechanisms that lead to these conditions.

demonstration of significantly higher frequencies of morphological abnormalities than those without joint hypermobility, raises the possibility of an important pathoaetiology residing in either an enteric or supporting pelvic floor abnormality of connective tissue' (Mohammed et al 2010)

Uterine prolapse:

Uterine prolapse - Occurs when the cervix or uterus slips from its normal position and drops into the vagina, pressing on the bladder. In some instances the cervix descends to a level just inside the opening of the vagina or sags completely out of the vagina. Uterine prolapse is often associated with loss of anterior or posterior vaginal wall support (Pocinki A.G. 2010), and hence often occurs alongside the forms of prolapse previously mentioned.

'In women with hypermobility, the ligaments supporting the uterus can be weak, leading to an increased risk of uterine prolapse, a condition where the uterus "slips" and presses on the bladder (Pocinki A.G. 2010)'

Symptoms often increase with prolonged standing, walking, coughing or straining, and may be relieved when lying down. They include:

- Backache and pelvic discomfort.
- Sensation of a bulge or pressure in the vagina or vaginal opening.
- Perineal pain.
- Abdominal cramping.

How is prolapse treated?
Many women with prolapse do not need treatment as the problem does not seriously interfere with their normal activities. In mild cases, changes to lifestyle, such as pelvic floor exercises and weight loss, are usually recommended.
If the symptoms do require treatment, then a device called a vaginal pessary may be offered, which is

inserted into the vagina to hold the prolapsed organ in place. For some women, surgery may be necessary to provide support for the prolapsed organ, or to carry out a hysterectomy (9/NHS.uk).

Reducing the risk
Females identified as having the defective collagen structure found in those with hEDS/HSD should be advised of the risk factors associated with pelvic floor weakening, in order that they can then make personal decisions to reduce their risk of pelvic floor weakness or injury. Risk can be reduced by maintaining a healthy weight or losing weight if required, eating a high-fibre diet with plenty of fresh fruit, vegetables and wholegrain bread and cereal to avoid constipation and straining when going to the toilet, avoiding heavy lifting and stopping smoking (9/NHS.uk).

Smith D.B. (2012) writes: *'From adolescence, females should be taught to incorporate pelvic floor exercises into their routine. Strengthening the pelvic floor muscles provides support for the pelvic organs against the forces of increased intra-abdominal pressures from activity or exertion. This can be particularly important if they are involved in sports such as ballet, gymnastics...'* Effective and consistent pelvic muscle exercises should be maintained throughout a females life.

Post childbirth, pelvic floor exercises should be started as soon as approval is given by the female's health care practitioner. It takes time, effort and practice to become good at these exercises (often between 12-20 weeks for noticeable improvement to begin to occur). In those with hEDS/HSD, it is important to ensure that all post-natal exercises are performed with greater care, taking any individual requirements into account, but pelvic floor exercises are particularly important to prevent possible problems such as a uterine prolapse in later life (Hakim A.J & Keer R. 2013h). If a female is uncertain whether they are carrying out pelvic floor exercises effectively, advice should be sought from their doctor, physiotherapist or continence advisor.

Other gynaecological aspects
Many of the gynaecological aspects of hEDS/HSD have been largely ignored in the past. However, it is now clear that women with hEDS/HSD commonly suffer from the following :

i) Vaginal dryness (vaginal dryness) - may be associated with autonomic dysfunction and related

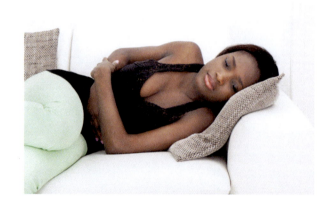

dehydration that is so often associated with hEDS/HSD (Castori M. 2012 and Bravo J. & Wolff C. 2006)

ii) Dysmenorrhea (painful menstrual cramps) - It is hypothesized that defects in collagen structure may result in the muscles of the womb having to contract much harder during a females's menstruation in order to shed the unused womb lining. In a 2012 study by Castori, 82.9% of the women included (who all had hEDS/HSD) were found to be affected by dysmenorrhea (Castori M. 2012b). This finding has recently been replicated by Hugon-Rodin et al, who found 72% of 386 women (each of whom had hypermobile Ehlers-Danlos syndrome) were affected by dysmenorrhea.

iii) Metrorrhagia (bleeding from the uterus between menstrual periods) - This condition affected 53.7% of women in a study of women with hEDS/HSD by Castori (2012b).

iv) Menorrhagia (consistently heavy periods that interfere with quality of life) - Menorrhagia was found to affect 53% of women in a study of women with hEDS/HSD by Castori (2012b). A more recent study by Hugon-Rodin et al (2016) found the percentage to be even higher; 76% of women as compared with 33.3% in the general population (16/NHS.uk).

(Also see: Sorokin Y. et al 1994 / Castori M. 2012b / Ainsworth S.R. & Aulicinio P.L. 1993)

v) Dyspareunia (Pain during intercourse) - Excessive stretchiness of the vagina itself and weakness of the muscles supporting the pelvis can make intercourse painful for some women with hypermobility. Vulvodynia or vaginismus, a painful spasm of the vagina, also may occur more commonly in the setting of hypermobility. (Pocinki A.G. 2010). Hugon-Rodin et al (2016), found 43% of the 386 women included to be affected by dyspareunia.

Male Urinary Tract Dysfunction

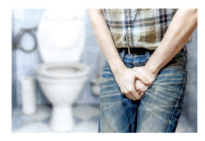

According to Peter Cuckow, Registrar in Urology, the most common EDS related problem seen in male urology is bladder diverticulum, probably resulting from an anomaly of the bladder wall.

Bladder diverticulum
In an article for EDS Support UK, he explains: *'The pressure inside the bladder remains low while it is filling but rises significantly when urine is passed. It is probable that this rise in pressure stretches the bladder wall in susceptible individuals and causes the diverticulum to form.'* Cases have been seen in several subtypes including the hypermobile and classical types. One explanation for the complete absence of diverticula in female patients is the significantly higher voiding pressures generated by male bladders (6/EDS Support UK).

Urinary tract disorders
As is the case with females, it is unclear whether those with hEDS/HSD are more susceptible to urinary tract disorders than the general population although some studies show a modestly increased risk (Hakim A. 2013f). Dysfunction of the urinary tract covers disorders such as:

- Frequency - the need to urinate frequently.
- Urgency - the need to urinate urgently, sometimes urine leaks before you have time to get to the toilet. It is usually due to an overactive bladder.
- Dysuria - painful or difficult urination
- Nocturia - the need to wake and pass urine at night.
- Urinary incontinence - defined as the involuntary loss of urine as a result of more pressure in the bladder than in the sphincter.
- Voiding symptoms - this can be due to nerve dysfunction, non-relaxing pelvic floor muscles or both. Voiding dysfunction is also classified as being caused by under-activity of the bladder. Symptoms include: difficulty emptying the bladder such as slow or weak urine stream, urinary hesitancy, dribbling of urine, and overflow incontinence (due to chronic urinary retention).
- Urinary tract Infections: were reported more frequently in boys with hypermobility, compared to controls (De Kort L.M. et al 2003 / Adib N. et al 2005 / Tinkle B.2010).

Treatment
Doctors may need to modify advice they give on treatments such as fluid intake and surgery, to take into account problems that tend to arise in the hypermobility syndromes. (Hakim A.J. 2013f HMSA / Cuckow P. EDS Support UK). Although instances are very rare, the possibility of bladder diverticular should always be considered during the diagnosis process for urinary infection / blood in the urine in males. Surgery to remove the diverticulum should be reserved for those cases in which symptoms are severe and poorly controlled with medication or in whom kidney function is threatened (6/EDS UK Cuckow P. / Levard G. et al 1989).

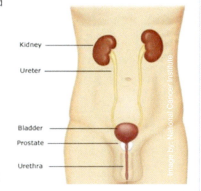

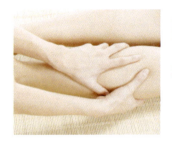

Restless leg syndrome

Restless Leg syndrome (RLS) is a common neurological disorder within the general population, characterised by an irresistible urge to move one's body to stop uncomfortable or odd sensations (Earley C.J. 2003) - about one person in 10 experience symptoms over a lifetime.

Often no cause for RLS can be found (this is known as idiopathic RLS) but, in some people, it can be linked to pregnancy, lack of iron, certain medications, problems with the kidneys or thyroid gland, having diabetes, or Parkinson's disease. It is also described in those who have hEDS/HSD with some 42% of 40 participants who took part in a questionnaire study, looking into the prevalence of sleep disorders in those with EDS, reporting symptoms of restless legs syndrome (Metlaine A. et al 2012).

What are the symptoms of restless legs syndrome?

Many people with RLS find it difficult to describe the sensation that they feel in their legs. According to Dr Sarah Jarvis, *'it may be like a crawling sensation, or like an electric feeling, or like toothache, or like water running down your leg, or like itchy bones or just fidgety, jumpy or twitchy legs, or just uncomfortable.'* Whatever the sensation, the result is an recurrent urge to move your legs every few few seconds or minutes (Jarvis S. 2013).

The severity of symptoms can vary from a mild restlessness of the legs on some evenings, to a distressing problem that occurs every evening and night (and, sometimes, during the daytime) which regularly disturbs sleep. Many people fall somewhere in between these extremes (10/patient.co.uk).

Many people find symptoms:

- are usually worse in the evening or at night, which can have a knock-on effect of causing poor sleep, and fatigue,
- are worse lying or sitting down,
- often start when in a restrictive space such as a car,
- usually affect both legs and, in some, the arms can be affected too,
- tend to ease briefly if you are able to stretch or massage your legs, but return shortly after resting again

Around three quarters of people with RLS also experience sudden jerks (involuntary movements) of their legs when they are asleep.

How is it treated?

If a GP suspects a patient's RLS is secondary to another disorder or attributed to side effects of particular medications, the appropriate tests / changes will be undertaken. If, however, the cause is idiopathic, some people find relief by cutting out caffeine, avoiding alcohol, massaging the affected limbs for a few minutes, trying to avoid sitting in confined spaces for long periods and taking some exercise early in the day.

Benign idiopathic nocturnal limb pains

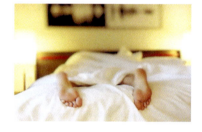

Benign idiopathic nocturnal limb pains (commonly know as growing pains) in children and adolescents are characterised by evening and night time aches and pains in the lower limbs (often the calves, shins and around the ankles, with no obvious cause and no visible signs such as swelling or bruising. The pains can often be relieved with massage or simple painkillers such as paracetamol.

The cause of growing pains is not understood, but it is hypothesized by some that they may occur during periods of rapid growth (hence the common name - 'growing pains'). As bone growth happens mainly at night, and requires the muscles, ligaments and tendons to lengthen to adapt to the new bone length, it would seem possible that (where the lengthening of these soft tissues happens more slowly than the increase in the length of the bones) it may give rise to pain. A diagnosis of growing pains can usually be made by clinical assessment, but a GP should first rule out other potential musculoskeletal disorders that may cause similar symptoms.

Growing pain-like symptoms have been linked to underlying joint hypermobility in some children. Of course, children who are hypermobile may experience nocturnal limb pains in the same way that children in the general population do. However, writing for the Oxford Journals in 2001, Murray postulates that, in those children and adolescents who are hypermobile, unusual or excessive exercise may lead to minor injury or repetitive strain to musculotendinous or ligamentous structures in the lower limbs. This in turn may lead to 'growing pain-like' symptoms which are noticed when children are at rest in the evenings.

A physiotherapist may be helpful in putting together a programme of gentle strengthening exercises to address weakness and reduce the strain placed on tissues and joints during daily activities. They may also suggest some gentle stretching techniques that the child may find helpful when carried out before bedtime, in order to address underlying muscular tightness.

Disorders of the Knee

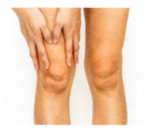

Chronic knee pain is one of the most common symptoms of hEDS/HSD, with one survey finding 85% of patients with the hypermobile type affected (Weinberg J. et al 1999). Patella instability is another common problem, thought to occur in around 57% of patients who have hEDS/HSD (Ainsworth S.R. & Aulincino P. 1993).

Patellofemoral pain syndrome
Patellofemoral pain syndrome primarily causes unilateral or bilateral pain in the front of the knee. It is particularly associated with pain when walking up or down stairs, prolonged sitting, squatting or kneeling. It usually described a deep, aching pain, but can become sharp or burning in nature. Some people describe a sense that their knee may give out on them, even though it doesn't actually do so, particularly when going down the stairs.

Fat pad impingement
Fat pad impingement occurs when the fat pad located between the patella and the femur gets pinched, causing inflammation.

Impingement can occur as a result of knee arthroscopy, trauma to the area, or micro trauma from repeated hyperextension of the knee when walking. People who stand with their knees hyperextended often suffer from fat pad impingement, which sometimes gets misdiagnosed as Patellofemoral pain (see above) (Eldridge J. 2014). It is important to get an accurate diagnosis, as the treatment for these two conditions is different. Symptoms may feel worse when walking down steps, or during prolonged periods of standing or walking.

Taping may assist initially in offloading the fat pad, but guided postural correction and corrective leg exercises from a physiotherapist are the best long-term approach to relieving fat pad impingement.

Patella malalignment syndrome
Those with hEDS/HSD are prone to patella malalignment and instability as a result of ligament laxity around the joint (Tinkle B.T. 2010 / Sheehan F.T. et al 2008). But patella malalignment can be caused by a number of contributing factors, for example:

- Tightness of the lateral retinaculum and ilio-tibial band.
- Abnormal positioning and contractions of the VMO muscle.
- Anatomic variations of the trochlea groove.
- A high-riding knee cap (patella-alta).
- Tibial tuberosity that is too far off to the outside.
- An elevated Quadriceps angle

(Grelsamer R. 2008).

If there is an imbalance in any of the muscular structures that stabilise the knee they may pull on the patella at different rates or strengths. This can cause the patella to become malaligned, allowing it to tilt and track abnormally, which can result in friction or rubbing of the patella on surrounding structures within the trochlear groove in which it sits. Accelerated wear between the surfaces of the bones can lead to the protective articular cartilage surface over the bone wearing away, leading to arthritic degeneration.

A malaligned patella can cause pain which can range from minimal discomfort, to acute and severe pain (Kramer P.G. 1986). Although pain is the main symptom, patella malalignment syndrome is also associated with patella dislocation or repeated subluxation, knee effusion, locking, grating, or weakness (Hughston J.C.1968/1979).

Miserable malalignment syndrome (MMS)

The series of malalignments that can occur in the area between the pelvis and feet are often referred to as rotational malalignment, or 'miserable malalignment syndrome'. When faced with a combination of imbalanced limb muscular strength, excessive soft tissue pliability and excessive stiffness, the body attempts to try and centre the knee under the hips and above the ankle (Robert-McComb J.J. 2014), compensating by rotating the hip joint inward while the tibia rotates outward, with either outward or inward (squinting) knee-caps, higher Q-angle and increased foot pronation. This condition can occur in one or both knees and can lead to instability or other patellofemoral symptoms affecting the position, movement and function of the knee joint (Robert-McComb J.J. 2014). Pain and discomfort are commonly experienced with this condition, and a person may also be at a higher risk of patellar joint dislocation or subluxation and arthritic change to the joint (Magee D.J. 2008). MMS can also have a knock-on effect to the upper body, contributing to back and neck pain.

Patella subluxation / dislocation

The patellofemoral joint is stabilised by ligaments and bones, and the extensor muscles. The patella (knee cap) should rest in a bony groove, known as the trochlear grove, at the end of the thighbone. When the knee bends or straightens the knee cap should move straight up and down within the groove. In those with hEDS/HSD, the ligaments, which act as 'guy ropes' holding the knee cap in place, may be lax, allowing it to slide too far to one side or the other. When this occurs, the knee cap can subluxate or dislocate. Repeated subluxations / dislocations, especially those which are traumatic, may cause significant damage to the structures around the knee including rupture of the medial patellofemoral ligament. This generally does not heal well and results in an increased risk of further dislocations. If the inherent ligamentous laxity found in those with hEDS/HSD is further complicated by anatomical abnormalities of the other structures that are supposed to stabilise the patella, dislocations become far more likely.

Some examples of such abnormalities are:

Trochlear dysplasia: The normally deep grove of the trochlea (in which the patella sits) is too shallow and does not adequately contain the patella when the knee goes through its range of motion, leaving the patella vulnerable to dislocation.

Patella alta: the position of the patella within the trochlear groove sits too high, meaning it does not properly engage the trochlea groove until the knee is in deeper flexion, allowing it to slide out more easily.

Increased Q-angle: The Q-angle is the angle of divergence between the line of pull of the quadriceps and the line of pull of the patella ligament. The wider this angle, the more likely the quadriceps muscle will pull the patella out of line, causing subluxation / dislocation.

Disorders of the foot/ankle

The association between underlying joint hypermobility and foot symptoms is incomplete, but HSD accounts for a large proportion of rheumatology referrals. It has been shown that people with HSD have greater foot impairment than matched controls and that the severity of symptoms correlates with severity of systemic hypermobility (Redmond A.C. et al 2006a / Redmond A.C. 2006b).

Sprains

Sprains occur when the ankle joint twists, rolls in or out, or is forced into an abnormal position, causing the ligaments that connect the bones to tear or stretch (Livestrong.com). Rombaut (2010) lists frequent ankle turning or spraining as common in hEDS/HSD and instability arises when the injured ligament fails to regain its structural elasticity, or has too much anatomic elasticity due to defective tissue proteins (as in hypermobility), causing the joint to move in atypical ways. Chronic low-grade swelling and pain may also be noted. Once sprained, the frequency of future ankle sprains is increased if long-term weakening of the joints occurs. It is, therefore, important to take steps to prevent this injury from occurring again, and treatment to strengthen the joint laxity should commence as soon as possible.

Peroneal nerve neuropathy

Lack of sensation in the top-of-the-foot (or foot and ankle) and motor weakness/pain, are the most common characteristics of dysfunction of the peroneal nerve. The peroneal nerve branches off the sciatic nerve just behind the knee, and goes down the outside of the front of the leg to the top of the

© Understanding hEDS and HSD by C. Smith

foot. It is responsible for supplying sensation over the outside front of the calf as well as most of the top of the foot and toes. Thought to be caused by excessive pressure of tissues surrounding the outer, lower part of the knee/upper calf, how symptoms present themselves and the severity of the symptoms, varies depending on which of its three branches are compressed and at what point. A possible link between Ehlers-Danlos syndrome and multiple-pressure sensitive neuropathy, that blocks conduction of the common peroneal nerve has been reported by Bell K.M et *al* and the condition is commonly seen in people who have had knee dislocations, surgery or trauma in this area of the body.

Over pronation

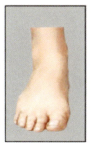 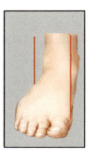

Pronation refers to a movement of the foot i.e. the lowering of the arch that occurs when weight is put on the foot in order to absorb shock. In a hypermobile foot/ankle there is often excess motion caused by over pronation, a biomechanical problem that occurs during the walking process when a person's arch *collapses* upon weight bearing (www.foot.com). This can cause extreme stress or inflammation on the plantar fascia, potentially causing severe discomfort and leading to other foot problems. Causes include muscle and ligament weakness in the ankle and calf, excess weight, knock knees, hyperextended knees, or other biomechanical distortions in the foot or ankle.

Pes plenus (flat feet)

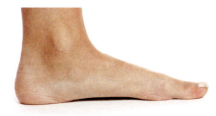

Pes plenus and over pronation often occur together, but they are two different conditions. Pes plenus occurs when the ligaments that normally support the arch of the foot are overly stretchy and unsupportive, allowing the arches to collapse under the body's weight and the feet to pronate inwards. This, in turn, can contribute to other lower extremity disorders such as foot pain, plantar fasciitis, ankle injuries shin splints, and knee disorders such as meniscal injury or ligament sprains. Pes planus may not be apparent unless an individual is weight bearing; it is, therefore, important that a patient is observed when standing up and/or walking.

Pes planus is a prominent feature in people who have heritable disorders of connective tissue.

Hallux valgus (Bunions)

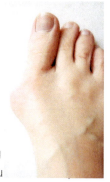

In some people, generalised laxity of the ligaments and the resulting over pronation can cause the first metatarsal bone in the big toe to become unstable and move upwards and turn inwards. This can lead to abnormal tension being applied by the adductor hallicus mu turn, subluxates the metatarsophalangeal joint and causes a bunion to form. Individuals with Ehlers-Danlos or Marfan syndrome, have also been shown to have a higher-than-average occurrence of bunions (Acfaom.org & 4/Patient.uk).

Plantar fasciitis

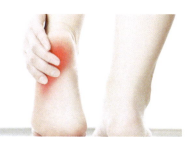

Plantar fasciitis (also mentioned on page 46), is usually caused by an inflammation of the plantar fascia, a long fibrous band that helps maintain the foot's long arch. It usually manifests as pain on the underside of the heel that feels worse when first standing in the morning or after a period of sitting during the day. For some, plantar fasciitis resolves without treatment, but for others it can persist for on average two years and be very resistant to treatment. In the early stages, home-based remedies are worth trying but, for resistant or long-standing heel pain, consultation with a GP, physiotherapist or podiatrist is required (11/ EDS Support UK).

Subluxation or dislocation of the toe

As with other joints in the body, people with hEDS/HSD frequently describe subluxations and dislocations of the toes. (also see page 61 'dislocations').

Note: *Additional information on management of the foot and ankle, and regarding the use of orthotics can be found on page 146.*

Photo attribution:
Page 111 by: imagerymajesticv - under Creative Commons Licence
Page 112 by: jk1991 - under Creative Commons Licence
Page 114 (pronation) author's archive
Page 114 (flat foot) Esther Max - under Creative Commons Licence
Page 114 (hallux valgus) - Lamiot - under Creative Commons
Page 114 (Plantar fasciitis) - Daniel Max - under Creative Commons Licence

© Understanding hEDS and HSD by C. Smith

Chapter 3

Diagnosis and Management of hEDS and HSD

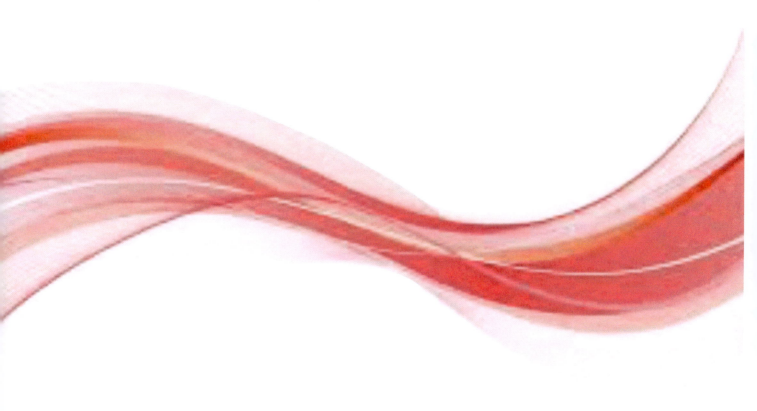

© Understanding hEDS and HSD by C. Smith

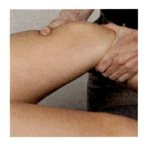

Initial diagnosis by clinical assessment

If a doctor suspects that a patient has a hypermobility related disorder, he or she may diagnose the patient themselves (using the criteria and scoring system shown on pages 121 and 122), or they may choose to refer the patient to a rheumatologist to undergo a clinical examination and assessment of their medical and family history. For some types of Ehlers-Danlos syndrome, genetic testing is also available to help confirm diagnosis but, at the current time, no genetic test is available for hEDS or HSD.

In this section, we will look at the route of 'diagnosis via clinical assessment', and at some of the services that may, in some instances, be involved in a patient's care.

A note to clinicians:

HEDS, and HSD are difficult to diagnose because patients often look well and present differently from each other. The severity of the wide ranging, multi-systemic symptoms, the joints that are affected and the level of pain and fatigue, experienced by those with hEDS or HSD, can vary greatly from day to day, or even hour to hour, and in each individual (3/HMSA 2014).

In terms of joint hypermobility, some individuals are very mobile, while others who were once mobile are no longer so. Patients generally fall into two broad groups: The first being those who suffer periods of pain and injury, usually lasting several weeks. After effective treatment, they can be relatively symptom-free for some time but experience symptoms intermittently. For patients in the other group, who may be more severely affected, each day is a struggle against pain and injury (Gurley-Green S. 2001). Patients from both groups report deterioration over time, which is contrary to much in the literature which suggests that symptoms decrease with age. Reported stiffening with age does not always bring less pain. On the contrary, many report increasingly painful symptoms as age advances ((1/Arthritis Research UK / 1/EDNF.org, Uptodate.com).

Pain is the most common symptom reported. For patients it comes in varying degrees, and is often quite unbearable (Levy H.P. 2012, Chopra P. et al 2017).

DIAGNOSIS

Persistent pain can affect cognition and clarity, which limits good communication between patient and doctor (Gurley-Green S. 2001).

With such complex disorders it is often difficult for patients to tell their doctors the impact that hEDS, and HSD is having on them and their loved ones. In some cases, the whole family may need treatment/guidance, as this disorder can affect every aspect of daily and family life.

Many patients have struggled for years with medical treatment that has made them worse, not better. Many receive fragmented and single-body-system, rather than holistic, care; something which is not only detrimental to their physical and psychosocial wellbeing but is also non-cost-effective for the health care provider. Inappropriate interventions and poor past experiences in these individuals have often resulted in increased psychological and physiological distress, and the understandable adoption of coping mechanisms that can sometimes become a barrier to further management. General practitioners often do not recognise that there may be a need to send their patients to specialised clinics. Patients are left feeling isolated and disbelieved; frustrated by the lack of effective treatment/service provider knowledge, and with no clear pathway available.

The route to diagnosis may depend on many factors, including the patient's GP's own knowledge of heritable disorders of connective tissue, and the original and 'presenting symptoms' for which a patient first attends a clinic. When taken individually, symptoms often lead down many dead ends and it is not until underlying hypermobility is recognised that the dots are finally joined and hEDS, or HSD is recognised. Unfortunately, it is not uncommon for patients to attend many appointments before this possibility is considered; in fact, the Hypermobility Syndromes Association state that for 55% of its members it takes more than 10 years to receive a diagnosis.

With this in mind, please remember:

- If the patient has struggled to obtain a diagnosis, the chances are that they may, in the past, have been made to believe that their symptoms are psychosomatic or that they may have injured themselves on purpose. This scenario is most common when the patient does not recall an 'accident', which would normally account for such pain or injury, or when their description of how an injury occurred could not (seemingly) account for such a severe injury in a normal patient.

Continued...

Box 1.

Quick questions designed to assist GPs

Due to demand on Services, many GPs are only able to offer 10 minutes for routine appointments. With this in mind, Dr Alan Hakim has devised the following list of questions to help GPs, faced with a patient describing multi-system dysfunction (who they may suspect has a hypermobility related disorder) elicit sufficient information to decide if further investigation would be beneficial.

The concerns with which patients typically present:
Clinical experience has highlighted that patients frequently present with the following complaints, which can be easily elicited by asking the following questions (Hakim. A. 2016 - correspondence)

- Hypermobility (see page 122, **Box 3**), joints that subluxate/dislocate,
- recurrent musculoskeletal injuries / pain / degenerative joint disease, neck instability without neuropathy, temporomandibular joint instability.
- Skin manifestations including mild stretchiness, atrophic scaring, bruising, varicose veins.
- Bowel dysfunction / hernia
- Cardiovascular autonomic dysfunction
- Anxiety, depression
- Fatigue

The questions to ask:
- Do your joints feel like they slip or pop in or out?
- Do you easily injure yourself?
- Do you bruise / scar easily (have stretched scars or varicose veins?
- Do you experience a lot of acid regurgitation or fullness/nausea, abdominal pain, bloating, constipation, sluggish bowel?
- Do you experience bladder concerns - difficulties passing urine, recurrent burning sensation during urination / prolapse front or back (bladder/vaginal/rectal)?
- Do you experience fast heart rate or feel faint / faint - on standing up or standing a long time?
- Do you feel anxious or depressed?
- Do you constantly feel very tired (unrefreshed after sleep) / can't think clearly (brain fog)?
- Is there anything like this in your family history? e.g. vascular, eye or bowel complications?

Please note:
In the UK a GP is a medical doctor who treats acute and chronic illnesses and provides preventive care and health education to patients. In other countries GPs may be known as 'family doctors' or 'primary care providers' (see page 133). The services they can provide and the referral route itself may differ from country to country (or even within) countries.

The full diagnostic criteria for generalised joint hypermobility and hEDS, can be found on pages 121 - 122.

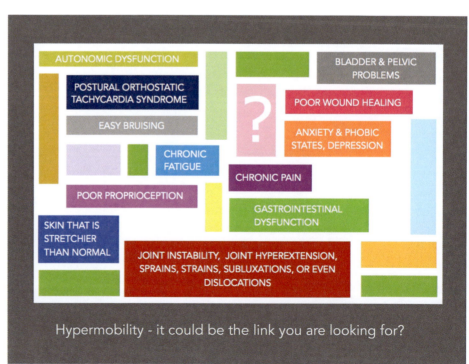

Hypermobility - it could be the link you are looking for?

Image: © Hypermobility Syndromes Association 2014 - All rights reserved. Design Redcliff-House Publications 2014

© Understanding hEDS and HSD by C. Smith

DIAGNOSIS

...continued

- He/she may have high expectations, having waited many weeks for an appointment to see the consultant and having invested in the hope that the specialist might be able to help.
- They may be depressed as a result of their pain and disability. In addition, they may seem desperate, willing to do anything to be free from the pain.
- The patient may appear to be angry at all medical professionals after years of inadequate or inappropriate care.
- They may be defensive and anxious to prove that they need help, and they may therefore appear to be exaggerating their problem.
- Finally, they may be unclear what symptoms to relate, as the problems may have been present throughout their life and have become 'their normal.'
(Gurley-Green S. 2001 / Hamonet C. 2017)

Patient–led management and self management are currently the best approaches for the long–term treatment of both hEDS and HSD (along with multi-disciplinary referral where required). Unfortunately, patient-led management and self management are particularly problematical for the hEDS/HSD patient because they are disorders that can rob patients of control over their lives. All chronic illness and chronic pain cause feelings of loss of control. The problem is exacerbated with hEDS/HSD because there is not always a clear link between an activity and the onset of pain or injury; making it difficult for the patient to lower the level of pain, or avoid injury, by behavioral modification. This lack of a clear cause-and-effect relationship between an event and subsequent pain can make patients unsure of their body's limits, and can promote self-blame and poor self–esteem, ultimately leading to a lowering of the patient's strength through progressive physical inactivity (Gurley-Green S. 2001).

For successful self management, it is important for patients to feel some internal sense of control, to feel that they can change their lives for the better. This self-empowerment is often made more difficult because many hEDS/HSD patients have to go from one doctor or alternative practitioner to another in search of help. Many have complained of having to see a different physiotherapist each time they are referred for treatment, often with serious consequences relating to lack of continuity and conflicting advice.

Another aspect of this problem is that because pain often occurs some time after the activity that caused it, exercise programmes are difficult to maintain. The lack of regular appropriate exercise, combined with self-blame, may lead to weight gain for some patients. The resultant lowering of self–esteem fuels the downward spiral, putting both patient and doctor in a difficult position. Doctors correctly suggest to an already vulnerable patient that the weight gain is making the problem worse. This fuels the self–blame and accentuates the downward spiral (Gurley-Green S. 2001).

To support patients, it is important to recognise the impact of hEDS, and HSD, on their lives; research into the development of strategies of management, including physiotherapy and drug and cognitive therapies; research into patterns of symptoms to determine why, for example, many people who are very mobile have no pain while others who are less mobile are suffering; respond to the needs of the patient, and if unable to answer a patient's question, *explain that* to the patient whilst providing reassurance that you will work with them to find the answer.

Diagnostic criteria

The pathway to EDS/HSD diagnosis starts with a physical examination, using the Beighton Scale to assess how mobile joints are, a search for abnormal scarring and testing the skin to determine what it feels like and how much it stretches, as well as any additional tests they physician feels are needed. There should also be a look into a patients medical history to look for conditions and problems associated with EDS/HSD, and a discussion about family to help determine if an EDS/HSD was inherited (1/Ehlers-Danlos Society 2017).

The 2017 International Criteria for hEDS (incorporating the Beighton Score for generalised joint hypermobility) has been laid out on page 121, **Box 2**. The criteria for other types of Ehlers-Danlos syndrome can be found on pages 127-128.

Please note that, when using the Beighton Score to diagnose generalised joint hypermobility, several additional points need to be taken into consideration.

These are shown in **Box 3** and include:

- The need for other symptoms to be present.
- Score adjustments that may need to be made relating to age, past surgeries etc.

Continued on p123...

Box 2. 2017 International Criteria for hypermobile Ehlers-Danlos syndrome

Incorporating the Beighton Score

Note: The clinical diagnosis of hypermobile Ehlers-Danlos syndrome (hEDS) requires the simultaneous presence of criteria 1 AND 2 AND 3.

Criterion 1

Generalised joint hypermobility (GJH) must be present

Using the Beighton Score (see page 122, **Box 3**) the cut-off for the definition of GJH is:

6 points or more (out of a total of 9) for pre-pubertal children and adolescents
5 points or more (out of a total of 9) for men and women post puberty up to 50 years of age
4 points or more (out of a total of 9) for men and women over 50 years of age

Important note:
Additional factors that **MUST** also be taken into consideration when using the Beighton score system are detailed on page 122, **Box 3 (points i - iii).**

Criterion 3

All of the following prerequisites MUST be met

1) Absence of unusual skin fragility, which should prompt consideration of other types of EDS
2) Exclusion of other heritable and acquired connective tissue disorders, including autoimmune rheumatologic conditions. In patients with an acquired connective tissue disorder (e.g. lupus, rheumatoid arthritis, etc.), additional diagnosis of hEDS requires meeting both Features A and B of Criterion 2. Feature C of Criterion 2 (chronic pain and/or instability) cannot be counted towards a diagnosis of hEDS in this situation.
3) Exclusion of alternative diagnoses that may also include joint hypermobility by means of hypotonia and/or connective tissue laxity. Alternative diagnoses and diagnostic categories include, but are not limited to, neuromuscular disorders (e.g. Bethlem myopathy), other hereditary disorders of connective tissue (e.g. other types of EDS, Loeys-Dietz syndrome, Marfan syndrome), and skeletal dysplasias (e.g. osteogenesis imperfecta). Exclusion of these considerations may be based upon history, physical examination, and/or molecular genetic testing, as indicated.

Criterion 2

Two or more among the following features MUST be present (e.g. A and B; A and C; B and C, or A and B and C)

Feature A - Systemic manifestations of a more generalised connective tissue disorder (NB/ a total of 5 must be present)

1) Unusually soft or velvety skin
2) Mild skin hyperextensibility
3) Unexplained striae such as striae distensae or rubrae (at the back, groins, thighs, breasts and/or abdomen in adolescents, men or prepubertal women without a history of significant gain or loss of body fat or weight
4) Bilateral piezogenic papules of the heel
5) Recurrent or multiple abdominal hernia(s) (e.g., umbilical, inguinal, crural)
6) Atrophic scarring involving at least two sites and without the formation of truly papyraceous and/or hemosiderotic scars as seen in classical EDS
7) Pelvic floor, rectal, and/or uterine prolapse in children, men or nulliparous women without a history of morbid obesity or other known predisposing medical condition
8) Dental crowding AND high or narrow palate
9) Arachnodactyly, as defined in one or more of the following: (i) positive wrist sign (Steinberg sign) on both sides; (ii) positive thumb sign (Walker sign) on both sides
10) An arm span-to-height ratio of equal to or greater than 1.05
11) Mitral valve prolapse (MVP) mild or greater based on strict echocardiographic criteria
12) Aortic root dilatation with Z-score greater than +2

Feature B - Positive family history
One or more first degree relative(s) must independently meet the current diagnostic criteria for hEDS (biological mother, father, brother, sister).

Feature C - Musculoskeletal complications
The patient must have at least one of the following three:

1) Musculoskeletal pain in two or more limbs, recurring daily for at least 3 months

2) Chronic, widespread pain for 3 months or longer

3) Recurrent joint dislocations or clinically evident joint instability, in the absence of trauma (a or b):

   a) Three or more atraumatic dislocations in the same joint, or two or more atraumatic dislocations in two different joints occurring at different times
   b) Medical confirmation of joint instability at 2 or more sites not related to trauma

General Comment: Many other features are described in hEDS but most are not sufficiently test specific or test sensitive to be included in formal diagnostic criteria, at the moment. These include but are not limited to: sleep disturbance, fatigue, postural orthostatic tachycardia, functional gastrointestinal disorders, dysautonomia, anxiety, and depression. These other systemic manifestations may be more debilitating than the joint symptoms, often impair functionality and quality of life, and should always be determined during clinical encounters. While they are not part of the diagnostic criteria, the presence of such systemic manifestations may prompt consideration of hEDS in the differential diagnosis.

(Criteria: Malfait F et al. 2017)

DIAGNOSIS

Box 3. The Beighton Score to diagnose generalised joint hypermobility

The Beighton Score has been used for many years as an indicator of generalised joint hypermobility (GJH).

- **Score 1 point** if you can you bend forward from the waist, with your knees straight and put your palms flat on the floor
- **Score 1 point** for each elbow that you can hyperextend backwards (see picture below)
- **Score 1 point** for each knee you can hyperextend backwards (see picture below)
- **Score 1 point** for each thumb back you can bend back to meet your forearm (see picture below)
- **Score 1 point** for each little finger you can bend back beyond 90 degrees towards the back of the hand (see picture below)

The International Classification 2017 defines the cut-off for the definition of GJH using the Beighton Score as:

6 points or more (out of a total of 9) for pre-pubertal children and adolescents
5 points or more (out of a total of 9) for men and women post puberty up to 50 years of age
4 points or more (out of a total of 9) for men and women over 50 years of age

Important notes:
As a clinical tool the Beighton Scoring System (above) can be a quick and straightforward thing to do **BUT** there are additional factors that **must** be taken into consideration :

i. A high Beighton score by itself does not automatically mean that an individual has a hypermobility related disorder - other symptoms and signs need to also be present. Patients with Hypermobility Spectrum Disorder usually experience one or more of the following musculoskeletal manifestations (Castori M. et al 2017):

Pain: Occasional, recurring pain is a natural result of the trauma, but chronic pain can develop—perhaps because of unusual sensitivity to pain (hyperalgesia), perhaps because of an impaired connective tissue function (as suggested by the discovery of small fiber neuropathy in adults with classical, hypermobile, and vascular EDS).

Musculoskeletal and/or soft tissue trauma: Macrotrauma includes dislocation, subluxations, and connected soft tissue damage (ligaments, tendons, muscles). It can cause acute pain and loss of joint function. Microtrauma are injuries too small for them to be noticed as they happen. Over time, they may make one susceptible to recurrent or persistent pain, and possibly early joint degeneration like osteoarthritis.

Disturbed Proprioception: Proprioception is the sense of the relative position of parts of the body and how much effort is needed for movement—can be reduced. Not understanding where our joints are and how much muscle strength it takes to use them can lead to a cycle that increasingly limits our abilities to manage every day life.

Other Musculoskeletal Traits: Those with GJH often have other minor musculoskeletal physical traits, which may be the result of the interactions between "softer" musculoskeletal tissues and mechanical forces during growth. These include flat feet (flexible type), misaligned bones in the elbow and big toes,

mild to moderate scoliosis (side to side curvature of the spine), kyphosis (outward curvature) of the upper spine and lordosis (inner curvature) of the lower spine. There may be an indirect association with mild reduced bone mass as a result of many factors—lack of proprioception, muscle weakness, and the resulting reduced activity (All above 5/Ehlers Danlos Society 2017)

ii. Score adjustments should be made for injury/trauma, past surgeries, wheelchair use, amputations and age etc. If a patient scores one point below the required total but answers 'yes' to two or more of the questions listed in the five-point questionnaire (see below), GJH can still be diagnosed (Malfait F. et al 2017).

1) As a child did you amuse your friends by contorting your body into strange shapes, or could you do the splits?
2) As a child or teenager, did your shoulder or knee-cap dislocate on more than one occasion?
3) Do you consider yourself 'double-jointed?
4) Can you now (or could you ever) place your hands flat on the floor without bending your knees?
5) Can you now (or could you ever) bend your thumb back to touch your forearm? (All above: Hakim A. 2017c HMSA).

iii. A low score should be considered with caution when assessing someone, as hypermobility can be present at a number of sites that are not counted in the Beighton Score. For example, at the jaw joint (the 'TMJ'), neck (cervical spine), shoulders, mid (thoracic) spine, hips, ankles and feet. Joints outside these scores should be assessed also, and in particular if they are sites of pain / injury. For example, the shoulder, hip and ankle are common sites of pain and instability but are not in the Beighton Score – in such a situation, only using the Beighton Score to decide whether hypermobility might explain a presentation is inappropriate (Hakim A. 2017c HMSA).

 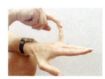 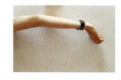
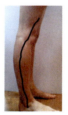 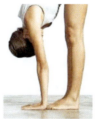

Pictures showing a patient touching their thumb to their wrist; bending their little finger back; a patient's knees and elbow in hyper-extension; bending forwards and placing their palms flat to the floor (all past the range of movement that is considered 'normal')

Additional comment: Establishing whether a joint is hypermobile or not is a relatively easy task and it is carried out by (i) using professional tools, such as the orthopaedic goniometer; (ii) following specific procedures (e.g. Juul-Kristensen B. et al., 2007; and (iii) comparing the measured range of motion (ROM) with normal parameters. (Tinkle B. et al 2017)

If there is any concern that a patient may have a connective tissue disorder other than HSD or hEDS, they should be referred for expert opinion, and further assessment might include genetic testing, vascular imaging and ophthalmic review.

...continued from page 120

- The need for all joints to be assessed (not just those described in the scale).

The latter is well illustrated by a parent of children diagnosed with HSD, who herself has the condition, she writes:

'My daughter can't touch her thumb to her wrist let alone her palms to the ground, but my son and I both can. My daughter's elbows, shoulder, hips and thumbs ARE hypermobile. My son scores very low number on the Beighton scale; he can't touch his thumb to wrist, but he can bend all his fingers together up to 90 degrees backwards, and also has hypermobile shoulders, hips, patella and other joints!'

Reaching a diagnosis

Hypermobile Ehlers-Danlos syndrome

Having clinically assessed a patient using the diagnostic assessment criterion shown in **Boxes 2 and 3** (pages 121 and 122), and considered and excluded all other differential diagnoses (criterion 3, **Box 2**), those who meet the criteria for hypermobile Ehlers-Danlos syndrome (hEDS) should receive this diagnosis. (NB/ An 'EDS Types Chart' showing each subtype, inheritance patterns, and genetic basis and the protein involved (where known) can be found on page 187.

As we have seen in the previous two chapters, there are a range of conditions which can accompany hEDS, although, as yet, there is not enough data for them to become diagnostic criteria (while they are clearly associated with hEDS, they are not proven to be the *result* of hEDS). Some of these include sleep disturbance, fatigue, cardiovascular autonomic dysfunction (such as postural orthostatic tachycardia); anxiety and depression; mechanical and neuropathic bowel dysfunction (hernia, reflux, sluggish bowel and constipation), chronic bowel inflammation (inc. mast cell activation); myopia, astigmatism; poor response to local anaesthetic; pelvic floor weakness, rectal and/or uterine prolapse, chronic bladder inflammation (inc. mast cell activation); influence of progesterone - worsening musculoskeletal symptoms; also heavy and painful menstrual cycle; musculoskeletal and pelvic complications of pregnancy; and anxiety disorders, such as panic disorder and agoraphobia (9/ Hakim (HMSA) 2017 / 2/Ehlers-Danlos Society 2017)

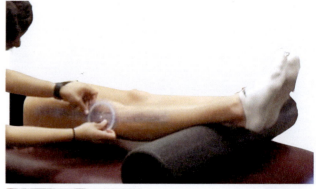
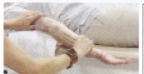

Assessing hyperextension in the hypermobile joint using an orthopaedic goniometer

For the patient, these other systemic manifestations may be more debilitating than the joint symptoms often impairing functionality and quality of life, and should always be determined during clinical encounters. While they are not part of the diagnostic criteria, the presence of such systemic manifestations may prompt consideration of hEDS in the differential diagnosis (2/Ehlers-Danlos Society 2017).

Hypermobility Spectrum Disorder

Those individuals with hypermobility-related problems that meet the Beighton Score criteria (see **Box 3**, page 122), and who experience one or more of the secondary musculoskeletal manifestations described in **Box 3** point (**i**), but who do not meet the full criteria for hEDS or any other heritable disorder of connective tissue, should be given the diagnosis of hypermobility spectrum disorder (HSD) (Castori M. et al 2017 / Hakim A. 2017c). The subtype of HSD is then distinguished based on *which* joints are hypermobile (see **Box 4**).

Cautionary points - hEDS and HSD

1) As stressed in Chapter 1, musculoskeletal manifestations fall within a wide spectrum of severity (both in terms of the physical signs and severity of symptoms).

2) As with the hypermobile type of Ehlers-Danlos syndrome, individuals with HSD may <u>also</u> be affected by one or more of the comorbid disorders commonly associated with joint hypermobility. For example, postural orthostatic tachycardia, fatigue, functional gastrointestinal disorders, pelvic and bladder dysfunction etc (a larger list of examples can be found on page 42). The 2017 Classification recognises that they are present in some people with EDS, and HSD, and that health care professionals should be looking for them and treating them (9/ HMSA 2017 / Castori M. et al 2017 / 3/Ehlers-Danlos Society).

3) *Where* a patient's diagnosis is placed within the spectrum of hypermobility related disorders (also see diagram and post-it note, page 32) does <u>not</u> necessarily represent *severity* of symptoms experienced, it represents the *range* of symptoms experienced. Indeed, one person's hypermobile Ehlers-Danlos syndrome joint pain may be less severe than another's hypermobility spectrum disorder joint pain. The overall spectrum isn't strictly linear from least to most severe, it represents the *range* of symptoms seen in patients from single joint issues through to the 'syndrome of disorders' seen in hEDS .

Type	Beighton score	Musculo-skeletal involvement	Notes
Asymptomatic GJH	Positive	Absent	
Asymptomatic PJH	Usually negative	Absent	JH typically limited to hands and/or feet
Asymptomatic LJH	Negative	Absent	JH typically limited to single joints or body parts
G-HSD	Positive	Present	
P-HSD	Usually negative	Present	JH typically limited to hands and/or feet
L-HSD	Negative	Present	JH typically limited to single joints or body parts
H-HSD	Negative	Present	Historical presence of JH
hEDS	Positive	Possible	

Source: 5/Ehlers-Danlos Society

'HEDS and HSD can be equal in severity, and both need similar management, validation and care.'
3/Ehlers-Danlos Society)

Is a formal diagnosis necessary?

The issue of whether or not a formal diagnosis is beneficial is a question often asked in patient forums.

As there is no definitive genetic test, and treatment is symptom based, doctors may advise against a formal diagnosis on the basis that, in many patients, symptoms can be effectively managed without a formal diagnosis. Some doctors also fear that 'labeling' patients with a diagnosis can lead to fear, anxiety, hypervigilism, and reluctance to exercise, resulting in a downward spiraling of health.

Where patients are left to find information themselves, and resort to searching the internet for answers or to creating their own (not necessarily beneficial) coping mechanisms, diagnosis without adequate support may be a risk. However, where a patient is signposted to appropriate educational sources after diagnosis (for example, to a charity whose information is accredited under NHS England's Information Standard), diagnosis may significantly reduce patient anxiety, be personally empowering and save NHS funding in terms of inappropriate tests and treatments.

Whether it's best to seek, or push for, a formal diagnosis is dependent on lots of factors, and is a very personal choice on the patients part. The

---

Box 4.

When symptomatic joint hypermobility is experienced but the symptoms do not meet the diagnostic criteria for defined syndromes or disorders that feature hypermobility (such as those described on page 18) a patient may be given a diagnosis of 'hypermobility spectrum disorder (HSD).

HSD form part of a single continuous spectrum ranging from asymptomatic joint hypermobility at one end, through the various hypermobility spectrum disorders, and on to hEDS (Castori M. et al 2017).

Four different HSD may be identified:

Generalised (joint) hypermobility spectrum disorder (G-HSD): Diagnosed where generalised joint hypermobility has been objectively assessed (e.g. by the Beighton score) plus one or more secondary musculoskeletal manifestations as identified in **Box 3 (point i),** page 122. In these patients, the pattern and severity of the involvement of the musculoskeletal system should be carefully assessed in order to explore the possibility of a hEDS. In this category usually fall most patients with GJH and additional musculoskeletal manifestations but who do <u>not</u> meet the full diagnostic criteria for hEDS.

Peripheral (joint) hypermobility spectrum disorder (P-HSD): Diagnosed where joint hypermobility is limited to hands and feet plus one or more secondary musculoskeletal manifestations identified in **Box 3(i)** page 122**.**

Localised (joint) hypermobility spectrum disorder (L-HSD): Diagnosed where joint hypermobility is found at single joints or group of joints plus one or more secondary musculoskeletal manifestations regionally related to the hypermobile joint(s) (see **Box 3(i)**, page 122).

Historical (joint) hypermobility spectrum disorder (H-HSD): Self-reported (historical) symptomatic generalised joint hypermobility (e.g., by the five-point questionnaire - see page 122, **Box 3, point (ii)** with negative Beighton score plus one or more secondary musculoskeletal manifestations as identified in **Box 3 (i)** page 122; in these cases, physical examination aimed at excluding the alternative diagnoses of G-HSD, P-HSD, and L-HSD as well as other rheumatologic conditions is mandatory.   (All above: Castori M. 2017)

© Understanding hEDS and HSD by C. Smith

main thing is that a patient gets the right treatment/management advice. If they are getting the support they need, then a formal diagnosis might not be needed. If problems are not being addressed however, then, again, a diagnosis may help.

Some of the many reasons patients seek diagnosis are listed below:

- The confirmation and validation a diagnosis brings can often be a huge relief to patients, many who have been seeking answers for many years or who have been made to feel disbelieved.
- A diagnosis helps doctors know to look for related, co-morbid conditions frequently seen with EDS and to have an idea where to look when new symptoms occur.
- An official diagnosis can alert surgeons and therapists to changes in how they do carry out procedures and potential problems with anesthesia and healing issues.
- A diagnosis can help a physiotherapist understand that alterations to "traditional or rehabilitative" physiotherapy may be required in order for it to work successfully for patients.
- The official diagnosis may be important to receive services from some specialists.
- A diagnosis can be helpful in order to obtain accommodations at work or for a child's requirements for PE or with sports activities to prevent injuries (ref: Supporting Pupils at school with Medical Conditions' Department of Education 2014).
- Outside of the UK, a diagnosis is helpful if you ever have to file for disability benefits (in the UK, disability benefits are based on symptoms rather than diagnosis).
- Some patients find that receiving diagnosis makes it easier to make appointments through private medical insurers.
- A diagnosis provides researchers with a better idea of the incidence of EDS.
- A diagnosis can help other family members understand what may be happening with them and help them to be diagnosed.
- A diagnosis can be important when advice is required to make informed decisions about family planning.

As discussed in Chapter 1, an international registry for EDS is planned and, over the next few years, it is likely that formal diagnosis will be encouraged in order to identify the global EDS population, raising

Diagnosing children

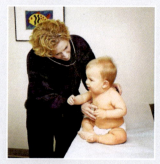

A baby is born with 300 bones which gradually fuse and strengthen as they progress through toddlerhood and childhood. By the time they reach adulthood they have 206. Due to this process (ossification), it can be difficult for clinicians to tell whether or not a child has excessive laxity in comparison to other children of the same age. In some instances, it may be necessary to wait until they are around 6 years of age or older (Tinkle B. 2010) and, even at that point, unless there is clear evidence that a strong family history or genetic family link is involved, it is unlikely that a child will be given a formal HSD or hEDS diagnosis - any such diagnosis would usually be reserved until the child reaches their teens or adulthood and a clear history can be established.

In the meantime, if the child is struggling with pain and other problems, a child's GP can refer to a paediatrician or direct to physiotherapy. They may also benefit from a referral to podiatry and occupational therapy. Additional support and/or adaptions may also be needed in school.

Image by: Jim Gathany, CDC - under Creative Commons Licence

awareness, standards of care, clinical trials, facilitating scientific identification of the underlying genetic cause(s) of hEDS and, in the future, a treatment or cure.

It seems clear therefore that, although not right for everyone, formal diagnosis has value that should certainly be considered.

Concerns relating to differential diagnosis

If there is any concern that a patient may have a connective tissue disorder other than HSD or hEDS, they should be referred for expert opinion. Further assessment might include vascular imaging, ophthalmic review and genetic testing; geneticists are most adept at distinguishing between the types of Ehlers-Danlos syndrome, as well as differentiating EDS from the more than 200 other heritable connective tissue disorders (1/ Ehlers-Danlos Society 2017).

> Management strategy and multi-disciplinary referral, physiotherapy; occupational therapy; joint protection; splinting, bracing, taping, compression-ware and orthotics; relief of severe pain, and using pain killers effectively; self management; cognitive behavioural therapy; complementary and physical therapies; making the most of your health care team; dental implications, and surgical issues are all discussed in the remainder of this chapter.

Summary of investigations and management of HSD and hEDS

This section has been written by Dr Alan Hakim and has been included with the kind permission of the Hypermobility Syndromes Association. It is aimed primarily at clinicians (Hakim A.J 2017c (HMSA).

A patients' concerns may be protean [ever-changing]. A long list of investigations and treatments is inappropriate for a summary of this nature. Detail regarding specific concerns can be found on the Hypermobility Syndromes Association website (see 'Resources') and in the cited reference literature at the end of this page. Many aspects of care should involve guidance over self-management, and likely include physical treatments, medicines, and therapies, often running in parallel and managed in a multidisciplinary way.

The more common areas of investigation include:

Musculoskeletal and fatigue blood tests:

- If there is any concern that joint and/or muscle pain may be due to an inflammatory or autoimmune disorder then the relevant blood tests should be undertaken.
- Blood tests may be required to exclude haematologic, endocrine, and metabolic causes for fatigue.

Neuro-muscular Imaging:

- Radiographs, Ultrasound, MRI : imaging of joints / soft tissue may help to determine whether mechanical or inflammatory damage is present, impingement at the joint or of a nerve has arisen, or whether subluxation/listhesis etc. is occurring.
- Neuropathic concerns might require central nervous system imaging; peripheral tests including NCS/EMG.

Echocardiography

Echocardiography should be carried out if there is any concern on examination, or as part of the diagnostic work up for hEDS and other HDCT.

Bowel and urogynaecologic investigations:

- Tests for helicobacter, coeliac, bacterial over-growth.

- Upper or lower GI endoscopy and functional bowel tests.
- Urodynamics and cystoscopy might be required to delineate a problem, as might hysteroscopy.

The more common areas of management include (recent reviews cited in brackets and shown at the end of this page):

- Physical therapies (Engelbert et al, 2017).
- Pain Management (Chopra et al. 2017).
- Anxiety and Mood management (Bulbena et al. 2017).
- Fatigue (Hakim et al. 2017b)
- Reflux, nausea, and sluggish bowel (Fikree et al. 2017)
- Cardiovascular autonomic dysfunction (Hakim et al. 2017b)
- Management of gynaecological concerns

Very recent literature reviews in this field of medicine detail the current understanding of the associations with hypermobility-related disorders (in particular HSD and hEDS) and the treatment options available. These are cited in the references below:

Bulbena A, Baeza-Velasco C, Bulbena-Cabré A, Pailhez G, Critchley H, Chopra P, Mallorquí-Bagué N, Frank C, Porges S. Psychiatric and psychological aspects in the Ehlers-Danlos syndromes. Am J Med Genet C Semin Med Genet. 2017 Feb 10. doi: 10.1002/ajmg.c.31544. [Epub ahead of print] PubMed PMID: 28186381.

Castori M, Tinkle B, Levy H, Grahame R, Malfait F, Hakim A. A framework for the classification of joint hypermobility and related conditions. Am J Med Genet C Semin Med Genet. 2017 Feb 1. doi: 10.1002/ajmg.c.31539. [Epub ahead of print] PubMed PMID: 28145606.

Chopra P, Tinkle B, Hamonet C, Brock I, Gompel A, Bulbena A, Francomano C. Pain management in the Ehlers-Danlos syndromes. Am J Med Genet C Semin Med Genet.2017 Feb 10. doi: 10.1002/ajmg.c.31554. [Epub ahead of print] PubMed PMID: 28186390.

Engelbert RH, Juul-Kristensen B, Pacey V, de Wandele I, Smeenk S, Woinarosky N, Sabo S, Scheper MC, Russek L, Simmonds JV. 2017. The evidence-based rationale for physical therapy treatment of children, adolescents, and adults diagnosed with joint hypermobility syndrome/hypermobile Ehlers Danlos syndrome. Am J Med Genet Part C Semin Med Genet 175C:158–167.

Fikree A, Chelimsky G, Collins H, Kovacic K, Aziz Q. Gastrointestinal involvement in the Ehlers-Danlos syndromes. Am J Med Genet C Semin Med Genet. 2017 Feb 10. doi: 10.1002/ajmg.c.31546. [Epub ahead of print] PubMed PMID: 28186368.

Francomano C and Bloom L. 2017. http://ehlers-danlos.com/2017-eds-international-classification-webinar/

Hakim A, De Wandele I, O'Callaghan C, Pocinki A, Rowe P. Chronic fatigue in Ehlers-Danlos syndrome-hypermobile type. Am J Med Genet C Semin Med Genet. 2017 Feb 10. doi: 10.1002/ajmg.c.31542. [Epub ahead of print] PubMed PMID: 28186393.

Hakim A, O'Callaghan C, De Wandele I, Stiles L, Pocinki A, Rowe P. Cardiovascular autonomic dysfunction in Ehlers-Danlos syndrome-hypermobile type. Am J Med Genet C Semin Med Genet. 2017 Feb 4. doi: 10.1002/ajmg.c.31543. [Epub ahead of print] PubMed PMID: 28160388.

Malfait F, Francomano C, Byers P, Belmont J, Berglund B, Black J, Bloom L, Bowen JM, Brady AF, Burrows NP, Castori M, Cohen H, Colombi M, Demirdas S, De Backer J, De Paepe A, Fournel-Gigleux S, Frank M, Ghali N, Giunta C, Grahame R, Hakim A, Jeunemaitre X, Johnson D, Juul-Kristensen B, Kapferer-Seebacher I, Kazkaz H, Kosho T, Lavallee ME, Levy H, Mendoza-Londono R, Pepin M, Pope FM, Reinstein E, Robert L, Rohrbach M, Sanders L, Sobey GJ, Van Damme T, Vandersteen A, van Mourik C, Voermans N, Wheeldon N, Zschocke J, Tinkle B. 2017. The 2017 international classification of the Ehlers–Danlos syndromes. Am J Med Genet Part C Semin Med Genet 175C:8–26.

Tinkle B, Castori M, Berglund B, Cohen H, Grahame R, Kazkaz H, Levy H. Hypermobile Ehlers-Danlos syndrome (a.k.a. Ehlers-Danlos syndrome Type III and Ehlers-Danlos syndrome hypermobility type): Clinical description and natural history. Am J Med Genet C Semin Med Genet. 2017 Feb 1. doi:10.1002/ajmg.c.31538. [Epub ahead of print] PubMed PMID: 28145611.

The 2017 Classification Criteria for 8 of the 13 Ehlers-Danlos syndrome subtypes

Box 6.

Diagnosis of an EDS subtype comes by finding the one that most matches the patient's symptoms. There are clinical criteria that help guide diagnosis; signs and symptoms should be matched up to the major and minor criteria to identify the subtype that is the most complete fit. There is substantial symptom overlap between the EDS subtypes and other connective tissue disorders including HSD, as well as a lot of variability between them. So a definitive diagnosis for all the EDS subtypes (except for hypermobile EDS) also calls for confirmation by testing to identify the responsible variant for the gene affected in each subtype. The information on these pages is taken from the Ehlers-Danlos Society website (www.ehlers-danlos.com) where more in depth details and information on subtypes and their criteria can be found.

Classical EDS (cEDS)

Major criteria are:
Skin hyperextensibility and atrophic scarring; and
Generalised joint hypermobility (GJH).
There are nine minor criteria. Minimal clinical standards suggesting cEDS are the first major criterion plus either the second major criterion or at least three minor criteria.
A final diagnosis requires confirmation by molecular testing. More than 90% of those with cEDS have a heterozygous mutation in one of the genes encoding type V collagen (COL5A1 and COL5A2). Rarely, specific mutations in the genes encoding type I collagen can be associated with the characteristics of cEDS. Classical EDS is inherited in the autosomal dominant pattern.
Notes:
Skin is hyperextensible if it can be stretched over a standardized cut off in the following areas: 1.5 cm for the distal part of the forearms and the dorsum of the hands; 3 cm for neck, elbow and knees; 1 cm on the volar surface of the hand (palm).
Abnormal scarring can range in severity. Most with cEDS have extensive atrophic scars at a number of sites. A minority are more mildly affected. The relevance of surgical scars should be considered with caution in classical EDS, they can appear normal in patients with classical EDS if well managed. Atrophic surgical scars can be found in the general population due to mechanical factors and site of the incision.
Joint hypermobility is evaluated according to the Beighton score; a Beighton score of >5 is considered positive for the presence of generalised joint hypermobility. Since joint hypermobility decreases with age, patients with a Beighton score <5/9 may be considered positive based on their historical observations.

Classical-like EDS (clEDS)

Major criteria are:
Skin hyperextensibility with velvety skin texture and absence of atrophic scarring;
Generalised joint hypermobility (GJH) with or without recurrent dislocations (most often shoulder and ankle); and
Easily bruised skin or spontaneous ecchymoses (discolourations of the skin resulting from bleeding underneath).
There are seven minor criteria. Minimal clinical standards suggesting clEDS are all three major criteria plus a family history compatible with autosomal recessive transmission.

A final diagnosis requires molecular testing; clEDS is caused by a complete lack of Tenascin XB (due to biallelic TNXB mutations, that lead to nonsense-mediated mRNA decay, or biallelic deletion of TNXB). TNXB is the only gene associated with clEDS. Classical-like EDS is inherited in the autosomal recessive pattern.
Note: skin hyperextensibility and joint hypermobility are defined as in cEDS.

Cardiac-valvular EDS (cvEDS)

Major criteria are:
Severe progressive cardiac-valvular problems (aortic valve, mitral valve);
Skin involvement: skin hyperextensibility, atrophic scars, thin skin, easy bruising; and
Joint hypermobility (generalised or restricted to small joints).
There are four minor criteria. Minimal clinical standards suggesting cvEDS are the first major criterion plus a family history compatible with autosomal recessive transmission, and either one other major criterion or at least two minor criteria.
A final diagnosis requires confirmation by molecular testing; cvEDS is caused by a complete lack of the proa2-chain of type I collagen due to biallelic COL1A2 mutations, that lead to nonsense-mediated mRNA decay. COL1A2 is the only gene associated with cvEDS. Cardiac-valvular EDS is inherited in the autosomal recessive pattern.

Vascular EDS (vEDS)

Major criteria are:
Family history of vEDS with documented causative variant in COL3A1;
Arterial rupture at a young age;
Spontaneous sigmoid colon perforation in the absence of known diverticular disease or other bowel pathology;
Uterine rupture during the third trimester in the absence of previous C-section and/or severe peripartum perineum tears; and
Carotid-cavernous sinus fistula (CCSF) formation in the absence of trauma.
There are twelve minor criteria. Minimal clinical standards suggesting vEDS diagnostic studies should be performed are: a family history of the disorder, arterial rupture or dissection in individuals less than 40 years of age; unexplained sigmoid colon rupture: or spontaneous pneumothorax in the presence of other features consistent with vEDS. Testing for vEDS should also be considered in the presence of a combination of the other "minor" criteria.

© Understanding hEDS and HSD by C. Smith

A final diagnosis requires confirmation by molecular testing. Patients with vEDS typically have a heterozygous mutation in the COL3A1 gene, with the rare exception of specific heterozygous arginine-to-cysteine substitution mutations in COL1A1 that are also associated with vascular fragility and mimic COL3A1-vEDS. In very rare instances, biallelic pathogenic variants in COL3A1 may be identified. Vascular EDS is inherited in the autosomal dominant pattern.

Hypermobile EDS

The diagnosis of hypermobile EDS (hEDS) remains clinical; there is no molecular, genetic cause yet identified, so there is no test available for almost all with hEDS.

There is a clinical spectrum ranging from asymptomatic joint hypermobility, through "non-syndromic" hypermobility with secondary manifestations, to hEDS (see pages 29-32 and 123-124) or, for further reading, see "A Framework for the Classification of Joint Hypermobility and Related Conditions" by Castori M. et al 2017 in this book's bibliography.

A diagnosis of hEDS should be assigned only in those who meet all of the criteria, which should help research efforts to discover the underlying genetic cause(s) which, in turn, may help clinical management. As this is a clinical diagnosis, it's important to be relatively confident that the diagnosis is not instead one of the many other disorders of connective tissue. Hypermobile EDS is inherited in the autosomal dominant pattern.

The clinical diagnosis of hEDS needs the simultaneous presence of criteria 1 and 2 and 3. This is a complex set of criteria, and there is much more detail than presented in this overview; please see page 121 for hypermobile EDS criteria.

Generalised joint hypermobility (GJH); and
Two or more of the following features must be present (A & B, A & C, B & C, or A & B & C):
Feature A - systemic manifestations of a more generalised connective tissue disorder (a total of five out of twelve must be present)
Feature B - positive family history, with one or more first degree relatives independently meeting the current diagnostic criteria for hEDS
Feature C - musculoskeletal complications (must have at least one of three); and
All these prerequisites must be met: absence of unusual skin fragility, exclusion of other heritable and acquired connective tissue disorders including autoimmune rheumatologic conditions, and exclusion of alternative diagnoses that may also include joint hypermobility by means of hypotonia and/or connective tissue laxity.
There is a range of conditions which can accompany hEDS, although there is not enough data for them to become diagnostic criteria. While they're associated with hEDS, they're not proven to be the result of hEDS and they're not specific enough to be criteria for diagnosis. Some of these include sleep disturbance, fatigue, postural orthostatic tachycardia, functional gastrointestinal disorders, dysautonomia, anxiety, and depression. These conditions may be more debilitating than the joint symptoms; they often impair daily life, and they should be considered and treated.

Arthrochalasia EDS (aEDS)

Major criteria are:
Congenital bilateral hip dislocation;
Severe GJH, with multiple dislocations/subluxations; and
Skin hyperextensibility.
There are five minor criteria. Minimal criteria for aEDS are congenital bilateral hip dislocation (major criterion 1) plus either: skin hyperextensibility (major criterion 3); or severe GJH (major criterion 2) with at least two minor criteria.
A final diagnosis requires confirmation by molecular testing; aEDS is caused by heterozygous mutations in either COL1A1 or COL1A2, that cause entire or partial loss of exon 6 of the respective gene. No other genes are associated with aEDS. Absence of a causative mutation in COL1A1 or COL1A2 that leads to complete or partial deletion of the exon 6 of either gene excludes the diagnosis of aEDS. Arthrochalasia EDS is inherited in the autosomal dominant pattern.

Dermatosparaxis EDS (dEDS)

There are nine major criteria and eleven minor criteria. Minimal criteria suggestive of dEDS include the two major criteria of extreme skin fragility and characteristic craniofacial features, plus either: one other major criterion, or three minor criteria.
A final diagnosis requires confirmation by molecular testing; dEDS is caused by biallelic mutations in ADAMTS2. It is the only gene associated with dEDS. Dermatosparaxis EDS is inherited in the autosomal recessive pattern.

Kyphoscoliotic EDS (kEDS)

Major criteria are:
Congenital muscle hypotonia;
Congenital or early onset kyphoscoliosis (progressive or non-progressive); and
GJH with dislocations/subluxations (shoulders, hips and knees in particular).
There are ten minor criteria, as well as gene-specific minor criteria (four for PLOD1 and four for FKBP14). Minimal criteria suggestive for kEDS are 1 and 2 of the major criteria —congenital muscle hypotonia and congential/early onset kyphoscoliosis—plus either: major criterion 3, or three minor criteria (either general of gene-specific).
A final diagnosis requires confirmation by testing. The majority of patients with kEDS harbor biallelic mutations in PLOD1; recently, biallelic mutations have been identified in FKBP14 in patients displaying a phenotype that clinically largely overlaps with kEDS-PLOD1. Laboratory confirmation should start with a urine test using high-performance liquid chromatography (to evaluate the ratio of lysyl-pyridinoline to hydroxylysyl-pyridinoline crosslinks; a normal ratio is ~0.2, whereas kEDS-PLOD1 range is 2-9). This method is fast and cost-effective and it can also be used to determine the pathogenic status of a variant of uncertain significance. Molecular analysis can follow if the urine test is normal. Whereas absence of an abnormal urinary LP/HP ratio excludes the diagnosis of kEDS-PLOD1, absence of the confirmatory genetic findings does not exclude the diagnosis of kEDS, as other yet-to-be-discovered genes may be associated with this phenotype; however, alternative diagnoses should be considered in the absence of PLOD1 or FKBP14 mutations. Kyphoscoliotic EDS is inherited in the autosomal recessive pattern.

What might a patient expect at a rheumatology clinical assessment?

If an individual thinks they might have one of the Ehlers-Danlos syndromes or hypermobility spectrum disorders, and particularly if someone in their immediate family has been diagnosed, a doctor should be consulted to see if a diagnosis fits their symptoms. If they choose to, any medical doctor is able to diagnose EDS/HSD; but it is most common to be given a referral to a rheumatologist (or geneticist; if there is any doubt or concern about the diagnosis or distinguishing between different disorders) (4/Ehlers-Danlos Society 2017). The following is an idea of what might be expected from a rheumatology clinical assessment.

Preparation

Either before or during the physical examination, the patient is likely to be asked questions about their medical and family history.   Before attending the appointment, it may be helpful to prepare by gathering together:

- a list of any symptoms or pain being experienced,
- a list of current medications taken, including over-the-counter drugs and any herbal supplements,
- the results from any recent or relevant tests,
- medical and surgical history,
- the names and contact information for other doctors seen recently,
- details of any hypermobility related symptoms or relevant diagnoses relating to first degree relatives,
- any additional questions one might like answered
- supporting information printed from reputable sources (the Hypermobility Syndromes Association and Ehlers-Danlos Support UK, both hold NHS England Information Standard Accreditation).

Physical examination

At the appointment, it may be necessary for the patient to change into comfortable sports clothing to allow easy examination of joints.

Assessment of the joints and skin:

Whilst thoroughly checking the patient against each of the appropriate criterion, the clinician may look at, feel, and move each joint; evaluating it for:

- the number and distribution of affected joints,
- the degree of hypermobility,
- any swelling or tenderness,
- the range of motion present in each joint,
- the presence of subluxations or dislocations.

Examples of questions the clinician might ask:

Do you suffer from/ have you ever suffered from:

- joint sprains and ligament and tendon injuries and, if so, do they take a long time to heal or become chronic?
- persistent and/or widespread pain?
- history of joint subluxation (partial dislocation),
- history of joint dislocation?
- do you experience persistent fatigue, above and beyond what would be considered normal?
- do you have poor proprioception?
- do your symptoms worsen around the time of your menstrual period (females)?
- weakness of the abdominal pelvic wall - herniation and/or prolapse (females)?
- have you ever experienced symptoms of cardiovascular and/or gastrointestinal autonomic dysfunction such as low blood pressure, feeling faint or fainting, symptoms similar to irritable bowl syndrome or even gastroparesis?
- do you experience the full effect of local anaesthetics?
- do you experience anxiety or depression?

In addition, patients are likely to be asked relevant questions about their family, work and sporting history. For example, a clinician will want to know whether either parents, grandparents, or any of your siblings are/were hypermobile and whether career or hobbies have been influenced by hypermobility.

Additional questions for those more advanced in years

Hypermobility itself tends to lessen with age (although the associated symptoms may worsen) (8/ HMSA 2014) so, if a patient is older, they may also be asked questions relating to symptoms they may have experienced in the past. These may include:

© Understanding hEDS and HSD by C. Smith

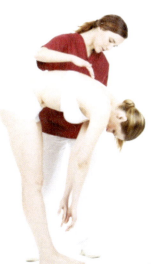

- Can you now (or could you ever) place your hands flat on the floor without bending your knees?
- Can you now (or could you ever) bend your thumb back to touch your forearm?
- As a child, did you amuse your friends by contorting your body into strange shapes, or could you do the splits?
- As a child or teenager, did your shoulder or knee-cap dislocate on more than one occasion?
- Do you consider yourself 'double-jointed?'

(Hakim A.J. 2016 - personal correspondence)

Other questions which could be asked include:

- Do you now (or did you as a child) go over on your ankles a lot?
- Did you have 'growing pains' in your legs?
- Did your joints click a lot?
- Did you fidget a lot as a child?
- Did you bump into things/fall over a lot as a child?

(Oliver J. 2005)

Assessment of the skin: An assessment of the skin will be made, to look for any of the more mild skin signs that can be seen in hEDS and to help rule out the presence of the more florid skin signs that could indicate a rarer form of EDS, such as classical EDS.

It is likely that the skin will be checked for:
- consistency and texture,
- translucency,
- extensibility,
- integrity.

A clinician may also ask questions about skin history, such as any problems experienced with:
- wound healing,
- easy bruising,
- unusual scarring,

DIAGNOSIS

> Unfortunately, there is little diagnostic data available to measure skin findings against, and findings are often only discernible to someone who has a great deal of experience working with those who have the condition. Testing for extensibility should not take place on areas of natural skin redundancy. For example, extensor surfaces such as elbows should be avoided. Similarly, parameters are not available for measuring velvety/smooth skin and, even for the experienced, one clinician's perception of 'stretchy' skin or 'soft' skin could be very different from another.

- development of stretch marks at a young age,
- history of varicose veins.

Gait Assessment: A gait assessment, to observe walking and check for over-pronation and pes planus (flat feet), knock knees, hyperextended knees, muscle weakness, ligament weakness, or other biomechanical distortions in the foot or ankle is deemed an essential part of the examination of the hypermobile patient (Helliwell P. 2011).

What to expect after the assessment is complete

After the assessment is completed, the clinician will discuss their findings with the patient and explain any further tests or investigations that they feel need to be carried out. At this point, the patient should also be given the opportunity to ask any questions they may have. If the assessment has taken place as part of a referral appointment, the clinician will write to the patient's GP, summarising their findings and detailing any further tests (should they be required). They should also suggest an appropriate plan for ongoing management of symptoms.

Most individuals with hEDS, and HSD, will be treated within primary health care (please see Chapter 3 page 133). However, where the diagnosis of hEDS is suspected but not confirmed; if the patient has particularly severe or complex symptoms, or if there are significant additional findings, aside from the diagnostic criteria, the GP may refer a patient to secondary healthcare for further tests and appropriate treatment.

An overview of Services that may be involved in patient care of those with hEDS or HSD can be found on page 131.

Image by: Flare- Freedigitalphotos.net

An overview of services that may be involved in patient care

Management of hEDS/HSD may include access to some, or all, of the services shown below, depending on an individual's diagnosis and the symptoms experienced (this is not an exhaustive list).

In alphabetical order:

Cardiology and/or autonomic dysfunction evaluation: Depending on the symptoms experienced, some patients with hEDS may be referred to a cardiologist in order to assess any possible complications involving the cardiac valve, aortic arch or a vascular disorder. Others may need to be seen in relation to symptoms of cardiovascular dysautonomia, including postural orthostatic tachycardia syndrome. Tests may include blood, cardiology or neurology, and a tilt-table test may be performed.

Charities: Patients who have recently been diagnosed should be provided with contact details for a charities such as the Hypermobility Syndromes Association or EDS Support UK, who are accredited by NHS England's Information Standard, and offer support, advice, and education on management of all heritable disorders of connective tissue, including EDS (all subtypes) and HSD (all aetiologies).

Cognitive behavioural therapy: (CBT): Many people with long term conditions feel overwhelmed by their symptoms and the effect their health may have on their partners, children, friends, family or employers (Wicks D. 2015). Psychological therapies, such as CBT, can help people to accept their diagnosis and to find ways to deal with it effectively (17/NHS.co.uk). It can help patients learn the skills needed to challenge negative thought patterns, feelings and behaviours. Being recommended for this form of therapy does not mean that the healthcare professional thinks your symptoms are 'all in your head'. Instead, it means that they recognise that things can be very difficult for those living with complex conditions and feel that CBT would be an effective way to help support you.

Gastroenterology: In most cases, gastrointestinal manifestations involved in hEDS/HSD (such as Irritable Bowel-like symptoms) can be managed with help from a patient's GP. However, where symptoms such as gastropareisis, diverticulitis, hiatal hernia, rectal evacuatory dysfunction or other unexplained symptoms are involved, a patient may be referred to a gastroenerologist.

Genetic testing (biochemical blood sampling and skin biopsy): If there is a concern relating to the possible presence of a rarer, or life threatening, form of EDS (or other form of heritable disorder of connective tissue), a patient may be referred for blood sampling and skin biopsy. Such services are usually reserved for those in whom significant additional findings aside from diagnostic criteria are found. As we have discussed in previous chapters, genetic testing to diagnose most patients with hypermobile Ehlers-Danlos syndrome is currently not available, although geneticists are working to change this. In recent years, some research studies have shown that, '*in a small portion of people with* [hEDS], *the low expression of a gene that controls the production of structural protein called Tenascin X has been found. However, this only seems to arise in less than 10% of families and, currently, this is not a routine or diagnostic test in use* (Hakim A.J. 2013a).

GP support: In the UK, family doctors (known as GPs) coordinate patient care, and can refer to other services they feel would be beneficial such as physiotherapy, occupational therapy, pain clinics, cognitive behavioural therapy or specialist consultants, should the need arise. They may also prescribe analgesics (painkillers) that might include anti-depressants and anti-epileptics at analgesic doses, and, where appropriate, muscle relaxants (Hakim A.J. 2013i).

If persistent pain is experienced, the GP can help the patient manage their condition by working out which treatments and management options work best for them. Pain is a complicated, hard-to-treat problem, and the answer may not necessarily always be stronger and stronger painkillers. GP's won't know everything, but they'll know where to find answers (2/arthritis research uk.org).

Gynaecological referral: A referral to a gynaecologist may be made if symptoms such as pelvic floor insufficiency, rectal or vaginal prolapse are present. The gynaecologist should be made aware of the underlying disorder of the connective tissue.

Haematological and immunological testing: These tests may be undertaken in order to exclude any other potential causes for the of the symptoms experienced (Hakim A.J. 2013c).

© Understanding hEDS and HSD by C. Smith

MANAGEMENT

Imaging: Following clinical assessment, a patient may be referred for X-rays / MRI's, if required.

In the HMSA's 'Clinician's Guide to JHS/EDS-H (HSD/hEDS) (Hakim A.J. 2013c), Consultant Rheumatologist, Dr Alan Hakim, writes:

'(In some cases) *Imaging may be undertaken, typically looking for:*

- *Evidence of early degenerative disease of the joints that may arise as a consequence of excessive mobility*
- *Presence of excessive hypermobility*
- *Concern over a rare form of bone disorder associated with collagen deficiency e.g. osteogenesis imperfecta*
- *Nerve root or cord compression consequent on hypermobility or nerve tethering*
- *Osteopenia or Osteoporosis*
- *Pneumothorax (collapsed lung)*
- *Cardiac valve, and aortic arch vascular disorder*

He goes on to say: '*It should be noted that most often imaging is normal. Joint instability may only be demonstrable by dynamic imaging with ultrasound or positioning joints at the limit of their extension or rotation'* (Hakim A. J. 2013c).

Occupational therapy: Occupational therapists work with patients to identify everyday activities and tasks that they find difficult e.g. bathing, cooking, writing, getting to the shops etc. They use a range of strategies, specialist equipment, splints and gadgets to help patients achieve/maintain independence and reach goals at home, work or school.

Orthopaedics: A specialty that primarily deals with the surgical management of musculoskeletal disorders (Hakim A.J. 2017 personal correspondence).

Pain clinics: If a patient's symptoms are not able to be well controlled by GP-led pain management, they may be referred to a pain clinic. Pain clinics focus on the diagnosis and management of chronic pain. Many clinics offer a variety of treatments aimed at relieving long term pain, such as painkillers; injections, acupuncture and hypnotherapy. They can also refer patients for further tests. Some clinics have large teams of experts. Some pain clinics also offer pain management programmes, (see below) or can refer patients to them.

Pain management programmes: help patients learn the skills needed to improve their quality of life despite their pain, rather than reducing their pain. They focus on the total person, not just the pain, and aim to help patients regain control. Some programmes are residential, whilst others run one day a week for around six weeks.

Physiotherapy: Physiotherapy is generally considered the most beneficial method of managing hEDS/HSD. Provided by a trained specialist, this form of therapy helps to keep joints and muscles moving, ease pain and keep an individual mobile. Advice may also be given on safe stretching and protecting joints from stress or injury. A holistic approach is required, i.e. assessing all areas of the musculoskeletal system for signs of weakness and deconditioning and working towards strengthening the body as a whole, as well as paying particular attention to specifically troublesome joints.

Podiatry/gait assessment: Assessment of biomechanical and gait deficiencies can be a useful tool in diagnosing causes of toe, foot, ankle, knee and hip pain or injury. Where appropriate, corrective orthotics may be provided.

Rheumatology: A medical specialty that deals with the diagnosis and treatment of musculoskeletal disorders, including the wide variety of organ and systemic problems that can arise from these disorders (Hakim A.J. 2017 personal correspondence).

Self management courses: focus on helping patients to develop skills that will help them take an active role in looking after their own health condition. The courses often include approaches used to cope with fatigue and pain, along with healthy eating and exercise. The courses also cover ways to cope with the emotional side of living with a long-term condition.

Several UK organisations run free self-management courses; for example, the Expert Patients Programme Community Interest Company, and the Pain Association Scotland. Unlike many services, it is not necessary to be referred by a GP or other healthcare provider; an individual can take part by contacting the organisations directly. Contact details for these organisations are shown in the contact list at the back of this book.

References:
Howard Levy 2010 'Ehlers-Danlos Syndrome, Hypermobility Type"
Marco Castori 2012 ' Ehlers-Danlos Syndrome, Hypermobility Type: An Under-diagnosed Hereditary Connective Tissue Disorder with Mucocutaneous, Articular, and Systemic Manifestations' .8
Brad Tinkle 2010 'Joint Hypermobility Handbook'
Hakim A.J. 2013i - Pain Medication and HMSs - hypermobility.org
Hakim A.J 2013c - Clinician's Guide to JHS - hypermobility.org
Hakim A.J.2017 - personal correspondence

© Understanding hEDS and HSD by C. Smith

Management strategy and multi-disciplinary referral (UK)

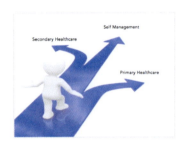

When deciding on an appropriate treatment pathway, it is important that patients are assessed on an individual basis and that a tailored plan for referrals, treatments and management is put in place. For some who are diagnosed, referrals for cardiac tests, or in-patient rehabilitation may be the most appropriate initial course of action. For others, imaging or surgical procedures may be necessary (see page 125). For the vast majority (in the UK), however, the appropriate treatment pathway can be successfully achieved through General Practitioner (GP) co-ordinated primary health care, combined with practical advice relating to long term self management. Note: In the UK a GP is a medical doctor who treats acute and chronic illnesses and provides preventive care and health education to patients. In other countries GPs may be known as 'family doctors' or 'primary care providers.' The services they can provide and the referral route itself may vary from country to country (or even within) countries.

Primary health care

GP co-ordinated primary care for those with hEDS or HSD, will typically encompass management of the physical, fatigue and pain manifestations of the syndrome. This is usually done through GP-led pain management, which may include referral for physiotherapy, prevention strategies, self-management education and perhaps cognitive behavioural therapy to help individuals come to terms with their diagnosis and the effect it may have on their life (Russek L.N. 1999/2000, Kerr A.J 2000). In some circumstances a patient may be referred to a pain clinic and/or a pain management course. Where necessary, occupational therapy may also be involved in order to recommend / provide assistive devices e.g. pens and ergonomic equipment to aid writing and posture braces to improve joint stability; a wheelchair or scooter to offload stress on lower-extremity joints or a suitable mattress to improve sleep quality. Some primary care doctors prefer to control most things, whilst others prefer to act as a central hub for communication and coordination (Tinkle B. 2010).

Secondary health care

A patient who has been provided with primary health care may also be referred to a secondary care healthcare professional or service, such as rheumatology, orthopaedics or other consultant-led services. Such referrals are usually reserved for more complex cases and/or diagnostic uncertainty. Appropriate referrals may also be made for related or comorbid symptoms such as postural orthostatic tachycardia, gastrointestinal disorders, stress incontinence etc., with services such as cardiology, gastroenterology and urology. Secondary care is usually (but not always) delivered in a hospital / clinic with the initial referral being made by the primary care professional.

Shortages in funding and centres for treatment in the UK mean that patients may need to be prepared to face a significant wait for referral appointments and other services, and to understand that, if needs are complex, their service needs may not all be able to be met locally.

Continuing care

Once primary or secondary healthcare referrals and any resulting treatment pathway are completed, it is normal practice for patients to be discharged from the consultant / services list, back to the ongoing care of their GP. Usually, a letter of discharge is sent to the patient's GP, outlining any recommendations for local referrals, such as occupational therapy, psychology support etc. The GP needs to make sure that effective support is provided and agree a plan of action where required. The severity and complexity of each patient's hEDS/HSD will vary, so it is important that physicians apply a flexible approach, regularly reviewing proposed management plans. Just because a GP has previously seen significant improvement following physiotherapy prescribed for several patients with hEDS/HSD, it does not necessarily follow that this will be all that is required for someone with more complex hEDS/HSD symptoms. It can take a while for a doctor or therapist to build a true picture of an individual's situation, and to find the best way to help; after all, no two patients are the same, and the variety of symptoms with which they present, and the subjective nature of pain and suffering varies widely.

> 'Although for many, the symptoms of [hEDS/HSD] will never be fully relieved, if the management guidelines that help prevent symptom onset and further deterioration are well managed by both the individual and the healthcare professionals who support them, stabilisation of symptoms with short periods of complete or partial relief can be achieved' (Castori M. 2012).

MANAGEMENT

Why patients must be assessed on an individual basis

Taking a 'seen one person with hEDS, seen them all' attitude to hEDS patients is not acceptable. The signs, symptoms and associated disorders which affect an individual with hEDS most profoundly can vary not only between different individuals, but also (during any given period) in each individual themselves.

'The severity of the wide ranging symptoms, the joints that are affected and the level of pain / fatigue experienced by those with HSD or hEDS, can vary greatly from day to day, or even hour to hour' (3/HMSA 2014).

Trying to categorise one individual as being more or less severely affected than another, in anything other than the extremes of severity, can also be futile. For example, how can someone affected by debilitating levels of gastrointestinal dysfunction, chronic fatigue, moderate levels of pain, but minor levels of joint instability (see **B**) be graded as more or less severely affected than someone who suffers with disabling levels of dislocations and soft tissue injuries and high levels of widespread pain and depression (see **C**)? In each case, the patient's most severe presenting symptoms are different, but can significantly interfere with their daily activities of living, including schooling or work.

When deciding on an appropriate treatment pathway for patients, such variations must be taken into account. Patients should be assessed on an individual basis and a tailored plan for referrals, treatments and management put in place and regularly reviewed.

Image © Claire Smith - All rights reserved

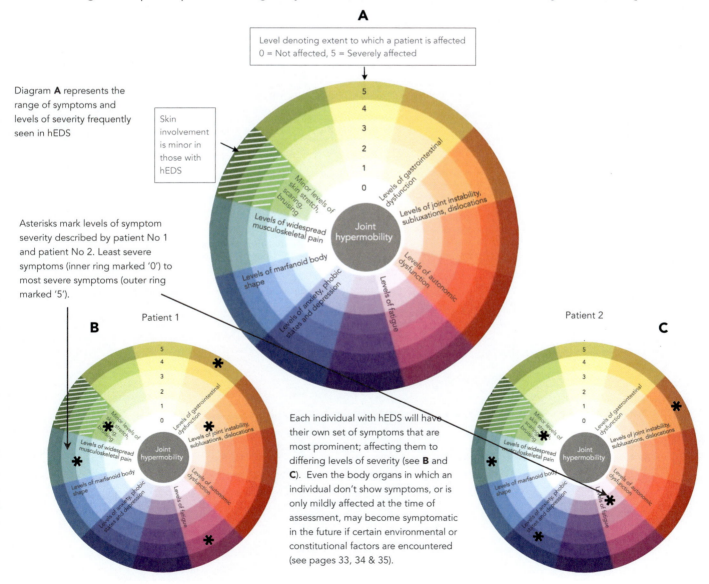

© Understanding hEDS and HSD by C. Smith

134

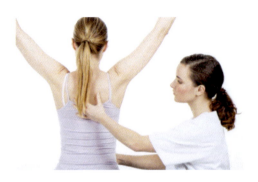

Physiotherapy

Introduction

Physiotherapy is the treatment, or management, of a condition through manual therapy, prescribed exercises and education. A physiotherapist may also use other methods such as the application of heat, cold, and electrotherapy. Physiotherapy may include work on proprioception, strength, balance, relaxing tight muscles, and building endurance. Depending on a patient's presentation of symptoms, treatment may focus on the musculoskeletal system, nerves, heart, blood vessels and lungs, or a combination of these systems. It is also likely to include education on preventing further problems from occurring in the future.

Physiotherapy is widely accepted as a mainstay of management for those who have hEDS or HSD. It is somewhat surprising therefore, to find that supporting evidence for this is scarce. According to Shea Palmer, Professor of Musculoskeletal Rehabilitation at the University of the West of England, there is a significant lack of high quality research available, and more studies are urgently needed in order for experts to determine which physiotherapy programmes are most effective (Palmer S. 2014). He and his team carried out a systematic review of available data and found that, although evidence suggests that people with HSD who undertake exercise improve over time, to date, the wide range of conditions and measurements used by researchers, when carrying out studies, can make it very hard to weigh up which exercise models produce the best results (also see Engelbert R.H. et al 2017).

To help address this, in 2015 Professor Palmer and his team undertook studies to develop an understanding of patient and health professional views and experiences of physiotherapy in the management of joint hypermobility syndrome (now known as hypermobility spectrum disorder), and used this information to design a physiotherapy intervention. The team found that the physiotherapy intervention showed evidence of promise in terms of both primary and secondary clinical outcomes. In the future, they hope to be able to secure funding to carry out a UK-wide, randomised controlled trial of physiotherapy for adults with HSD, with the aim of studying the effectiveness of physiotherapy for HSD and hypermobility related disorders across the UK.

In the meantime, anecdotal evidence from patients and those in clinical practice make it clear that to achieve the best outcome in hEDS/HSD, it is important that the physiotherapist to whom a hypermobile person is referred has a good working knowledge of hypermobility, along with the level of limitations and pain with which a hypermobile patient can present (Tinkle B. 2010). Working in partnership with the patient, listening to their symptoms, and, where necessary, researching the effects that associated conditions, such as postural orthostatic tachycardia and persistent fatigue, can have on a patient's needs and progress, is likely to lead to more achievable goals being set, and greater trust in the physiotherapist and the proposed treatment/management plan.

Ideally, physiotherapy sessions should be conducted on a one-to-one basis to allow for close supervision and feedback, while the patient is learning new movements (Melson P. & Riddle O. 2010). In reality, many patients are more familiar with physiotherapy programmes that involve a more 'consultative' approach, where, after one or two initial consultations, patients are required to carry out exercises at home, following instructions provided on photocopied sheets that are periodically updated by the therapist (Tinkle B. 2010). Regardless of whether sessions are one-to-one or more consultative, physiotherapy exercises should always be specifically tailored to the individual, and a clear, hands-on demonstration of exercises, joint positioning and postural alignment is necessary, as poor proprioception is common in those with hEDS/HSD (see page 57 and 140) (Simmonds J.V. 2015).

A holistic approach should be practiced, considering all the joints in a patient's body. On too many occasions, patients only receive physiotherapy for a particular joint that has been injured, rather than as a front-line form of management for their condition as a whole. This leads to absurd situations, such as that where a patient's left knee is being treated because it dislocates badly, but their right knee and left shoulder, which have subluxated since the initial referral was made, are left untreated. It is crucial that a holistic physiotherapy plan is specially created for each patient, depending upon the signs and symptoms of that patient (Palmer S. et al 2015 & 2016). Physiotherapists should also anticipate that patients with hEDS/HSD may take longer to treat, because they have complex presentations and pain at several sites (Levy H.P. 2004). Patients themselves must be prepared to persist regardless of setbacks, because keeping the body strong and active will always be fundamental in the ongoing management of musculoskeletal symptoms, as well as benefiting mood and cardiovascular fitness.

Why is physiotherapy considered the main form of management for hEDS/HSD?

'*Referral to a physical therapy specialist is expected for all JHS-EDS-H* [HSD-hEDS] *patients in order to identify the need for specialised intervention, choose the best suited sport/fitness activity, and educate the patient to "joint" health.*' (Castori M. 2012)

In Dr Brad Tinkle's Joint Hypermobility Handbook (2010), it explains that, in those who are hypermobile, the laxity of ligaments and other joint structures allows joints to rest in extreme positions and to rely on the stretched structures for support instead of using muscle strength and controlled movement to provide stability to the body. The aim of physiotherapy is to correct this (see **Box 7**, page 137).

Muscle strength promotes joint stability and, together with postural awareness and correction, is the starting point for improving many symptoms of hEDS/HSD. This is particularly true for symptoms such as joint injury and pain, both of which have been shown to improve by strengthening weak muscles (Pacey V. et al 2014, Maillard S. 2012). In addition to providing mechanical stability to joints, muscles contribute to the sensory feedback mechanisms associated with the joint structures themselves, known as proprioception (Blasier R. B et al 2014). This means that by improving muscle function, better feedback will be provided to the joint which, in turn, increases stability and awareness of where the joint should be best positioned (Olson T. 2005).

Exercise is also key in promoting strength and the integrity of other supporting structures such as tissue tendons, ligaments and bone (Kjaer M. 2006). The extracellular matrix enables 'linking' to other tissues, and plays a key role in force transmission and tissue structure maintenance, whilst collagen found in connective tissue provides its tensile strength. The

MANAGEMENT

Jess Glenny, a yoga teacher and therapist with a specialism in hypermobility, and member of the International Somatic Movement Education and Therapy Association, writes: '*While developing strength is clearly desirable for hypermobile people, it should be remembered that* [hEDS] *is a genetic condition of the collagen. This means that, while muscle strength can compensate to some degree for lack of tensility in the fascia, it may never create the kind of stability that is inherently present for non-hypermobile people. The compensatory form of stability achieved by those who have* [hEDS] *is not automatic and must be consciously turned on and maintained. Therapists should be aware that, for this reason, stabilising their body can be physically and mentally exhausting for hypermobile people.*'

turnover of extracellular matrix and the synthesis of collagen is significantly influenced by the level of physical activity carried out by an individual, and the resistance/weights involved; physical exercise increases turnover and synthesis, whereas inactivity significantly *decreases* turnover and may lead to collagen atrophy / wasting of the connective tissue (Keer R. 2003 / Kjaer M. 2005 / Kjaer M. 2004). Inactivity also impedes the blood flow necessary for tissue recovery. The constricted blood flow, in turn, reduces the supply of nutrients to the muscles and the removal of acids and other waste products away from the tissues (Keer R. & Grahame R. 2003 / Steering Committee for the Workshop on Work-Related Musculoskeletal Injuries).

Focuses of physiotherapy intervention in hEDS/HSD

Dependent on patient's symptoms, physiotherapy for those with hEDS/HSD will be focused on long term '*Graded Exercise*' or '*Progressive Resisted Exercise*'. Where patients are already in pain, or struggling with persistent fatigue, exercises may need to start very gently before progressing to dynamic and resisted work (Simmonds J.V. & Keer R. 2007). The aim is to improve control of the joints and muscle strength, using exercises which minimise trauma to joints and help to reduce pain (Simmonds J. V. 2014).

Graded exercise
Graded exercise therapy (GET) is commonly used to manage the symptoms of persistent fatigue and

© Understanding hEDS and HSD by C. Smith

Box 7. Physiotherapy in hEDS/HSD should aim to:

- provide education, reassurance, advice and pain management, and to develop problem solving,
- take a *global* rather than regional approach to the patient's body,
- take into account the pre-injury 'greater than normal' range of joint movement (Hakim et al. 2010),
- take into account fear of movement (kinesophobia), which is often associated with pain and fatigue (see page 142). If present, this should be assessed and managed (Celletti et al. 2013a & 2013b),
- restore muscle strength and function throughout the full range of movement,
- restore normal joint motion and effective movement patterns,
- enhance joint stability, proprioception and muscle endurance around hypermobile joints,
- improve proper body mechanics including skeletal alignment and muscular imbalances (when a muscle becomes weaker or stronger than its opposing muscle) through gentle stretching and strengthening exercise programmes, deep tissue massage and posture education,
- provide advice on suitable, controlled stretches to restore and maintain muscle length,
- provide advice on activities which are vital to maintain strength and stamina and improving general fitness,
- provide advice on core strengthening exercises which are helpful for strength, stability, balance and posture.

Box 8. Closed chain exercises: The term 'chain' refers to the kinetic chain of the body; all of your bones and muscles are connected in a 'chain' therefore the movements you make are also part of a that kinetic chain. In closed chain exercises the extremity remains stationary and in constant contact with an immobile surface e.g. the floor. A squat is an example of a closed-chain exercise because the feet stay stationary while the quadriceps do the work. Closed chain exercises are typically weight-bearing exercises, where an exerciser uses their own body weight and/or external weight.

In an open-chain exercise, the body is stationary while the limb moves. A seated leg extension is an example of an open-chain manoeuvre because the series of body parts in the limb (hip, knee, ankle, and foot) are moving freely; it might be recommended as part of a plan to increase strength in the quadricep muscles at the front of the thigh. Open chain exercises are typically non weight-bearing (Martin S.D).

In general, closed chain exercises are considered to provide greater muscle protection of the joint, and are able to better simulate daily functional demands of an extremity. However, non weight-bearing 'open chain' exercises also play a very useful role; allowing specific targeting of muscles that are weak and that are required to control the joints into their hypermobile range, reducing strain on injured ligaments, enhancing proprioceptive feedback, and optimising muscle action . For example, they can be very effective for achieving particular therapeutic goals such as increasing quadriceps strength after a patella dislocation. (BSPR, Palmer S. 2014, Russek L.N. , Michael M.A.J.)

physical deconditioning, progressively building up tolerance and confidence for daily activities. GET allows patients to start slowly, establishing a baseline for the amount of exercise that can be tolerated without causing significant repercussions. Once a level that is comfortable to the individual has been established, the level of exercise is gradually increased in frequency, duration, and intensity. GET allows the body time to make the coping changes necessary to deal with the increased amounts of activity.

Dr Simmonds explains that: '(with GET) *you agree a baseline for an individual's fitness/activity level based on a bad day. This level of activity should be carried* out for two weeks, then increased by no more than 10% for a further two weeks. For example, if an individual starts by walking for 30 minutes each day, this would then be increased to 33 minutes per day for the following two weeks and so on, until a patient is back to full activities. Where the aim is to increase muscle strength, set slow goals, building up tiny areas of muscle each time. Start with 'anti-gravity' movements, moving your limbs upwards without pain.'

Progressive resisted exercise

The progressive resisted specific exercise programme (PRSEP) consists of exercises prescribed to target specific muscles that are found to be weak, during a detailed physical assessment. These muscles are then strengthened individually; starting with low repetitions (around 5) but a constant and gradual increase to 30 repetitions - and progressed further with the use of specific weights. The PRSEP approach is designed to ensure that each muscle is strengthened so that the joints are protected and the hypermobile range used effectively in order to reduce pain and fatigue, and to ensure the body is fit enough that complex activities such as sport and physical activities can be completed safely (see **Box 7**). (Maillard S. 2012).

Exercise programmes may consist of a combination of both open chain and closed chain exercises (see **Box 8**) and should commence at a level where the patient can perform in a pain-free and stable manner. Initially, there is a need to establish internal core stability and teach appropriate recruitment of pelvic floor and transverse abdominus muscles (10/EDNF.org / Keer R. 2010).

> 'Stability always precedes mobility in coordinated action... it is extremely important to ensure stability before directing a person outwards into mobility' (Barber J. 2012).

Then, as stability improves, exercises progress from static to weight bearing, gently building muscle tone, helping patients control joints into their hypermobile range, correcting posture and improving stability, with functional activities being encouraged as the patient progresses (Russek L.N. 2000, Simpson M.R. 2006, Olson T. 2005, Simmonds J.V. & Keer R. Masterclass).

Other forms of physiotherapy

Hydrotherapy

Hydrotherapy is a form of treatment frequently used in rehabilitation of those with hEDS/HSD, along with other musculoskeletal disorders. It involves

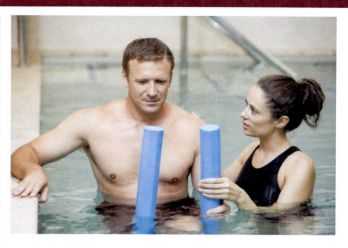

physiotherapy exercises that you carry out in a pool, which usually has a water temperature of between 33–36°C (warmer than a typical swimming pool). Hydrotherapy is normally carried out within a hospital's physiotherapy department. Exercising in the water challenges balance and core strength, whilst simultaneously supporting a persons weight. Weak muscles can be strengthened by carrying out exercises against the resistance of water, and overly tight muscles can relax in the warmth of the water, easing joint pain and allowing normal range of motion to be restored.

Pelvic physiotherapy

Training and strengthening the pelvic floor muscles (the muscles that support the bladder and urethra) is recommended as first-line management for women with stress, urge or a mixture of stress and urge urinary incontinence (Chartered Society for Physiotherapy). Physiotherapists can also provide therapies which may improve dyspareunia, abdominal pain, back pain, and sometimes radicular lower-extremity pain. (Levy H.P. 2004). More on pelvic floor weakness can be found on page 106.

Setting Goals

Discussing and setting goals is vital, in order that both patient and therapist know what they want to achieve from treatment, and what is reasonable to expect for the future. Goals might be quite small, such as being able to increase stability in a particular joint, or something much bigger like going back to work. In some cases, goals are aimed at maintaining function and independence rather than gaining anything more. Goals should not be thought of as being 'set in stone'; they should be progressive and achievable, and adjusted as time goes on. Any potential barriers need to be identified and individuals helped to overcome them. (Simmonds. J. Masterclass).

The life-long commitment

According to the British Society for Paediatric and Adolescent Rheumatology, patients need to understand that a life-long commitment to exercise is needed for all those with hEDS/HSD. For some patients, physiotherapy shows its benefits very quickly. For others, however, progress can seem slow and may be peppered with setbacks. In his guide to physiotherapy management of the hypermobile patient, Terry Olson stresses the importance of persisting, writing: '*Just as it often takes years for joint laxity to cause significant pain and instability, it can take at least months, or even years, to gradually reverse the process via muscle toning exercise* (10/ EDNF.org).

Progressing to general exercise

When sufficient progress has been made, patients should be encouraged to try more general exercise alongside targeted physiotherapy exercises, and to consider this to be an essential part of long-term treatment. Research carried out by Celletti et al (2013a) concluded that, in order to keep range of motion and muscle tone (and to reduce pain, fatigue, and fear of movement) regular day-to-day physical exercise combined with cognitive therapies (see page 156) appear to be beneficial. Focusing on activities which promote control of movement, coordination, graduated strengthening of muscles, stability of joints and careful cardiovascular fitness is often helpful (Simmonds J. V., 2/HMSA 2015). Suitable activities might include swimming, walking and Pilates, rather than contact sports where sharp cutting, acceleration, deceleration and change of directions increases the risk of injury. Rest breaks should be factored in and, where necessary, appropriate joint protection, such as splints and strappings considered (see page 146). The key is to build up stamina and strength gradually, allowing time to rest and recover. Activities such as these are important because they can be incorporated into daily life and, most importantly, enjoyed.

Using compensatory exercises

Repetitive movements involved in exercise can sometimes lead to *over strengthening* of particular muscles. For example, in cycling the action involved in pedaling can cause the muscles down the outside of the thigh and knee to become much stronger and tighter than the less-used medial muscles found on the inside of the knee/thigh. This can cause the patella to be pulled subtly off-kilter (towards the outside of the knee), increasing the likelihood of pain,

subluxations and dislocations. Regular progress checks should pick up such senario's and, where necessary, physiotherapists can prescribe compensatory exercises. In the case of cycling exercises may be provided to strengthen the inner medial areas, thus balancing out the stabilising forces of the knee.

Other considerations when planning physio-therapy:

Range of motion

'*Many patients who are hypermobile do not exercise their full range of motion - they do not have the control to do so.*' (Olson T. 2005) '*Improving joint proprioception, and building sufficient muscle strength around a joint to allow patients to control the full range of motion that is normal for them, is the goal.*' (Simmonds R & Keer R. - Masterclass)

The idea of teaching patients to exercise into their full range, in a controlled way, is a relatively new one and differs from the traditional approach, which taught that hypermobile patients should avoid using their 'additional range' of movement and should, instead, try to keep their joints within what would be considered 'normal' range in the general population. For example, when teaching leg exercises, a physiotherapist would often place their hand behind a patient's knee, acting as a stopping point to mark the maximum range they should extend into. Patients were often told that they should learn not to extend into their hypermobile range when carrying out exercises because they would risk injury to the joint.

In day-to-day activities, it is indeed prudent not to over-extend weak/loose joints, but in order to strengthen and protect those joints from future injury, physiotherapists at Great Ormond Street Hospital's Rheumatology Unit (GOSH), which specialises in joint hypermobility and fatigue in children, have adopted a new approach. In severe cases, GOSH will admit a child for a two-week 'in-patient' intensive physiotherapy rehabilitation programme. During the programme, they are encouraged to exercise fully into their maximum range *in a controlled manner*, gradually building up use of resistance weights. The child may be discharged at the end of the fortnight, having achieved the ability to carry out the prescribed exercises using a weight of 3lb and will then be set the goal to reach 8lb by continuing the exercises at home over the following 6 months. The belief is that for a hypermobile person, the extra range given to them is 'their normal'. If this extra range is not strengthened, it will remain unprotected and then, when they accidentally slip back into this extra range whilst carrying out day to day activities, the extra range, which has been left weak and unprotected, will inevitably suffer injury.

This approach appears to be backed up by the 2014 study into joint proprioception in hypermobile children by Pacey V. et al, which states: *'Even if advised to avoid the hypermobile range, it is likely a child with JHS [HSD] will inadvertently use their knee joint hyperextension when walking. If the treating clinician incorporates proprioceptive training within a treatment programme for a child with JHS [HSD], this training should not be limited only to neutral knee extension. ...By performing these exercises through full hypermobile range, physiotherapists do not need to provide children with close supervision to prevent movement into hyperextension, or provide physical stops to knee hyperextension, such as bracing or taping, when undertaking proprioceptive exercises.'*

Intensive physiotherapy programmes, such as the one held at GOSH, may be particularly effective where hypermobile children are primarily suffering from deconditioning related fatigue, and need an intensive programme to strengthen all the muscles in their body. A conservative approach to treatment, through physiotherapy and pain management, is promoted within such programmes, and surgical intervention is usually discouraged due to the potential for poor outcomes. This form of programme may not be suited to those who are affected by more complex symptoms, such as repeated dislocations, and such patients may wish to consider undergoing appropriate investigations (e.g. x-rays and or MRI's) prior to commencing similar programmes, in order to establish, from the outset, whether the underlying cause is purely inadequate muscle strength, or whether their weakness and laxity is complicated by issues such as ruptured ligaments, or skeletal abnormalities (such as severe trochlear dysplasia and patella alta). In the later case, bony surgical interventions, such as trochleoplasty, may still need to be considered. (NB/ Programmes like the ones held at GOSH are generally only available via consultant's referral).

Targeting Proprioception
As we saw in Chapter 2 (page 57), patients with hEDS/HSD may have altered proprioception; the body's ability to transmit a sense of position, analyse that information and react. This makes it harder for them to carry out exercises correctly on their own. According to Melson P. (2010), unless provided with appropriate instruction, patients often fail to use the most effective combination of muscles and joint positions to accomplish a task. Physiotherapists need to watch closely as exercises are performed, in order to correct poor positioning that can result in exercises being ineffective or damaging. Patients need to be encouraged to be aware of their bodies and to increase their core strength, endurance and muscle tone, particularly in relation to postural muscles. Altered proprioception in these patients means that considerable proprioceptive input is likely to be required from physiotherapists, in order to help patients understand how to effectively increase strength, particularly in the mid-range of the joint (Hickmott R. 1987).

In their guide for professionals managing young people with hEDS/HSD, the BSPR state that exercises to enhance proprioception can include the use of mirrors, bio feedback and balance boards as well as strengthening exercises.

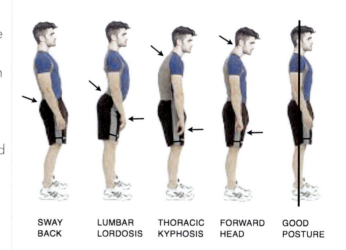

SWAY BACK | LUMBAR LORDOSIS | THORACIC KYPHOSIS | FORWARD HEAD | GOOD POSTURE

Considering postural alignment
Good posture involves training the body to stand, walk, sit and lie in positions where the least strain is placed on supporting muscles and ligaments. It can be overlooked in the battle to manage other symptoms, but left untreated, the long term effect of poor postures can cause significant muscle pain and contribute to injury. Postural alignment should always be taken into consideration when assessing patients with hEDS/HSD and planning physiotherapy interventions (Booshanam D.S. et al 2011 / Em S. et al 2014). Patients may need more help than most in learning correct posture, as many also struggle with poor proprioception (see previous paragraph and page 57).

For many hypermobile people, proper assessment and targeted exercise, prescribed by a podiatrist, gait analyst and/or physiotherapist may also be of great benefit.

Practicing good postural alignment:

- helps to protects supporting structures against injury,
- reduces the abnormal stresses on joint surfaces.
- helps to keep bones and joints in the correct alignment so that muscles are being used properly,
- reduces fatigue because muscles are being used more efficiently, allowing the body to use less energy,
- provides optimum positions for thoracic and abdominal organs,
- decreases the stress on the ligaments holding the joints of the spine together,
- prevents the spine from becoming fixed in abnormal positions,
- reduces backache and muscular pain,
- contributes to a good appearance.

(Cleveland Clinic / Mayfield Clinic)

Poor posture is not something that can be fixed overnight; after all, it will have taken many years to develop, but through a combination of specifically targeted exercises, determined conscious effort and sustained practice, great improvement can be made.

Hypermobile individuals should also try to avoid holding postures that force their joints to remain at the extreme range of movement (Simmonds J.V. & Keer R. 2007). Examples of this include:

- sustained standing with the knees pushed back i.e. hyperextended,
- holding weight on one hip when standing,
- sitting in a slumped position,

(www.hypermobility.org)

Patients will need to learn to recognise and constantly correct posture throughout the day and to carry out prescribed exercises to strengthen targeted areas of weakness.

Core Strengthening

Core and specific muscular strength is vital for patients with hEDS/HSD in order to reduce joint instability, minimise pain and facilitate good posture. Exercises are aimed at improving stability, balance

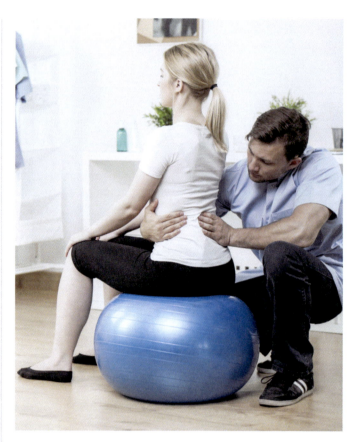

and coordination (BSPR 2013). Core strengthening exercises should start in basic, gravity eliminating positions and progress to sitting, standing and finally, dynamic activities (Melson P & Riddle O. 2010) using equipment such as balance boards, wobble cushions and gymnastic balls as well as specific exercises (BSPR 2013).

Stretching

'Many hypermobile people like to stretch, but have been advised not to by health professionals for fear of damaging their tissues or joints through over-stretching.' (Keer R. & Butler K. 2010)

In fact, hypermobile people need to stretch; everybody does. In a hypermobile body, tight, contracted muscles often become so because they are compensating for weaker muscles or have been injured in the past. Many have some muscles in a state of *chronic* contraction and, despite their obvious flexibility, describe feeling as stiff as a 90 year old (Glenny J. 2013 / Keer R. & Butler R. 2010). Stiffness around the joint, especially after waking, may arise as the result of fluid gathering in the joint to try to heal the damage caused by overuse the previous day. This feeling may take several hours to dissipate, or sometimes it may last all day (Rotstein R. 2011). According to Keer et al, it is not yet clear what produces this feeling of stiffness in the muscles, but it is possible that hypermobile individuals are more likely to use their global muscles for stability (rather than their local / deep muscles) and are therefore subject to more increased muscle tension and spasm. Keer considers stretching exercises to be useful for reducing muscle tension, maintaining muscle length and joint range, and to stretch out old injuries or muscle spasms. However, she cautions against *over-stretching*, which is potentially easy to do. *Controlled*, safe stretching of the tight areas, combined with progressive strengthening of the over-extended ones is the aim.

In order to facilitate safe stretching, those who are hypermobile need to be taught to differentiate between the kind of stretching that is carried out in order to regain and maintain muscle length, relieve muscle tension and restore and maintain joint range, and the kind of stretching that may inadvertently increase an already hypermobile range (Keer R. et al 2010 / Russek L.N. 2000 / BSPR 2013).

A daily routine of somatic exercises (slow gentle movements that mobilise the deep, intrinsic muscles and ligaments) can be helpful, as can lengthening restricted tissues by applying direct, myofascial or deep tissue therapies (Levy H.P. 2004).

While the duration of benefit that hypermobile patients experience from therapies such as myofascial release may be fairly short lived and may need to be repeated frequently, the pain relief achieved can be crucial in facilitating a patient's ability to participate in the toning and strengthening exercise required for joint stabilisation (Levy H.P. 2004).

Stretching out and lengthening contracted muscles needs to be taken very slowly and combined with appropriate strengthening exercises, so that the hypermobile individual's body can adjust to the muscle rebalance and so that there is sufficient time to learn to use the correct muscles properly.

'I do this by having 30 mins Fascial Stretch Therapy followed by 30 mins Pilates - otherwise it is like loosening all the elastic bands holding you together and you get off the couch and resemble a pile of jelly on the floor!' (Jones B. - HMSA volunteer Coordinator)

Concerns regarding symptom aggravation

Exercising with postural orthostatic tachycardia
Increasing muscle strength is beneficial in fighting many of the symptoms associated with POTS; strengthening the calf muscles and tissues that surround the blood vessels helps to support them, reducing dilation / blood pooling in the legs and helping blood be pumped around the body more effectively (PoTS UK 2017).

As discussed in Chapter 2 (page 76, column 1), exhausting exercise should be avoided by those who have the common comorbidity postural orthostatic tachycardia, but it is important to avoid becoming deconditioned as this, in itself, can exacerbate symptoms.

Take regular, appropriate aerobic exercise. Initially, exercise should be restricted to non-upright exercises including the use of (where suitable) rowing machines, recumbent cycles, swimming, lower leg resistance training and (where carried out horizontally) Pilates, to minimise orthostatic stress on the heart. Upright exercises such as riding a stationary upright bike or walking on a treadmill can be gradually worked toward over a month or more. The challenge with exercise in POTs, is that it can be difficult to stick with it long enough to see benefits. In a study by Dr Fu and Dr B. Levine (2015) the researchers found it could take about 5 weeks of exercising 4 times per week before any symptomatic improvement was noted. In the short-term, many/most of these patients felt worse.

Kinesiophobia
Kinesiophobia is described as an excessive and irrational fear of movement and physical activity that is (wrongly) assumed to cause re-injury i.e. the belief of patients that painful activity can result in damage and can increase pain, suffering and/or functional loss (Bunzli S. 2015). It is regularly seen in patients following surgical procedures, and in many different pain conditions and musculoskeletal disorders including fibromyalgia, chronic fatigue syndrome, and arthritis (Vlaeyen J.W.S. et al 2000, Nijs J. et al 2004, Mielenz T. J. et al 2010).

Individuals who experience feelings of vulnerability to painful injury or re-injury often develop maladaptive pain avoidance strategies. In the case of kinesiophobia, this fear can lead individuals to stop or reduce a wide range of activities in the belief that they could generate pain or injury. However, this progressive limitation of mobility (also see 'Are hEDS/ HSD progressive, page 36) can be counterproductive, itself playing an important role in the transition from acute to chronic musculoskeletal pain and disability (Houben R.M.A. et al 2005).

Kinesiophobia and hEDS/HSD:
Of course, those with hEDS/HSD are as susceptible as the next chronic pain patient to developing pain

avoidance strategies such as kinesiophobia (Castori M. 2012 Celleti C. 2013b), and repeated musculoskeletal trauma exacerbated by joint hypermobility may lead to individuals with hEDS/HSD using prolonged periods of rest as a way to avoid potential pain and damage (Celletti C. 2013b). Such avoidance can play a significant role in declining conditioning and exacerbating some forms of fatigue associated with hEDS/HSD (Castori M., 2011c, Vlaeyen J.W.S. et al 2000, Voermans N.C. et al 2011). However, it could be argued that for this group of patients, describing their fear of movement as 'excessive' and 'irrational' is somewhat overly simplified and unfair. After all, it should be remembered that people with hEDS/HSD have often found, from a very early age, that movement/activity actually _can_ result in damage and function loss. They may, for example, have regularly experienced dislocations, subluxations and falls just by walking on a level surface (that others would take for granted) or suffered soft tissue injury just by turning over in bed; it is perhaps not necessarily 'catastrophic thinking' or an irrational fear therefore, for them to believe this will happen again - it is their reality.

In this group, being told by a physiotherapist or other clinician "_You are kinesiophobic_" during what is often a very short physical assessment, without an explanation that puts it into perspective for their condition, can lead to their feeling misunderstood, disbelieved and reluctant to participate further.

EDS/HSD patient forums frequently describe those who have previously had their symptoms made worse by inappropriate physiotherapy interventions or who have experienced doctors who do not believe or understand the symptoms they relate. It is not uncommon, for example, to hear of clinicians who move a patient's patella without permission and are then surprised at the patients 'extreme' reaction. What examiners may be seeing when trying to carry out tests, such as the patella apprehension test, may not always be kinesiophobia in the true sense, the fear may actually be justified and rational. It may also be enhanced by the patient's fear (understandable once you know their history) at being examined by, or asked to perform an exercise by, a clinician in whom they do not yet have trust; one who has not demonstrated that he/she understands connective tissue disorders and the impact they have on a patients daily life.

Establishing Trust:
Trust is everything for hEDS/HSD patients. By really listening, and recognising that what may be 'irrational beliefs' in some patients, are quite possibly legitimate concerns for these individuals, a productive relationship can be forged. The clinician needs to demonstrate that they truly understand the potential implications on the patients health or plans, should the requested movements/exercises cause increased pain, or dislocation, and be able to explain to the patient why it is still in their best interests to carry them out anyway.

Clinicians also need to be prepared to reassure patients that, should the need arise, they will be in a position to take a holistic approach to treating any resulting symptoms; committing to continue working with them despite any setbacks.

Patients, in turn, need to understand and accept that, despite the risks of injury and pain, maintaining movement and exercise (in forms that are adapted to their needs) is crucial in order to prevent further loss of muscle tone, flexibility, and aerobic capacity. Such degenerations can happen more rapidly in those with hEDS/HSD, due to underlying hypotonia and laxity, and may lead to psychological and physical disability (Celletti C. 2013b). Studies also show kinesiophobia can lead to anxiety, depression, and somatosensory amplification (a tendency to perceive normal sensations, such as touch, pressure, pain, temperature, position, movement, and vibration, which arise from the muscles, joints, skin, and fascia as being intense, disturbing and harmful) (Baeza-Velasco C. 2011, Celletti C. 2013b).

Acceptance of the fact that there may well be some pain and some risk with movement/exercise in hEDS/HSD, but that it shouldn't be avoided just because it hurts, is very important (please note: extreme pain or worsening of symptoms should always be reported, investigated and, if necessary, the activity ceased).

Overcoming kinesiophobia:
It is necessary to make sure a patient's pain is adequately under control before commencing exercises. Taking any prescribed pain medications prior to attending and practicing relaxation techniques such as deep breathing exercises, and other passive interventions can decrease the intensity of any pain, while judicious use of braces and supports may help prevent dislocations.

MANAGEMENT

'Beginning with non-invasive treatment such as stretches and breathing exercises helps the patient regain confidence in being able to move again. The smallest bit of movement every day is a major crucial step in breaking the vicious cycle of kinesiophobia. By enabling the patient to move with caution, and by enabling the patient to self-mobilise their body's soft tissue, the physiotherapist, in turn, shows the patient that they have control over their fear.'
(Dommerhault J. 2016).

Helping patients understand the causes and effects of symptoms such as delayed onset muscle soreness (DOMS, see below), and helping them make wise choices such as opting out of high-impact pursuits in favour of lower-impact activities such as swimming, and learning to pace (see page 154) are also helpful.

Zina Trost et al (2007) found that patients experiencing high levels of kinesiophobia predicted pain levels much higher than the actual experience when embarking on a given exercise, and that, when the movement was performed for the second time their pain ratings reduced significantly. However, although their fear was less the second time doing the same activity, their fear went right back up when starting any new (even slightly different) activities. They were unable to apply what they learned about specific movements to general movement.

Overcoming this fear for patients with hEDS/HSD, bearing in mind their propensity for injury, is therefore likely to require time and patience from both parties, before they can progress to a slow, graded, and progressive rehabilitation programme.

Delayed onset muscle pain
When starting a new exercise programme, deconditioning often means that the point at which a person with hEDS/HSD reaches their limit of effort before succumbing to exhaustion, when performing exercise, is low, and may result in them experiencing pain and fatigue the following day (BSPR 2013).

This kind of pain and fatigue is usually triggered by 'delayed onset muscle pain' (DOMS) caused by specific muscle imbalances, and joint discomfort. Patients sometimes misinterpret this type of pain and fatigue as a sign that the prescribed exercises have worsened their symptoms, resulting in a reluctance to carry on. Any significant symptoms should always be discussed by the patient with their physician, but for most people, DOMS is actually a completely normal response to an increased level of exercise. As long as the exercise programme is taken slowly and has been appropriately tailored to the hypermobile patient, such symptoms are unlikely to be an indication of damage. (As mentioned earlier in this section, extreme pain or worsening of symptoms should always be reported, investigated and, if necessary, the activity ceased). Although soreness is unlikely to be avoided altogether, by allowing the muscles time to adapt to new stress, patients should find that the severity of their symptoms is minimised (Palmer S. 2017).

Please remember:
The content of this book cannot and should not replace advice from the patient's healthcare professional(s). Any person who experiences symptoms or feels that something may be wrong should seek individual, professional help for evaluation and/or treatment. This book is for information only and is not intended to provide individual medical advice.

Image atribution (page 135) : Flare- Freedigitalphotos.net

© Understanding hEDS and HSD by C. Smith

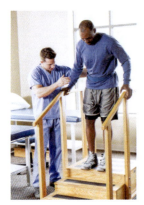

Occupational Therapy

What is occupational therapy?
'*Occupational therapists (OTs) are health and social care professionals who take a holistic, client-centred approach to physical and mental health and wellbeing*' (Southall J. 2016).

Many people with long term health conditions have difficulty in carrying out everyday activities. The primary goal of occupational therapy is to enable people of all ages to participate in the activities of everyday life which matter to them and are essential for health and wellbeing.

How can occupational therapy help?
Occupational therapy differs from other therapies in that it isn't necessarily about '*treating*' an individual's medical condition; it's about helping people to *live well* with that condition. An occupational therapist works with individuals to identify strengths and difficulties and then help find strategies to meet the individual's goals, allowing them to maintain, regain or improve independence. For example, they may suggest practical solutions such as learning new ways to do things or modifying the living, working or school environment in which the activity takes place. They can assess individuals for specialist equipment such as wheelchairs and seating, and recommend other aids such as splints or adaptive cutlery along with other equipment or assistive technology. OTs also provide advice on joint care, improving posture and pacing, and coping with pain and fatigue. They can teach alternative methods of doing things such as bathing and getting dressed, which put less strain on unstable joints.

How is Occupational Therapy delivered?
Occupational therapy usually forms part of Primary Health Care (see page 133) provision, accessed via referral from a patient's GP. It is also possible to 'self refer' privately by contacting a qualified member of a recognised body, such as the British Association of Occupational Therapists. Traditionally, OTs work in hospital wards or outpatient departments, or through social services, in the community and client's homes (Southall J. 2017). However, it is becoming increasingly common to find OTs working in other areas like businesses and schools, or in specialities such as hand therapy, paediatrics or pain management.

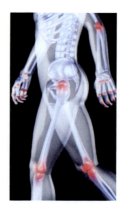

Joint Protection

Joint protection is a very important aspect of managing hypermobility. Repetitive movement, overtraining, carrying excessive weights, poor pacing, and focusing on joint flexibility rather than stability may all exacerbate joint pain and the risk of injury (Simpson M.R. 2006).

Protecting joints should not be confused with not using joints. In fact, joint protection and exercise go hand in hand. The aim is to use the body in ways that reduce pain and strain on joints, and to incorporate exercise to strengthen the muscles that protect them.

It is important to become more aware of how joints are used during day-to-day activities at home and at work. Hannah Ensor, Hypermobility Syndromes Association Patron and author of Stickman Communications, explains: '*Exercise equals controlled, good posture and movement. The important thing isn't how many repetitions of an exercise a person does, or how much weight they can lift, but how well they can keep their joints in good positions throughout the movement. Even doing housework can be exercise, but only if it is done with a focus on keeping good posture and using joints well. For example, when making a cup of tea, ensure that core muscles are engaged, and knees are soft (not forced backwards into hyperextension) then lift the kettle with shoulder, elbow and wrist all well positioned - this not only reduces subluxations and dislocations, but also allows joints to be strengthened slowly and steadily. Activity carried out in the floppy desperation of 'I must get this finished before I collapse' kind of way, which is so familiar to many of us, doesn't count!*'

Tips to help reduce strain on joints
- Spread the load over several joints; for example, by using two hands instead of one.
- Use labour-saving gadgets when possible.

continued...

...continued
- Don't grip things too tightly or for too long.
- Avoid actions that push your joints into awkward positions.
- Use your joints in more stable positions
- Carry a shoulder bag instead of a clutch or handbag.
- Hold heavier objects in your arms, close to your body. Don't let them dangle.
- Hold small items in your palms instead of your fingers.
- Use both hands, or your shoulder to open heavy doors.
- Keep to your ideal weight to reduce pressure on your joints; particularly your hips, knees and feet.
- Do exercises most days to improve your strength. Occupational therapists, physiotherapists and hand therapists can help you with exercises to improve your grip.
- Try to keep as fit as possible, and build up muscle stamina through regular exercise. You may, however, want to avoid contact sports.
- Unless advised otherwise by a healthcare professional, it's better to do a little at a time, with plenty of rest breaks, rather than give up something you enjoy.

Occupational therapists, physiotherapists and hand therapists can all advise on joint protection techniques, and individuals might find it helpful to discuss their own ideas about reducing the strain on their joints with them.

By learning to incorporate joint-protecting strategies regularly, rather than just when joints are hurting, people report less pain and stiffness in the morning, and fewer flare-ups.

Note: For many individuals with hEDS/HSD protection is also sometimes required in the form of splints, braces, taping or orthotics, in order to allow participation in sports, or to facilitate recovery after surgery or injury (for more on this subject, please see next section).

Image attribution:
1st image, page 145: Istock purchased
2nd image, page 145 by: Esther Max under Creative Commons Licence
Image 3, page 146 by: Pixabay free images

MANAGEMENT

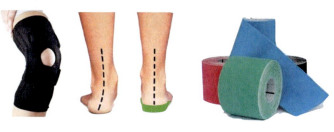

Splinting, bracing, taping, compression wear and orthotics

The benefits of using splints and braces often causes impassioned debate. In fact, many health care professionals advise not to splint or brace, as it can cause decline in the long run.

The range of symptom combination and severity within the hEDS/HSD spectrum is so wide, however, that in reality, it is unrealistic to be dictatorially prescriptive over the use of bracing. For an individual whose joints are so loose that they cannot get out of bed without dislocating, or who subluxates three joints in the space of any hour just sitting at their keyboard, the advice not to brace can seem intolerant and impractical.

One Facebook user writes:

> *'For me, bracing is sometimes essential just in order to get out of bed. Surgery is not always the best option in terms of outcome and anaesthetic risk. I for one would rather be upright and mobile, but looking like a 'mummy' under my clothes, than confined to bed.'*

In most cases, however, it is not necessary to wear a brace all the time, and it may well be detrimental to do so. Splints and braces should be used judiciously to avoid over-dependence and deterioration of muscle strength (Simmonds J.V. 2013 & 2016). The danger is that the wearer becomes reliant on the support, wearing them all of the time instead of only at the most vulnerable times, and muscle strength declines as a result. Braces and splints should therefore be worn for the shortest time possible and used primarily to facilitate participation in things that an individual wouldn't otherwise be able to do (Morrison J.). For example, many hypermobile individuals wear ring splints or wrist braces when carrying out tasks such as preparing vegetables or typing; others wear protective braces to enable them to take part in sport, or to provide temporary support during the process

© Understanding hEDS and HSD by C. Smith

of healing, should injury occur. If braces are used, the muscles need to be kept strong, so extra compensatory exercises may need to be performed. With appropriate physiotherapy and exercise, increased muscle strengthening should reduce the need for braces.

Taping

In recent years, taping, particularly with products such as Kinesiology tape, has become more commonplace. Such taping is frequently used by physiotherapists to promote awareness of posture and to aid in joint proprioception, as well as being used to support muscles, ligaments and joints, and reduce pain. An individual's skin sensitivity or allergies should always be considered when taping. As with splinting and bracing, it is important that, where possible, reliance and dependency is avoided. (Keer & Simmonds, 2011 / Macgregor K. et al 2005, Aminaka N. & Gribble P.A. 2008 / Callaghan M.J. et al 2002, 2008 / 11)EDNF.org).

Proprioceptive garments / compression wear

Many individuals find proprioceptive garments and compression wear an effective tool in increasing awareness of joint positioning, and for maintaining increased blood return to the heart in postural orthostatic tachycardia syndrome.

Proprioceptive garments aim to increase sensory and proprioceptive feedback, as well as provide musculoskeletal support. They provide constant, consistent compression, stretch, support and sensory (proprioceptive) information for the time that the garment is worn. The garments can be specially made lycra medical garments, prescribed by an occupational therapist or, if that option is not available, sports compression garments or compression support tights can also be very effective. At the time of writing, trials are being held at one of the UK's leading hospitals where patients (with conditions complicated by poor proprioception including hypermobile Ehlers-Danlos syndrome and Cerebral Palsy) are trying out tailor-made proprioception garments.

As with splinting, bracing and taping, the use of proprioception garments can be a double edged sword and the same care should be taken to ensure that muscles do not become deconditioned.

Orthotics, and management of the foot/ankle

In the section on disorders of the foot and ankle, we discussed flat feet (pes plenus) and pronation (page 114). In those with flat feet, the arch of the foot appears flattened and there may also be hallux valgus deformity. Flat feet are also commonly associated with a leaning inward of the ankle bones, known as pronation (see page 114). Such disorders can alter a person's gait (see pages 130 & 132), which can go on to adversely affect other areas of the body.

'Evidence-based guidelines suggest that children with flexible flat feet presenting with pain or impaired function, particularly in the presence of GJH, such as that commonly seen in children with JHS/hEDS, should use orthotics and/or sensible footwear [Evans A.M. & Rome K. 2011]. Preliminary findings of a small randomised control trial suggests that use of orthotics may improve the efficiency of gait of children with generalised joint hypermobility and developmental coordination disorder [Morrison S.C. et al., 2013].' (Englebert R.H. et al 2017)

Treatments are aimed at improving muscle strength, reducing muscle tightness and improving proprioception. The appropriate choice of footwear can provide control for overly flexible feet and can improve ankle stability, so shoes such as trainers or Dr Martin boots may be recommended. Products such as shock absorbing insoles can reduce the impacts on joints and soft tissues.

When exercises and footwear changes are not sufficient to improve stabilisation, or where a person's gait is being significantly affected, orthotics are sometimes recommended (Napolitano C. et al 2000), Although unlikely to prevent the ankle from turning, orthotics may limit the extra stress that can be placed on the joints of the foot, knee, hip and lower back as they try to compensate. These orthoses, which fit inside the shoe, are shaped to improve joint positioning and stability (3/Arthritis Research UK). It should be remembered that orthotics support, rather than correct, dysfunction. They may improve joint mechanics as well as improved nervous system function, but the underlying problems with movement and function still need to be addressed.

Mobility Aids

The provision of walking and mobility aids such as crutches and wheelchairs requires careful consideration and discussion between the hypermobile individual and medical team. The aim of these devices is to facilitate independence, participation, and quality of life. Each case needs to be individually assessed, and carers and hypermobile individuals require education to ensure appropriate use.

© Understanding hEDS and HSD by C. Smith

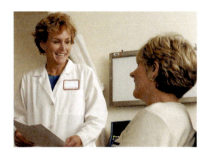

Relief of severe pain, and using pain killers effectively

Please note: The information on these pages has been kindly provided by the Hypermobility Syndromes Association, based on recommendations written by Professor Howard Bird MA MD FRCP and edited by Dr Alan Hakim MA FRCP. Professor Bird is Emeritus Professor of Pharmacological Rheumatology, University of Leeds, and Dr Hakim is Consultant Acute Physician and Rheumatologist at the Hypermobility Unit, Hospital of St John and St Elizabeth, London. The original source can be found in the HMSA's 2016 self-management publication, entitled 'Living well with heritable disorders of connective tissue' (version 3.4).

The precise cause of pain in hEDS/HSD is uncertain, but experience suggests that analgesics (pain killers) may help. GPs will be able to help patients decide which analgesics to try, based on symptoms and any contra indications which may be involved.

There are many options to choose from when trying to control pain such as different dosages, medication combinations, changing medications, or routes of administration. If one option is not working out, a patient should talk with their doctor and find out about the other choices available. It is important that those treating patients with hEDS/HSD understand the severity of the patient's pain and the impact it is having on their life. If the things tried are not working, or the help received seems inadequate, it is important that the patient talks this through with their GP and alternative measures are introduced where required.

'When dealing with the often complex array of symptoms seen in hypermobility syndromes it is most important to be aware of how different drug treatments may interact. For example, some pain medications can cause interactions with anxiety relieving medications. If you are seeing several different medical professionals, be sure to tell them what medications you are taking, and where necessary, ask them to consult with one another to ensure you're getting the most appropriate treatments.' (Living Well with an HDCT - HMSA, 2014)

MANAGEMENT

Obtaining the best from your pain medications

- Keep a diary of your pain – where it is, when it begins, when it peaks, when you take medications, and what helps relieve the pain.
- Inform your doctor or nurse that you are experiencing pain. Don't wait to be asked! Pain should be evaluated at every visit.
- Pain can be very hard to describe; don't be afraid to use words like sharp, radiating, aching, pounding, prickly, tight, deep, stabbing, dull, pinching, and tingly.
- Report the severity of your pain. On a scale from 0 to 10, where 0 is no pain and 10 is the worst pain you can imagine, how would you rate it before treating it and then after treating it?
- Take your medication exactly as prescribed. You may be taking several medications. Be sure you understand when and how to take them, and report any side effects.
- Find out how you can get advice on pain control when you need it. Know how to reach your doctor or nurse and when you should contact them.
- Take medication before pain builds up. Pain control is harder to achieve if it is allowed to build to a severe level.
- Use the same pharmacy. They will know which pain medicines to keep on hand, and can answer questions about the medicines and side effects.
- Consult members of your health care team (nurse, social worker, and physiotherapist) for help with the above.

Pain Killers

Take strong enough analgesia to relieve pain and muscle spasm. Paracetamol is a good painkiller, and a sensible one to start with. If these are inadequate, the compound 'generic' analgesics, co-codamol and co-dydramol, should be tried (probably in that order). That still leaves meptazinol and tramadol in reserve. A very small dose of a muscle relaxant (such as diazepam), can be helpful in the early stages of an

Continued...

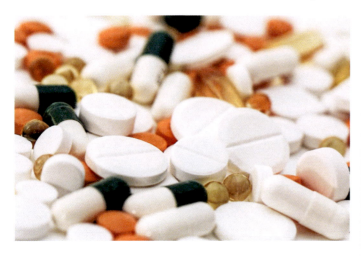

acute episode of pain with marked muscle spasm. Patients should discuss these with their GP. Each drug should be tried for an adequate period of time before being discarded as ineffective.

Non steroidal anti-inflammatories
Non-steroidal anti-inflammatory drugs (NSAID) can be helpful when there is an acute injury, such as a pulled ligament, subluxation or dislocation, and where the tissues have become inflamed and swollen. Ibuprofen tablets and gel can be bought over-the-counter (in the UK), and a number of other types of NSAID can be prescribed. Care needs to be taken in following the instructions, and in not taking an NSAID for too long as it may cause stomach pain and ulcers, high blood pressure, kidney problems, and trigger an attack in those who are asthmatic.

Antidepressants (inc. nocturnal antidepressants)
In parallel, antidepressants can be effective for their muscle relaxant property and can promote good sleep. A nocturnal antidepressant, used in doses lower than those used for the treatment of depression, seems to improve pain tolerance during the day. The more common antidepressants used as pain killers include Amitriptyline, Venlafaxine and Duloxetine.

Neuropathic analgesics
Medications such as gabapentin and pregabalin are prescribed to try and control either local nerve pain or widespread pain where the body is very sensitive, even to light touch.

Topical drugs
Oral medication can be supplemented by topical drugs, placed over the affected joints. These could be analgesics (e.g. Traxam gel), NSAIDs (although a proportion of these will still be absorbed and can cause side effects, even by the topical route) or counter irritants (e.g. Capsaicin). Lidocaine local anaesthetic plasters might also help.

Hydrocortisone Injections and Physiotherapy
For very severe, painful episodes, hydrocortisone injections and intensive physiotherapy may be necessary.

Non-pharmaceutical interventions
In addition to taking pain medications, there are many other things that can be tried in order to reduce pain levels including distraction, relaxation techniques, use of heat and cold, massage, and light exercise. More tips and techniques for the relief of persistent pain, muscle stiffness and fatigue can be found on Pages 151-155.

Please note:
With respect to any drug or pharmaceutical products identified, lay readers are advised to always seek advice from their general practitioner or healthcare provider. Practitioners are advised to check the most current information provided (i) on procedures featured or (ii) by the manufacturer of each product to be administered, to verify the recommended dose or formula, the methods and duration of administration, and contraindications.

Image attribution
Page 148 (consultation) - NCI under Creative Commons Licence
Page 149 (tablets) - Pexels.com

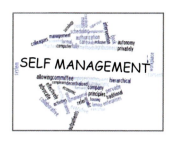

Self Management

What is self management?

The term 'self management' covers a wide range of things an individual can do to help themselves if they live with a long-term health condition. Self management does not mean having to do it alone. On the contrary, it is very important that a patient and health care professional work in *partnership* to manage a long-term condition. However, with estimates suggesting that most people with long-term conditions spend an average of only three hours per year with their healthcare team; it is important that education in self management is made available, so that patients gain a sense of control, have the confidence to manage their own set of symptoms, treatments, and day-to-day life in a way that is realistic for them. By taking responsibility, playing their part and following advice, those who self manage tend to do better in the longer term than those who rely solely on their health care providers (College of Medicine.org.uk).

Educational interventions

Self management education can come in many different forms. Doctors may provide self management literature, recommend online resources, or suggest local groups that patients may find helpful. In addition, self management courses, such as those run in the UK by the Hypermobility Syndromes Association and Ehlers-Danlos Support UK, and organisations such as Self Management UK, provide individuals with the opportunity to consider, adopt, and maintain the self-management skills and behaviours needed to improve their wellbeing. Such courses usually cover self management strategies such as practicing healthy lifestyle behaviors related to physical exercise, taking medications as prescribed, reducing stress and anxiety, relaxation, pacing, goal setting, problem solving and seeking medical care as appropriate (all of which are discussed over the following pages). Information may be provided on the nature of the disorder, as well as the positive and negative consequences of not adopting health recommendations, and they also teach useful skills to help individuals communicate better with family, friends, colleagues and health professionals.

MANAGEMENT

Self management encourages individuals to:

- Find out more about their condition
- Take charge of their health care and choose what is right for them
- Get support from other people in a similar situation
- Learn new skills and tools to help them manage their health
- Work better, and in partnership, with healthcare professionals
- Set goals and make action plans
- Solve problems
- Manage emotions
- Manage relationships with family, friends and colleagues
- Communicate better with health and social care professionals
- Learn to pace daily activities - manage fatigue, sleep, pain, anger and depression
- Understand the importance of exercise, keeping active and eating a healthy diet
- Get the best out of medications

(Ref: Self Management UK)

In this section, we look at some of the areas of everyday life in which self management can be useful when living with a long term health condition such as hEDS/HSD.

Challenges in a relationship

Although relationships may change because of hEDS/HSD, not all changes will be negative. Many couples find that they become closer by discussing things openly and that their relationship is stronger as a result. Sometimes, however, pain and fatigue can bring relationships under increased pressure.

Adjustments such as reconsidering roles within a relationship, changes to work and social lives, and to who does what around the home, can take some getting used to (2/HMSA 2015). Work-related changes may also lead to financial worries, increasing a couple's level of uncertainty and stress. Try to talk about the changing situation and any challenges that arise, so solutions can be arrived at which are right for both partners.

'It takes a non-affected partner time to adjust when their partner is newly diagnosed, or if existing symptoms significantly worsen.. The individual may be used to 'fixing things', but hEDS/HSD cannot be fixed. It can be difficult for partners to accept they cannot fix things and not feel like failures. It's also really tough to be the person who is hurting, and to realise that their condition is causing their partner to feel this way. It's tough all around. Give them time. Let them know that you don't expect them to fix it; you expect them to try to be with you on the journey.
(Anonymous advice - Inspire.com)

Donna Wicks, HMSA CEO, agrees and adds that long-term health conditions can also affect how partners see each other. *"Some partners describe feeling helpless and scared, uncertain as to the best ways to provide help and support. Others find themselves feeling resentful or frustrated if a joint social life has ceased or they find themselves having to help more around the house after long days at work."* She explains that it is crucial for partners to make time to talk to one another about how symptoms affect their relationship, and to be as open and honest as possible with each other. *"Try not to assume you know what's going on in your partner's head before you start a conversation, give each other a chance to explain how you feel"* (2/HMSA - 2014).

Physical Intimacy

Physical intimacy is another area where talking in a comfortable, relaxed environment is important. Some couples find it difficult at first to talk openly but, once open communication has started, it can be a great relief for both partners.

The worry, pain, discomfort and even medications that can be associated with long term conditions such as hEDS/HSD can dampen the desire for intimacy. Although sex itself won't make hEDS/HSD worse, fatigue and painful joints may cause discomfort or reduced enjoyment of sex. In his 2010 publication, 'Joint Hypermobility Handbook', Dr Brad Tinkle recommends taking pain medications before intercourse, and arranging the room with pillows or other comforts to support the body and joints. If vaginal dryness is a problem (also see page 109), he suggests the use of lubricant.

Where symptoms involve dislocations or subluxations, it is quite common for one partner to fear accidentally hurting the other during intercourse, or for the affected partner to fear being hurt. In this situation it is important that partners talk openly about their fears, in order to arrive at a solution that's right for both of them. Discuss limitations and try to agree on positions that are least likely to cause problems.

For some couples counselling may be beneficial, helping them relearn how to relate to each other post diagnosis (2/HMSA 2015).

Stress and anxiety

Although it is not healthy to avoid all stressful situations, particularly if they relate to things that really need to be addressed, it is a good idea to learn some techniques that can help reduce the levels of stress in everyday life. Some suggestions for this might include:

- Learning to be okay with '*good enough.*' Many people set themselves up for failure by demanding perfection. Instead, it may be better to adjust standards instead.
- Considering taking a course to learn the art of mindfulness or meditation.
- Learning to say "*no.*" When an individual feels they are continuously taking on more than they can handle it is a recipe for stress. Many people find it very difficult but it is important to learn how to say "no", whether it relates to personal or professional relationships. It can be helpful to try and distinguish between things that really '*must*' be done and things that, in an ideal world, '*should*' be done; working out limits and then sticking to them.
- Limiting the amount of time spent with people who consistently cause stress in life, or, if necessary, end relationships entirely.
- Questioning how important the stressful situation will be in the long run. Will it matter in a few months time? By looking at the bigger picture it may be possible to see that it is not worth getting stressed over.

When stress is unavoidable, remember to be kind to yourself, and allow yourself time to recover.

If symptoms of stress and anxiety persist, or if depression is suspected, it is important to seek advice from the GP as soon as possible.

Persistent pain

Pain is a complicated, hard-to-treat problem which doctors and other clinicians need to take seriously. Relief of severe pain, and using analgesics (pain killers) and other medications effectively is discussed on page 148. However, the answer may not

© Understanding hEDS and HSD by C. Smith

necessarily always be stronger and stronger analgesics. There are a variety of medicinal and non-medicinal strategies, along with lifestyle modifications, which can be considered when trying to reduce pain. In fact, it is usually *necessary* to use a combination of treatments (the so called 'tool box approach') in order to keep pain under control.

Kenneth Goldschneider MD, FAAP, Director of Pain Management at Cincinnati Children's Hospital writes: '*Medications can help, but cannot change the joints, only lessen the symptoms. [In the case of acute pain, for example] a fast acting, short-lasting pain medication can be helpful during a painful dislocation. A muscle relaxant to help reduce muscle spasm after a dislocation can help get the joint back into position. Some anti-seizure and antidepressants can help with widespread pain, or nerve-related pain.*' [But, ultimately a 'tool box approach is needed], and *no medication can take the place of proper physiotherapy, occupational therapy, and psychological therapies.*'

The 'tool box' approach

The importance of using multiple strategies to manage pain, even if each one only makes a tiny difference, should not be underestimated. It may not be possible to eliminate pain altogether but, when added together, the difference made can be significant. It may be helpful to consider each strategy as a tool in a 'pain tool kit'. Below, Dr Clair Francomano (2011) gives an example:

> '*Say, for instance, that your medications take care of 20% of your pain relief. Then you use your TENS unit for another 10% reduction. Some Tiger Balm on your painful joints brings another 5% of pain relief. Maybe you could pull out your heat pad too for another 5% of pain relief. Then you decide upon a warm soak with Epsom Salts for another 10% pain relief. Deep breathing and some physiotherapy exercises combine for another 10% of relief. And then, you watch a great movie to distract you for another 15% of pain relief. So now you have 75% of your pain managed effectively.*'

'Tool boxes' can be adapted to suit all ages, for example, children and adolescents may want to crate their own collection of activities and interventions that can be used to reduce the pain. These can be items that facilitate distraction (e.g. DVDs, toys, music or spoken word stories) as well as positive coping statements, relaxation scripts, helpful exercises, things that bring back memories of wonderful days out, and comforting objects such as favourite photos, postcards, treasures and keepsakes or pictures they have drawn.

Physical activity in everyday life

In addition to helping increase and maintain strength and stability, carrying out targeted physiotherapy exercises on a regular basis and integrating general exercise into every day life plays a crucial role in the self management of pain in hEDS/HSD. The HMSA publication, 'Living well with a heritable disorder of connective tissue' explains: '*It is very important to keep moving. When we are in pain, our bodies react by tightening the muscles – which can make pain in hypermobile joints worse. So, although lying on the sofa all day can feel nice at the time, it can make pain worse in the long term. Change your way of life – the way you move; when you exercise; continually correct your posture; keep your joints moving without over-stretching; take rest breaks. If you are having a bad pain day, use gentle slow rhythmic self-mobilisation and local stretching techniques, incorporating any exercises you have been given by your physiotherapist.*

As soon as it is possible, it is also a good idea to gradually introduce regular low impact exercise. This should be based on advice given by the individual's physiotherapist or other health care professional, and adequate joint protection should also be taken into consideration. Kenneth Goldschneider writes: '*We have found several effective treatments for pain relief, but physical therapy (PT) is the most important intervention. The right kind of PT emphasises "proprioception," which is the sense of where one's joints are in space. Patients with EDS lose some of the sense of where their joints should be, which causes misalignment. And this is a large factor in their pain.*'

Keeping weight under control can help to reduce stress and load on joints. Activities should be chosen that fit in with lifestyle, abilities and taste. If the exercise chosen is too difficult to stick to, too expensive to maintain, or makes an individual feel awkward, it is unlikely to be continued in the long run.

Thought should also be given to modifying any daily activities or repetitive movements that induce symptoms and, if required, these should be avoided or modified. Excessive loading of weight bearing joints should also be avoided and, where necessary, adaptive equipment utilised to accomplish daily activities without triggering, or worsening, symptoms (Pocinki A. 2010 2/HMSA 2015, 2/Physiopedia).

Ergonomics and posture at work and at home

Try to be aware of, and correct, posture and body positioning throughout the day and night, to avoid exacerbation of pain. This involves thinking about the way we hold ourselves and the positioning of our joints, as well as maintaining good ergonomic hygiene. Examples of ergonomic hygiene include choosing chairs and equipment that specifically suit body dimensions and the tasks that must be performed; choosing pillows and mattress firmness to provide appropriate support to the neck and knees and maintain spinal alignment etc. Where necessary, an occupational therapist (see page 145) can visit to make an assessment and to help solve difficulties by providing aids and adaptations, or to demonstrate how something can be done in a different way.

Keep a symptom diary

Keeping a diary can help a patient and their health care provider to build up a picture of how symptoms such as pain, fatigue or dislocations are affecting the patient's life. By listing the symptoms experienced and when they occur, and making a note of things that seem to trigger or increase these symptoms, this information can also help establish if there are any patterns relating to the symptoms. Noticing, for example, that dislocations increase around the time of mensuration could help the patient and doctor implement a plan to protect the patients joints around this time. Braces could, for example, be prescribed for use in the days immediately prior to, during and following menstruation. Realising that fatigue is regularly experienced on the day following a particularly busy event could lead a patient to re-assess pacing their activity.

The downside of keeping a diary is that constantly having to assess pain levels and what hurts, can cause a patient to focus on their pain, reinforcing the pain-cycle that pain-management teams try so hard to help patients break. Because of this, pain management clinics often advise that diaries are only kept in the initial stages of treatment.

Using your mind

The mind is a powerful tool in the battle against pain. Chronic pain is strongly influenced by the ways in which the brain processes the pain signals. In fact, chronic pain can provoke strong emotional reactions, such as sadness, fear and anxiety depending on what an individual believes about his or her pain signals. With practice, the brain can, to a certain extent, learn how to decrease the sensation of pain using a combination of deep focus, breathing, and imagery techniques.

Katherine Puckett, the National Director of Mind-body Medicine, says: *'Guided imagery is a way of using the mind to imagine or visualise oneself in a different situation. Use your mind to create a special place where you would feel your best, both physically and emotionally, and spend time in this place. When we use our physical senses to imagine what we would see, hear, feel, smell and taste in a situation, we can feel as if we've really experienced it,"* she explains. *'We can also use the mind to instruct the body to feel reduced pain and to feel calm, peaceful and relaxed.'* (Puckett K. / Myers W. 2012).

(5/Spine-Health.com).

Pain and sleep

Please see Chapter 2 - 'Sleep problems' (page 56), 'nocturnal antidepressants' (page 149).

Managing pain flare-ups

With appropriate treatment and management, pain can usually be kept under control, but there may be times when the levels experienced suddenly worsen and additional interventions will be needed. This is known as a 'flare-up' (2/HMSA 2014).

Although these flare-ups don't usually last very long, they can come on very quickly with little warning. Donna Wicks, HMSA CEO explains : *'Flare-ups can be a common experience for those suffering from a chronic pain condition and, whether they are short-lived or so severe you can hardly get out of bed, a flare can be painful, bewildering and frustrating. It can be helpful to devise a Flare Up Plan, that is personal to you. It should cover what you need to do to reduce the length of any flare up by incorporating techniques you know work for you. Check that your pain levels are under control, your sleeping pattern is healthy, any autonomic issues are dealt with and that the impact of anxiety and depression are also considered. Where possible, clearing your diary for a week at least, in the beginning, can help as it allows you to adopt these strategies without interruption.'* Coping with flare-ups is a skill which will improve with time and experience. Of course, if symptoms persist, it is important to see a GP for blood tests to rule out any sudden physical changes.

Managing pain flares can involve a number of different strategies, such as taking any prescribed pain medication, practicing relaxation and distraction techniques, keeping well hydrated, trying complimentary therapies such as gentle massage and using aids such as a TENS machine, or splints and

© Understanding hEDS and HSD by C. Smith

supports. The key is to use a multi-targeted approach, be open to ideas and not to give up.

Persistent (chronic) fatigue

Although not yet fully understood, the most likely contributor to symptoms of persistent (chronic) fatigue associated with hEDS/HSD, is dysautonomia of the cardiovascular system, often combined with one or more of the following factors:

- Muscle weakness
- Unrefreshing sleep / sleep disturbance,
- Malabsorption in the intestines related to gastrointestinal dysfunction
- Respiratory dysfunction including nocturnal cough or wheeze, and dyspnea
- Reactive depression and/or anxiety.
- In some instances, analgesic overuse.
  (Above: Castori M. 2012 & 2012a / Mathias C. J. 2011 / Harris J.G. 2013)

Many of the factors listed above have been discussed in more detail within the symptoms section of this book, and should be properly investigated in any hEDS/HSD patient displaying a disabling fatigue (Castori M. 2012).

Self management lifestyle steps that may help to minimise the effects of persistent fatigue are discussed below:

Pacing

Learning to pace the amount of activity carried out is a fundamental aspect of fatigue management. By the time they are diagnosed, some individuals may have already learnt to limit how much they do each day in order to make sure they have sufficient energy reserves to get through the following day. Others make the mistake of doing as much as they can when they are 'feeling up to it' and then paying for it by 'crashing' later or the following day. *'Wherever possible, try to spread out physically demanding tasks over a more manageable period, establishing what you can realistically achieve without exhausting yourself '* (2/HMSA 2014). When planning activities, factor in sufficient time to rest before further activities are undertaken.

The key to self management of fatigue through pacing is to establish a baseline level of activity that can be repeated each day with no exacerbation of symptoms. It is important to understand that this does not necessarily equate to a symptom-free day. The aim is to avoid the typical boom (high-activity day) and bust (low-activity day with exacerbation of

symptoms) pattern.

Goal Setting

Whether considering day-to-day activities or setting longer-term targets that need to be achieved, it is important to try to minimise fatigue by breaking goals down into small, progressive, more manageable steps, and working out what it is realistically possible to achieve. It may be helpful to ask a health care professional to help set realistic targets; the skill is to make sure that the goals (both the overall goal and the smaller steps) are achievable (2/HMSA 2014).

Relaxation and mindfulness

As with pain management, learning and practicing relaxation techniques, such as progressive muscle relaxation, breathing training and creative visualisation, can bring numerous potential benefits, including decreased sleep problems, lowered blood pressure, reduced levels of pain, fatigue, stress and anxiety, and decreasing impulsive behaviours (Bonfil A.). The concept of mindfulness (see page 158) encourages individuals to relax by focusing their full attention on the 'here and now' rather than multitasking or ruminating on the past or possible future events. Relaxation and mindfulness techniques also form part of cognitive behavioural therapy (see page 156).

Sleeping

Disrupted sleep not only contributes to feelings of fatigue, research has demonstrated that it can exacerbate chronic pain, triggering a vicious cycle in which pain disrupts sleep, and difficulty sleeping makes the pain worse, which in turn makes sleeping more difficult. This, in turn, can increase levels of stress, and affect mood and mental functions like memory and concentration (Alhola P. et al 2007).

As we saw on page 55, the persistent fatigue commonly associated with hEDS/HSD is not fully alleviated by sleep, but it is still important to practice good sleep hygiene in order to maximise the quality of sleep and avoid it exacerbating the existing symptoms. In an open letter to his patients, Dr Alan Pocinki explains that treatment of sleep problems begins with the basic rules of good sleep hygiene, such as trying to sleep the same hours each night, and avoiding using the bedroom for work or watching television. He suggests avoiding eating heavy meals or having caffeine, nicotine or alcohol late at night, as well as not checking the clock or looking at phones and other similar devices throughout the night. HMSA CEO Donna Wicks agrees, saying: "*Establishing a new sleeping pattern can take several weeks. So keep persevering. Try not to sleep during the day, or, if this is impossible, have a nap of only 15 minutes. Set an alarm to wake you, so that you don't sleep longer. Make sure your bedroom is the correct temperature for you, that it is dark, and that you have a comfortable mattress. Take sleep aid medications as prescribed and only for short periods of time. If your mind is racing with things to remember or do, jot them down so that you don't have to worry about forgetting them. Don't worry if your mind wanders, just keep bringing it back to focussing on your breathing and practice this for 30 mins.*"

When these measures fail, then medication may be indicated, because virtually every system in the body is strained when you don't get a good night's sleep (Pockini A. 2010). If sleep is disturbed by generalised pain and stiffness, medications such as the antidepressant amitriptyline can be effective for their muscle relaxant property, helping to promote good sleep. It should be realised, however, that medication is only suitable for the short term. Donna Wicks explains: "*It can be helpful in starting off a sleeping pattern, but is more effective when used in conjunction with other changes, which will be for the long term.*" Patients need to discuss poor sleep with their GP, who can suggest lifestyle changes and, if necessary, prescribe appropriate medications.

Being prepared for medical emergencies

Medical emergencies can happen to anyone, but when living with a variable and often under-recognised disorder such as hEDS/HSD, it can be particularly prudent to be as prepared as possible.

Medical identification tags

A medical identification tag is an engraved disc or emblem worn on a bracelet or neck chain bearing a message that the wearer has an important medical condition that might require immediate attention. Although attractive medical alert jewellery is now readily available through many websites, perhaps the best known worldwide is 'Medic Alert' (see the resources section at the back of this book).

Medic Alert are able to store detailed information on an individual's medical conditions, symptoms and medications, and provide these to those in charge of a person's care in an emergency situation. Their emergency response line can be accessed 24/7 from anywhere in the world.

Hospital bag

Being prepared by keeping a ready-packed hospital grab bag can help reduce the stress of dealing with emergency visits to hospital for everyone involved. Useful items may include:

- A personal information folder, including a concise, chronological, bullet point list of medical history and the results of any tests or imaging undergone to-date; details of any doctors or consultant providing existing care, details of treatments, medications and doses; details of any medications that have caused a bad reaction in the past; a list of family and friends' contact numbers; where necessary, a list of any mobility aids required and a description of the amount of assistance usually needed with personal care etc.
- A pen and paper to write down information you are told.
- Nightwear and lightweight dressing gown
- Underwear.
- Self-activating ice or heat packs.
- Toiletries and hairbrush.
- Plastic bag for soiled clothing.
- Small pillow or blanket.
- Reading material.
- Music or media player with earphones.
- A small amount of cash.

Care plans

If an individual has chosen to inform their school, college or employer of their condition, it may be prudent to prepare a care plan with them, outlining what needs to happen in case of medical or other emergencies, such as fire etc.

This may, for example, include a description of what happens when symptoms are experienced (e.g. symptoms of dysautonomia such as fainting, or musculoskeletal symptoms such as dislocations) and how people can best help during and afterwards e.g. providing fluids, fetching prescribed medications, ice packs, mobility aids etc. If symptoms are generally short-lived, then the provision of a quiet place to rest before returning to work may be all that is required. The care plan should say where this rest should take place. If recovery usually takes a long time, the care plan should say how an individual will get home and who will travel with them if necessary.

In respect of environmental emergencies, such as fire or power failure, a plan for the evacuation of a building needs to be put in place if the individual's mobility is affected.

Image on page 155 by: David Castillo Dominici - Freedigitalphotos.net

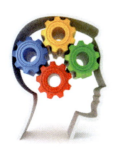

Cognitive Behavioural Therapy (CBT)

What is CBT?
Chronic conditions are notoriously difficult to treat. Although there are no cures for hEDS/HSD, a combination of psychological and physical therapies appear to provide significant benefits. One such psychological therapy is cognitive behavioural therapy (CBT). Although perhaps best known for its results in treating anxiety and depression, it has also been shown to be helpful in the management of chronic pain and other physical health problems (Hofmann S. G. 2012 / Morrison J.).

CBT is a talking therapy which combines examining the things patients think (cognitive therapy) and the things patients do (behaviour therapy) along with examining social and environmental factors; helping patients to address how these may be impacting on the pain and other symptoms they experience (Day M.A. et al 2012).

In essence, the approaches it incorporates aim to improve the way that an individual manages and copes with their pain, either in addition to other therapies or medications, or when alternative forms of treatment have been found to be ineffective.

Does this mean it's all in my head?
Instead of being thought of purely in physical terms, it is now recognised that persistent pain is made up of both physical *and* psychological factors combined (Grant M. 2012). Healthcare professionals recognise this and may suggest that a chronic pain patient would benefit from a psychological therapy such as CBT. Unfortunately, the way this is communicated to those in pain often causes a great deal of anxiety and stress on the patient's part. It is likely that patients with hEDS/HSD will have previously encountered practitioners who have expressed skepticism that their pain is real, and they may well have become hypersensitive to not being believed. To these patients, being referred for a psychological therapy such as CBT, without a clear explanation of the benefits, can lead them to believe that their GP thinks their symptoms are 'all in their head.' In fact, CBT is widely implemented as a standard treatment for chronic pain, including musculoskeletal pain, visceral pain and headache; therefore, cognitive-behavioral therapy is indicated in hEDS/HSD patients with debilitating pain not adequately treated by standard care (Castori M. 2012). Although often poorly communicated, its recommendation is actually an acknowledgement on a GPs part that they really understand that things are difficult for their patient, and feel that psychological therapy could be one of several useful tools in helping them cope.

How does it work?
A typical CBT programme might introduce an overview of a theory of pain control and promote assertive communication, structured relaxation, and pacing of behavior to avoid exacerbation of pain flares. It can be used at the same time as prescribed medication or on its own.

Therapists also understand that many people with long-term conditions feel overwhelmed about their condition, and hopeless about the future. A patient may feel guilty about the effect their condition has on their partner, children, friends, family or employer and feel they are letting people down (2/ HMSA 2014).' CBT works by providing individuals with the tools that allow them to challenge negative thought patterns, feelings, actions and behaviours, and replace them with thoughts that are oriented towards adaptive behavior (practical skills to help them function better in their daily lives) and positive functioning (shifting the focus of therapy from what is wrong with clients to what is right with them, and from what is not working to what is).

In short, CBT can help individuals develop coping skills intended to manage pain, improve sleep patterns, reduce other stress factors and improve psychological functioning. It enables them to better accept their diagnosis and to find ways of dealing with it effectively.

How is CBT delivered?
According to Freidberg F. (2016), effective practitioners ensure that the patient feels 'accepted and believed'; that the patient accepts their diagnosis; and that the model of treatment offered matches the model of illness held by the patient; avoiding ascribing the symptoms to a physical or somatic cause (given the lack of consistent medical findings or objective tests for diagnosis that are currently available).

CBT is available in a wide range of settings, including hospitals, clinics and private therapy centres, either on a 1-1 basis or in a group format. In some areas of the country, it is provided in the form of written or computer-based packages.

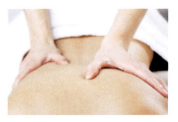

Complementary and physical therapies

A great deal of interest is currently being taken in the potential benefits of complimentary and physical therapies such as massage therapy, myofascial release, Pilates, the Alexander technique and mindfulness, for those affected by joint hypermobility. Pilates, in particular, is being studied in order to ascertain whether the benefits, anecdotally reported by hypermobile individuals and their teachers, may be encompassed into more established principles of managing hypermobility. This list is by no means exhaustive, and could go on to include chiropractic therapy, osteopathy, Tai Chi, acupuncture, trigger point therapy, Yoga and many more. Hopefully, over the next few years, more studies will be carried out into their efficacy, but as with all such therapies, individuals with hEDS/HSD who choose to participate should proceed with caution and make sure that the therapist is fully aware of their diagnosis and how it affects them. Below, we will look briefly at gentle massage therapy, Pilates, the Alexander technique, and mindfulness.

Gentle massage therapy, and myofascial release

Gentle massage therapy is the gentle manipulation of soft tissues of the body including, muscles, connective tissues, tendons, ligaments and joints. When writing on the subject of massage therapy for those with hEDS/HSD, Dr Brad Tinkle (2010) writes:

'(In hEDS/HSD) *the muscles will attempt to stabilse the joints that cannot stabilse themselves, causing muscle tightness* (and) *leading to long-term severe muscular tension that is extremely painful...*'

Where it can be tolerated, for hypermobile individuals, massage therapy may help ease tense muscles, relieve stress and anxiety (Armstrong V. 2016). A knowledgeable therapist who has been trained in a wide variety of techniques should be able to adapt to an individual client, working with them to gradually increase the individuals tolerance to pressure and muscle manipulation, rather than applying a set routine to treat all.

Myofascial release therapy focuses on reducing pain by easing the tension and tightness in soft tissues and the fascia, releasing 'trigger points'; the name given to tender areas which cause local and referred pain (also see Chapter 2, page 49). Myofascial tissues surround and support the muscles throughout the body. Habitual poor posture, repetitive stress injuries and traumatic events, such as falls or surgery can have a cumulative effect on the fascia, leading to tightening and the formulation of trigger points. As the fascia tightens, it can exert excessive pressure, producing pain or restriction of motion, influencing the comfort and the functioning of the body and affecting flexibility and stability. In addition to manual manipulation, myofascial release therapy aims to improve symptoms through education in proper body mechanics and movement, the enhancement of strength and flexibility, and postural and movement awareness.

Although research studies into the treatment of muscle and fascial pain in hEDS/HSD are still scarce, in a talk given by Dr Pradeep Chopra (leading EDS/pain expert) he recommends consideration of the following manual techniques in relation to muscle and myofascial pain:

- Controlled stretching (see page 141).
- Relaxation techniques.
- Muscle energy technique (utilises positioning of the body and using active muscle contraction to relax muscles and align joints).
- Strain–counterstrain (a positional technique to help relax tight muscles).
- Craniosacral massage therapy (a gentle technique to help balance the nervous system).
- Myofascial release (gentle techniques to improve the mobility of the muscles by mobilising the fascia tissue connecting and surrounding the muscle).
- Trigger point therapy (All above: Chopra 2013b).

The Alexander technique

The Alexander technique is a method that works to change movement habits in individual everyday activities. Its goal is to improve ease and freedom of movement, balance, support and coordination, and to help a person discover a new balance in the body by releasing unnecessary tension. The technique teaches individuals to use the appropriate amount of effort for a particular activity, which should in turn help increase their energy for all their activities. It is not a series of treatments or exercises, but rather a re-education of the mind and body. The Alexander technique is a method which can be applied to sitting, lying down, standing, walking, lifting, and other daily activities.

Image attribution, page 157: Nenelus - Creative Commons Licence

MANAGEMENT

In an article for the Hypermobility Syndromes Association, Dr Philip Bull, Consultant Rheumatologist and advocate of the Alexander Technique (AT), says: 'If your body is like a car, a physiotherapist is like a mechanic, while the AT teacher is equivalent to being a driving instructor [teaching how the body is designed to function so that you can work with the design rather than against it].'

Alexander teacher, Julie Barber (MSTAT), says: 'At least half of the people I see in my practice have some degree of hypermobility, ranging from general hypermobility to full blown EDS.... Sometimes hypermobility leads to reduced proprioception (our body awareness sense). Through Alexander work, people become more in touch with their bodies in a useful way; they can learn the difference between tense and free muscles so that they can look after themselves better. It helps prevent misuse and overuse, such as over-stretching when doing exercises or chronically tightening [the] muscles around joints in an attempt to produce stability (the classic paradox of being both 'too loose' and 'too tight' at the same time). As tension reduces, balance and co-ordination improve. Confidence grows in one's ability to move well and efficiently, with less risk of injury.'

Pilates

Pilates exercise focuses on using both the mind and body to achieve optimum performance. Using sequences of movements that use gravity, body weight and specially designed resistance equipment, the deep stabilising muscles of the body are conditioned and strengthened. Pilates trains the mind to maintain a constant level of awareness of the way the body moves, resulting in a greater control of motion.

Jessica Moolenaar contributed a chapter on Pilates and EDS to Isobel Knight's acclaimed book, Managing EDS (Type III) - Hypermobility Syndrome (2013). Jessica, a Pilates Foundation teacher and Director of Mindful Pilates, who herself is hypermobile, says: 'Gentle movement is helpful for people with EDS, but static work and repetitive movement are tiring and often lead to pain. Pilates helps by taking clients through gentle movements into smooth, coordinated recruitment patterns of the muscles.' Pilates can help build stabilisation by strengthening the structures around the joints and increasing proprioception and balance. It also promotes relaxation and good breathing techniques to combat fatigue and anxiety. Jessica says that Pilates Foundation teachers understand '...how to coordinate the body so that hypermobile clients get the distribution of force through the whole system instead of 'hanging' in certain areas and 'locking' in others. 'You don't push into the end range of movement ever because that's just not beneficial. ...Very good Pilates practice never pushes into the end range or locks any joints. There's always the flow of the in and out breath so you never stop moving or lock into position or push beyond your capabilities.' (Knight I. 2013 / Moolenaar J. / Pilates Foundation)

Mindfulness

Mindfulness-based therapies help individuals focus on their thoughts and feelings without becoming overwhelmed by them. By becoming more aware of the present moment, a person can begin to experience afresh things that they have been taking for granted, and to notice signs of stress and anxiety earlier and deal with them better.

'Mindfulness allows us to become more aware of the stream of thoughts and feelings that we experience, and to see how we can become entangled in that stream in ways that are not helpful. (It) lets us stand back from our thoughts and start to see their patterns. Gradually, we can train ourselves to notice when our thoughts are taking over and realise that thoughts are simply 'mental events' that do not have to control us. We can ask: 'Is trying to solve this by brooding about it helpful, or am I just getting caught up in my thoughts?' (Williams J.M.G.)

Research shows mindfulness can change the structure of the brain, thickening the cerebral cortex (the area associated with attention and emotion regulation) and dampening the amygdala's activity (the area that activates anxiety and depression) (Lazar SW. et al 2005 / Desbordes G. et al 2012 / Williams J.M.G. 2013 / Kok B.E. et al 2013). The National Institute for Health and Care Excellence has gone as far as recommending the use of mindfulness-based cognitive therapy for preventing relapse of depression. Mindfulness training has also been shown to strengthen the vagus nerve which is made of thousands of fibres that communicate with the brain about what is happening with the body's organs and autonomic nervous system.

As well as helping individuals notice their thoughts, mindfulness can also teach them to notice posture and the way that they move, which some people find reduces their levels of chronic pain. It teaches people to be curious about the intensity of their pain, instead of letting their minds jump into thoughts like "This is awful," said Elisha Goldstein Phd, author of 'The Now Effect' - stress reduction workbook. It also teaches individuals to let go of goals and expectations. Goldstein explains: '*When you expect something will ease your pain, and it doesn't, or not as much as you'd like, your mind goes into alarm-or-solution-mode. You start thinking thoughts like "nothing ever works." What we want to do as best as we can is to engage with the pain just as it is.*" It's not about achieving a certain goal - like minimising pain - but learning to relate to pain differently' (11/NHS.uk and article by Smith C. written for the HMSA Journal Issue 5).

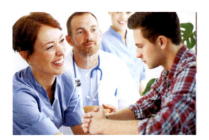

Making the most of your health care team

When dealing with a condition that is so poorly understood by so many, the need to be a proactive patient becomes even more necessary than normal. It is also important to remember that a healthcare professional can only do so much without the patient's cooperation.

> '*Working in partnership with your healthcare professionals and sharing in the decision making process are key elements of ensuring that you are all working towards shared goals to improve or maintain the quality of your life in ways that are relevant to you. Although some medical professionals still practice a more authoritarian approach (and not all patients wish to be an equal partner in decision making), many patients, and those working with them, find that this newer style of collaborative partnership leads to the best results and increased service-user satisfaction.*
> (Living well with an HDCT Guide - HMSA, 2014)

Making an appointment
In the UK, the average General Practitioner (GP) appointment lasts between 7 and 12 minutes, and many National Health Service (NHS) physiotherapy appointments are restricted to a 30 minute initial consultation with 15-20 minute follow up appointments. When making an appointment with a GP, thought should be given to how much time is likely to be needed and, if there are new symptoms or concerns to discuss, whether a 'double' or 'triple' appointment may need to be booked.

When seeking an appointment related to a long-term health disorder, it is usually best to see the same healthcare professional. This helps ensure continuity of care and saves time in the appointment that may, otherwise, be spent covering old ground. If an appointment is no longer needed, remember to cancel it.

The appointment and beyond
Better preparation and communication between patients and healthcare professionals helps both parties get the most out of what is often a brief interaction.

Tips to help achieve this goal include:

<u>Be prepared for appointments</u>
Before seeing the healthcare professional, it can be useful to make a list of problems and questions in order of their importance. Describe what the symptoms are, what limitations they have caused, when they happened, how long they lasted, and if there were specific triggers. Information like this helps a doctor see any patterns that might help them make a diagnosis or formulate a treatment plan. Although it may truly describe a patients feelings, when it comes to describing pain doctors may find descriptions such as 'I just hurt everywhere' or 'I feel like I'm old' vague and difficult to understand. Where possible, try to think in advance which words could best help a doctor to understand the pain. For example, is the pain dull and aching, pounding, sharp, spiky, radiating, tingly, tight, pinching, constant, intermittent, deep, stabbing or spasming?

<u>Take along any relevant information</u>
Include a concise, chronological, bullet point list of medical history and details of treatments or any medications, the results of any tests or imaging undergone to-date, any changes in symptoms and when those occurred, and any patterns observed (also see 'Hospital Bag' on page 155).

<u>Don't be rushed</u>
If the healthcare professional is running behind schedule and a patient feels they are being rushed through their appointment, they may need to be assertive, sticking to their list and continuing to ask

questions until their concerns are addressed. When being assertive, always be polite. Don't argue, and don't interrupt; wait for them to finish so it doesn't become confrontational and then, when they've finished, repeat the request.

Be clear
Patients should try to be clear about what they would like their healthcare professional to do, such as prescribe a different medication or refer on to a physiotherapist or hEDS/HSD specialist etc.

Ask questions
Ask the doctor to repeat and explain anything that is unclear. 'When a healthcare professional recommends a form of treatment, suggests surgery or prescribes a medication - a patient should ask questions until they feel satisfied that they understand, for example: '*You are recommending surgery, but are any more conservative treatments that I could consider first? 'How will this medication interact with others that I'm already taking?'*

Asking the doctor to write down any complex medical terminology can also be beneficial, as it can be then be looked up by the patient later if desired, and more easily explained to family and friends.

'Further clarification should be sought if a patient doesn't understand their diagnosis, treatment, or the outcome of any tests undergone. Remember, healthcare is a service industry and a patient is the customer - although it can seem daunting, they shouldn't hesitate to ask doctors questions, or, where necessary, to request a second opinion; they have a right to be involved in decisions about their healthcare (HMSA Living Well with an HDT 2014).'

Be prepared to ask for a referral if necessary
If a healthcare professional believes that a referral should be made for specialist treatment or tests, a patient usually has the right to choose the hospital they go to. The complexities of hEDS/HSD are often misunderstood. It is unsurprising therefore, that many patients with hEDS/HSD have, at some point, experienced a medical appointment which left them feeling frustrated, angry, disappointed or confused. It is important to remember, however, that a general practitioner is 'a physician whose practice is not oriented to a specific medical specialty.' They may be able to help a great deal, but may not have an in-depth knowledge of a particular condition, or have all of the answers a patient hopes for. It is important the patient feels they are in 'safe hands' and are under the

care of a doctor who believes them or is, at least, prepared to look into the most recent information on hEDS/HSD and its treatment. If this is not the case, the patient may wish to consider changing doctors, or asking for a referral to a centre specialising in hEDS/HSD (see 'Centres for Patient Referral' listed at the back of this book).

'Most of the clinics specialising in hypermobility syndromes now need a consultant referral. This means your GP needs to encourage a consultant to make the referral. For those clinics where referral criteria is not consultant based, a GP can continue to refer.'
(HMSA, Living well with an HDCT Guide 2014).

Leave with a plan
At the end of an appointment the patient should leave with a plan for the immediate future and an idea of what they should do if, after the period of time agreed upon ends, the plan is not working. What happens next? Do they need to come back and see the doctor? Who should they contact if things get worse? Does the doctor have any written information they could take for reference? Where should you go for more information? Is there a support group or any other source of help?

A step in the right direction
Try not to invest all of your hope into one particular appointment with a doctor or specialist, it is better to see each appointment as a possibility to take your treatment another step in the right direction. '*Take what you can from the appointment, even if it was not as beneficial or as informed as you would have hoped. Even one small piece of information or advice can be added to your arsenal of understanding.'*
(Ensor H. - Patron of the Hypermobility Syndromes Association).

Keep a diary
Keeping a symptom diary is discussed on page153. It is a way for patients and their healthcare professionals to monitor symptoms and learn how they affect their everyday life. A diary can be kept on a daily, weekly or monthly basis, and can help identify trigger factors and patterns. Once these are established, medications, activities and rest periods can be planned more effectively so symptoms can be better managed.

Using the Internet (with caution)
Use of the internet has become part of everyday life, and for many, it is now second nature to use it as a resource to search for answers or research a diagnosis. The important thing is to understand its limits.

There is nothing wrong with conducting background research before going to the doctor, as long as reputable sources are consulted. Internet searches should not, however, replace consultation with medical experts, and the limitations in the accuracy of online information should be kept in mind. Do not panic based on information learned online; notes of any concerns should be made and discussed with a GP or appropriate professional. While not all websites are reliable, many are managed by very reputable charities, such the Hypermobility Syndromes Association, Ehlers-Danlos Support UK, the Ehlers-Danlos Society (previously known as Ehlers-Danlos National Foundation), or entities such as the National Health Service and Patient.info.
Research carried out via such sources can enable patients to ask the right questions and to discuss their symptoms more intelligently, leading to more productive and satisfying visits with health care providers. An open mind should be kept and consideration given to any alternative information that the GP suggests.

Creating a health care team

Actively seeking out and building a team of medical professionals, who are knowledgeable about hEDS/HSD, or who are willing to learn, can be a necessary part of self management for many. These are the kind of health care professionals to whom patients feel they can take research and information specific to how they are affected, and who will help them self manage their condition by supporting them in their goals. Preferably, each member of the team should be prepared to make contact with one another, combining wisdom, training and experience to reach the best outcome for the patient. In an ideal world, such a team could be found in the locale of the patient, but, in reality, lack of provision and knowledge often means patients having to travel, which can have significant financial implications.

The best recommendations often comes from fellow patients who are coping with hEDS/HSD themselves, and who have navigated through treatment for themselves or their families. Asking around for good practitioners through local support groups, Facebook and blogs, is well worth the effort; most people are happy to share their experience when they come across healthcare professionals who they have found to be understanding and supportive. GPs can also recommend reliable websites, books and additional resources.

Of course, everyone with hEDS/HSD is different and will find certain forms of treatment more, or less, helpful than others. Recommendations or warnings should be taken into account, but ultimately patients need to make their own decisions on what works and what does not. Some, for example, find massage very helpful, others could not stand to be manipulated in such a way and may only be able to tolerate very gentle treatments such as the Bowen technique; by cherry picking the ones they find most effective, individuals can create a plan that works for them.

Personality clashes, second opinions and complaints

There may be occasions where a patient genuinely cannot build a relationship with a particular healthcare professional, and this can cause a great deal of emotional distress and anxiety. Donna Wicks, CEO of the Hypermobility Syndromes Association explains:. *Such situations are unhelpful in the management of symptoms and can jeopardise an individual's ability to self manage effectively. In this situation, the best option may be to ask to see a different team member, or a different doctor or consultant. If you are unhappy with the actual medical care or treatment that you have received, you might want to make a complaint. It is often best to try and resolve the situation in person, speaking directly to the health care provider and explaining the reasons for your dissatisfaction to them. Doing so gives them the opportunity to look at your case again and to discuss these matters with you.'* Staff should be open to hearing a patient's views, both positive and negative. If applicable, a second opinion can be requested, where another doctor examines a patient's medical records and gives his or her views about their condition and how it should be managed. Alternatively, in the United Kingdom, users of the National Health Service can complain to the commissioner of that service – either NHS England or the area clinical commissioning group. The NHS Patient Advice and Liaison Service, known as PALS, represent patient views. Their local office may be able to help resolve things informally. PALS provide a point of contact in hospitals for patients, their families and their carers. They offer confidential advice, support and information on health-related matters and can also provide information on NHS complaints procedures and how to make a complaint (see 'Useful Resources' on page 184).

Image attribution, page 159: Selmaemiliano - Creative Commons Licence

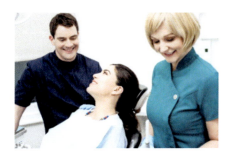

Dental management in hEDS, and HSD

The most common dental manifestations arising from hEDS, and HSD, are described in Chapter 2, page 86. The appropriate management is described over the following pages.

Visiting the dentist

When joining a new dental practice, consider asking for an initial consultation with the dentist or dental hygienist before scheduling an appointment. This will help develop a rapport and open communication about symptoms and any oral manifestations arising from hEDS or HSD (also see **Box 1**). It also provides the dentist and/or hygienist with an opportunity to discuss their proposed treatment plan and the types of procedures that can be expected during future appointments.

Existing patients should be sure to inform their dental team of any changes in their medical or dental history as well as current medications, (including over-the-counter medications).

The dental professional should familiarise themselves with the oral health and dental care implications of hEDS, and HSD, and be willing to work with and listen to the patient and their concerns. Alternatively, if a patient has complex disease or possible oral manifestations of EDS that warrant further investigation or treatment, they may chose to refer them to an appropriate specialist for advice (Porter S. 2016).

Regular dental cleanings, of minimal length, are recommended for those with hEDS, and HSD, with the aim of detecting issues early, preventing complications and the need for long, or difficult treatment sessions, which may be more likely to arise if visits are infrequent (Mitakides J. et al 2017). Determining whether tooth decay is an increased risk is important and should be discussed with the dental team. It is thought that the high plaque index of many patients with EDS may be related to difficulties with oral self-care from chronic pain in the hands or arms, restricted joint mobility, or concern of excessive bleeding from fragile mucosa. (De Coster P.J. et al 2005a & 2005b). EDS and HSD patients should be given instruction by their dentist on meticulous and gentle oral hygiene care, using modified brushing techniques with ultra-soft toothbrushes. For some patients, a dental procedure may trigger or increase manifestations such as Temporomandibular joint dysfunction (also see Chapter 2, page 86, and Chapter 3, page 163).

Box 1.

Before, during and after an appointment:

- Consideration should be given to the positioning of the patient in the dental chair according to their needs and comfort.
- Caution should be used when keeping the mouth open, to avoid overextension and possible hypermobility, which sometimes lead to subluxations, dislocation or locking of the TMJ if the mouth is opened too widely. (Utilisation of a mouth prop or device may help protect the jaw during a dental visit).
- A signal should be prearranged, which the patient can give the dental provider (such as holding their hand up) to indicate a break needs to be taken / the jaw rested.
- Rolled-up towels or pillows can be placed behind the neck or back to avoid discomfort.
- If teeth are sensitive, let the dental provider know; it may be possible to use a desensitising agent and make adaptations to water temperature or application of air.
- If swallowing difficulties are a problem, positioning the chair in a semi-upright position may be more comfortable.

After a dental visit the following should be considered:

- Ice or heat applications to the jaw.
- Medications to relieve inflammation, muscle spasms and pain.
- Scheduling of the next cleaning appointment to help maintain oral health.

(The TMJ Association 2016)

Image attribution, page 162: Stockimages - Freedigitalphotos.net

Preoperative cardiac consultation and antibiotic prophylaxis

Although still considered a potential clue for hEDS (and included in the diagnostic criteria, Mitral Valve Prolapse (MVP) is no longer considered a common manifestation (Dolan A.L. et al.1997 / McDonnell N.B.et al 2006 / Atzinger C.L. et al., 2011 / Tinkle B. et al 2017). Patients in whom MVP is suspected or confirmed require pre-operative cardiac consultation and antibiotic prophylaxis cover prior to any major dental operations (Abel M.D. et al 2006 / Ansari G. et al 2015).

Local anaesthetic

Topical anesthetics and, if needed, local anesthesia can be requested to lessen pain. Many patients with hEDS, and HSD, report being less responsive to local anaesthetics during dental procedures [Arendt-Nielsen L. et al. 1990 / Hakim A.J et al., 2005 / Tinkle B. et al 2017) (also see pages 25, 65 & 165). If this arises, patients are likely to be referred to a specialist in oral and maxillofacial surgery who will be able to ensure that a suitable technique or agent is used to provide effective anaesthesia (Porter S. 2016) (Also, see pages 65 & 165).

Soft tissue

To avoid tissue trauma during appointments, careful use of dental instruments and minimal use of ultrasonic scaling instruments are recommended for those with EDS (Pacak D.K.). Forces used in orthodontic treatment should be lighter than usual, given the fragility of the periodontal ligament (Létourneau Y. 2001). Orthodontic appliances should be smooth and relatively simple in spring design, so that the tongue and tissue lining of the mouth are not abraded (Norton L.A. for EDS Support UK, Mitakides J. et al 2017). Some patients may develop mouth ulcers due to the trauma of orthodontic appliances such as braces. This can be lessened by use of protective wax over the brace and possibly an occlusive paste placed over any sites of ulceration (Porter S. 2016). As some patients with EDS are more liable than others to develop mouth ulcers due to trauma from a loose denture it is essential that dentures are well fitting and regularly reviewed by a dentist (Porter S. 2016).

The teeth may move into the correct position faster than would be expected and may also be prone to relapse once appliances are removed. There may, therefore, be a need for patients to wear an appliance for many months to ensure that the teeth remain in position. Suturing should be done with great care due to the possible fragility of the tissues and oral mucosa (Gosney M.B. 1987, Barabas G.M. 1967,

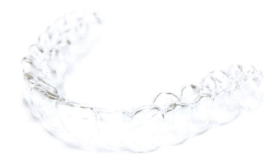

Dental appliances such as braces and retainers may need to be worn for longer than usual to ensure that the teeth remain in position

Hughes C.L. 2015, Mitakides J. et al 2017)

Temporomandibular joint dysfunction (TMD)

Pain and dislocation of the temporomandibular joint (TMJ) may arise in adults and children due to laxity of the lower jaw joint (mandible) (Adair S.M. & Hecht C. 1993). This is known as temporomandibular joint dysfunction (TMD). The TMJ in those with hEDS can be more mobile and may dislocate from its fossa in the temporal bone (the base of skull) causing the jaw to deviate and the patient to become unable to close their mouth. 'Sometimes the mandible will spontaneously relocate, while some patients develop a method by which they are able to easily relocate the lower jaw into its fossa. Unfortunately sometimes this is not possible and relocation must be undertaken by a clinician (e.g. in an Accident and Emergency clinic). Repeated dislocation can damage the bones of the joint causing pain and, paradoxically, limited movement. Similarly, even if the joint is not repeatedly dislocating the increased movement of the joint in normal activities can cause pain of the joint(s) and surrounding areas of the face and head' (Porter S. 2016).

'While proper diagnosis and precise treatment of TMD is always complex, it is far more so in the EDS patient. Even practitioners highly trained in the area of TMD can face unexpected challenges in diagnosing and treating an EDS patient if they do not have an in-depth understanding of EDS. Some symptoms are obvious to the practitioner familiar with the disorder, and some are very subtle'. (Mitakides et al 2017)

Prevention and treatment of TMD

Prevention of TMJ injury is multi-faceted. Changes to lifestyle may be suggested including alteration of chewing patterns, diet, stress reduction techniques, and management of physical activities (Mitakides J. et al 2017). Postural alignment as well as upper back and cervical spinal issues may also need to be addressed, with research showing that 90% of the patients with cervical spinal pain also had TMD (In^es M. et al. 2008), and concluding that the postural positioning of the cervical spine impacted TMJ function.

'As the neck and especially the upper cervical spine are often involved in EDS patients, their interaction, recognition, and potential co-management should be taken into consideration'. (Mitakides et al 2017)

Depending on the type and source of symptoms a patient is experiencing, multiple treatments are available for management of pain and TMD-associated problems. All the muscles of the body are prone to contracture and spasm in those with hEDS/HSD, including those in the jaw. *'Eliminating or reducing muscle spasms is often the first step in reducing pain, and is considered a conservative treatment option appropriate for the EDS patient'* (Mitakides et al 2017).

Further suggestions for care and management of TMD can be found in **Box 2**.

MANAGEMENT

Box 2.

Conservative, focused and highly informed care for TMD, taking into account the multiple manifestations of EDS:

The 2017 International Consortium of Experts on EDS recommend the following techniques as helpful:

- Deep heat has the ability to relax muscle fibres and decrease spasms. The usual protocol is 10 min of warm, followed by 3 min of cold, and 10 min of warm.
- Cold laser (Superpulsed Low Level Laser Therapy) has been shown to be effective in pain management of TMD (Marini I. et al., 2010).
- 'Friction muscle massage' stretches and relaxes the muscle fibres. A muscle is relaxed when it is a full length.
- Custom splints to stabilise the TMD have proven effective over time. Such appliances, when carefully created to target appropriate anterior repositioning, provide stabilisation, limit joint injury, and help maintain physiological posture.
- Prolotherapy, also called regenerative injection therapy, is a non-surgical alternative medicine treatment for ligament and tendon reconstruction. Injections of a combination of dextrose and local anaesthetic have proven promising (Hakala R.V. 2005).
- Medications offer a variety of options, such as muscle relaxants, mood elevators, anti-inflammatories, and pain medications. In the EDS patient, care must be taken to consider other medications and possible additional effects of any medication.
- Botulinum toxin to relax muscle or at trigger points can provide almost immediate relief for some patients. Botulinum toxin is injected into specific trigger points, particularly for the purposes of relieving migraines, muscle spasms, involuntary positional motions, and structural physicality.

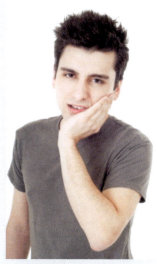

TMD may arise in adults and children due to laxity of the lower jaw joint.

- Physiotherapy can assist with muscle integrity, posture, and can maintain ranges of motion and physiological structural position for function. It is vital that the physiotherapist understand the special needs of the EDS patient, including the attendant increased fragility.
- Surgical options should be limited to extreme cases, such as physical damage to the TMJ. EDS patients in particular face unique surgical challenges, making them less than ideal candidates for surgical TMJ stabilisation. Surgical repairs heal slowly and often with unpredictable results.

(All the above bullet points: Mitakides J. et al 2017)

Image attribution page 164: artur84, Freedigitalmedia.net

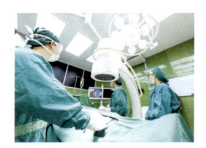

Surgical issues

'Many patients with hEDS/HSD are able to undergo the full range of surgical operations which may be offered to the general population, as long as their surgeon has been made familiar with their disorder, understands any possible complications this may cause, and is prepared to make any necessary alterations to their operating technique.' (Hakim A. 2015 - HMSA LWW Guide).

Each person and their symptoms / pre-existing and comorbid conditions are different. For that reason, it is very important that full details of medical history are made clear to all of the medical team involved in an individuals care, and appropriate measures to avoid complications, put in place.

When planning surgery, particular consideration should be given to:

- Instability of the cervical spine and/or temporomandibular joint. In the latter, intubation may need to be carried out more carefully due to temporomandibular joint dysfunction and the possibility of a slightly more fragile mucosal lining of the mouth (Castori M. 2012).

- The need for surgical and nursing staff to be prepared to take extra precautions when moving or positioning a patient with hEDS/HSD, in order to prevent injury, subluxation, or dislocation (Johnston B.A. 2006)

- Delays in wound healing are experienced by some with hEDS/HSD, and should be allowed for when planning for the removal of stitches and post operative movement. Experts recommend leaving sutures in place for longer than normal and/or brief immobilisation (Beighton P. 1969 / Shirley E.D. et al 2012 / Burcharth J. 2012 / Tinkle B. et al 2017); multilayered closure techniques with sufficient numbers of sutures (prefer nylon sutures over staples), deep stitches, and the support of wound closure strips (Weinberg J.et al 1999 / Tinkle B. et al 2017).

- The effects of muscle deconditioning may impact on recovery times and rehabilitation should be individualised (Castori M. 2012). For example, post-operative exercises designed to restore range of motion may need to be less aggressive than standard protocols, because the stiffness does not typically develop post-operatively in those with EDS, and there is a need to avoid stretching of repaired or reconstructed tissue (Shirley E.D. et al 2012)

- In patients who also have the common comorbidity, cardiovascular dysautonomia, it may be considered prudent to carry out cardiac evaluation with a possible echocardiogram before surgery. The anaesthetist involved in the patient's care should be made aware of the patient's cardiovascular dysautonomia diagnosis to allow them to plan for any increased risk of hemodynamic changes, such as a lowering in blood pressure, whilst under anaesthesia (Castori M 2012).

- Post operative orthostatic headache may occur in some patients as a result of spinal anaesthesia (Tinkle B. et al 2017).

In the case of minor surgeries (those which don't involve anaesthesia or assisted breathing), for example: dental procedures, tissue biopsies, mole removal etc., consideration should be given to the frequently reported resistance to topical EMLA cream and intradermal (situated or applied within the layers of the skin) lidocaine injections in hEDS/HSD patients (Arendt-Nielsen L. 1990 / Hakim A.J. 2005). According to Castori (2012), a double dose of anesthetic by intradermal injection may be an effective first choice option.

Although evidence is lacking, local anaesthetic resistance is also reported in those with hEDS/HSD in respect of epidural analgesia. This may result in insufficient or ineffective analgesia during instrumental or caesarean deliveries or other surgical procedures (Castori M. 2012, Hakim A.J. 2005).

If a patient's medical history shows potential for local anaesthetic resistance, then alternative methods of analgesia, for example, patient controlled analgesia (PCA), may be set up early, or in addition to other prescribed pain relief to enhance their action (Kochharn P.K. 2011).

NB/ Anesthetic issues are also discussed on pages 25, 65 and 104.

Bibliography

Abel M.D.& Carrasco L.R. 2006 - Ehlers-Danlos syndrome: classifications, oral manifestations, and dental considerations. Oral Surg, Oral Med, Oral Pathol, Oral Radiol, Endod. 2006;102:582-590. www.oooojournal.net/article/S1079-2104(06)00196-X/fulltext

About Us - International Foundation for Functional Gastrointestinal Disorders - The Low FODMAP diet approach:- Dietary Triggers for IBS symptoms. www.aboutibs.org/site/treatment/low-fodmap-diet/

Abu Jar Gifari Papon S.M. - Deviated Nasal Septum : Def, Causes, Clinical Features, Investigation, Treatment In Otolaryngology (ENT) / June 17, 2013

Acasuso-Diaz M. 1998 - Joint hypemrobility in patients with fibromyalgia syndrome Arthr Care Res 11:39-42

Acfaom.org - American Collage of Foot and Angle Orthopaedics and Medicine. www.acfaom.org/information-for-patients/common-conditions/bunions

Adair S.M. & Hecht C. 1993 - Association of generalized joint hypermobility with history, signs, and symptoms of temporomandibular joint dysfunction in children. Pediatr Dent. 1993 Sep-Oct;15(5):323-6.

Adib N. et al 2005 - Joint hypermobility syndrome in childhood - A not so benign multisystem disorder? Rheumatology 44:744-750

Afrin L. - Presentation, Diagnosis, and Management of Mast Cell Activation Syndrome (pp. 155-232) Division of Hematology/Oncology, Medical University of South Carolina, Charleston, SC, USA). www.novapublishers.com/catalog/product_info.php?products_id=42603

Afrin L.. & Molderings G.J. 2014 - A concise, practical guide to diagnostic assessment for mast cell activation disease. World J Hematol 3(1):1-17.

Agarwal S. 2002 - Textbook of Ophthalmology Volume 1 page 1086 - ISBN 81-7179-884-5

Ainsworth S.R. & Aulincino P. 1993 - A Survey of Patients with Ehlers-Danlos syndrome. Clin Orthop Relat Res. 1993 Jan; (286):250-6. PubMed

Akeson W.H. & Woo et al - Biomechanical and biochemical changes in the periarticular connective tissue during contracture development in the immobilized rabbit knee. Connect Tissue Res. 1974; 2(4):315-23. PubMed

Akin C. et al 2010 - Mast cell activation: proposed diagnostic criteria. The Journal of Allergy and Clinical Immunology 126 (6): 1099–104. doi: 10.1016/j.jaci.2010.08.035.

Akin C. updated 2014 - Mast Cell Activation Disorders. www.uptodate.com/contents/mast-cell-activation-disorders? source=search_result&search=mast+cell+activation +disorders&selectedTitle=1%7E44).

Aktas I. 2008 - The relationship between benign joint hypermobility syndrome and carpal tunnel syndrome - Clinical Rheumatology, vol. 27, no. 10, pp. 1283–1287, 2008.

Aktas I. et al 2011 Relationship Between Lumbar Disc Herniation and Benign Joint Hypermobility Syndrome - www.ftrdergisi.com/sayilar/212/ buyuk/85-88%20--.pdf

Alexander G.M. 2011 - The use of ketamine in complex regional pain syndrome: possible mechanisms Author(s): Source: Expert Review of Neurotherapeutics. 11.5 (May 2011)

Alexander G.M. 2012 - Changes in plasma cytokines and their soluble receptors in complex regional pain syndrome. J Pain. 2012 Jan;13(1): 10-20. doi: 10.1016/j.jpain.2011.10.003. Epub 2011 Dec 14.

Alexander G.M. - American College of Sports Medicine - Delayed onset muscle soreness - www.acsm.org/docs/brochures/delayed-onset-muscle-soreness-(doms).pdf

Alford W. 2005 - Mast Cells and GI Motility Disease alford.grimtrojan.com/Mast_Cells_GI_Motility_Disease.htm

Alhola P. et al 2007 - Sleep deprivation: Impact on cognitive performance www.ncbi.nlm.nih.gov/pmc/articles/PMC2656292/ Neuropsychiatr Dis Treat. 2007 Oct; 3(5): 553–567.

All about vision.com - Kertatoconus (steep corneas) www.allaboutvision.com

Al-Rawi Z.S. 2004 - Joint mobility in people with hiatus hernia - Rheumatology Rheumatology.oxfordjournals.org/content/ 43/5/574.full.pdf by Z.S. Al-Rawi - 2004

Alvarez-Twose I. 2010 - Clinical, biological, and molecular characteristics of clonal mast cell disorders presenting with systemic mast cell activation symptoms. J Allergy Clin Immunol. 2010; 125: 1269–1278 (e1262)

Alvarez-Twose I. et al 2012 - Validation of the REMA score for predicting mast cell clonality and systemic mastocytosis in patients with systemic mast cell activation symptoms. Int Arch Allergy Immunol. 2012; 157: 275–280

Aminaka N. & Gribble P.A. 2008 - Patellar taping, patellofemoral pain syndrome, lower extremity kinematics and dynamic postural control, Journal of Athletic Training 43:21–28, 2008.

Amir D. et al 1990 - Pulled elbow and hypermobility of joints. Clin Orthop Relat Res. 1990 Aug;(257):94-9.

Anderson B.C. 2014 - Multidirectional instability of the shoulder. www.uptodate.com/contents/multidirectional-instability-of-the-shoulder_

Andreotti L. & Cammelli D.1979 - Connective tissue in varicose veins. Angiology. 1979 Dec;30(12):798-805.

Ansari G. et al 2015 Article Type: Case Report; Received: Aug 1, 2014; Revised: Jan 6, 2015; Accepted: Jan 29, 2015; epub: Feb 20, 2015; ppub: Mar 2, 2015 - Journal of Comprehensive Pediatrics. 2015 March; 6(1): e22463 , DOI: 10.5812/jcp.22463

Anstey A. 1991 - Platelet and coagulation studies in Ehlers-Danlos syndrome. Br J Dermatol. 1991 Aug;125(2):155-63.

ARC (Arthritis Research Campaign - now known as Arthritis Research UK) 'Fatigue and arthritis' booklet, ,p.6, 2014

Archambault J. et al 1995 - Exercise loading of tendons and the development of overuse injuries, a review of current literature. Sports Med 1995;20:77-89.

Arendt-Nielsen L. et al 1990 - Insufficient effect of local analgesics in Ehlers Danlos type III patients. Acta Anaes Scand 1990; 34: 358-61

Arendt-Nielsen L. et al 1991 -The response of local anaesthetics (EMLA cream) as a clinical test to diagnose between hypermobility and Ehlers Danlos III syndrome. Scand J Rheumatol 1991; 20: 190-5

Armstrong V., 2016 - Bristol Massage Therapy. www.bristolmassagetherapy.co.uk/tips-articles/massage-and-hypermobility

Arnasson O. et al 1987. Surgical and conservative treatment of cervical spondylotic radiculopathy and my-elopathy. Acta Neurochir 84:48–53.

1/Arthritis Research UK - Joint hypermobility. www.arthritisresearchuk.org/ arthritis-information/conditions/joint-hypermobility.aspx - Content Contributor Prof H. Bird

2/ Arthritis Research UK - Where can I get treatment and advice - General Practitioner. www.arthritisresearchuk.org/arthritis-information/arthritis-and-daily-life/pain-and-arthritis/pain-report/where-can-i-get-treatment-and-advice/general-practitioner.aspx#sthash.wJX2nMYY.dpuf

© Understanding hEDS and HSD by C. Smith

3/ Arthritis Research UK - The foot and ankle in rheumatology. www.arthritisresearchuk.org/health-professionals-and-students/reports/topical-reviews/topical-reviews-spring-2011.aspx

Arulanandam S. et al 2016 - Laryngological presentations of Ehlers-Danlos syndrome: case series of nine patients from two London tertiary referral centres. Clin Otolaryngol. 2016 Jul 19. doi: 10.1111/coa.12708

Arunkalaivanan A.S. et al in 2009 - Prevalence of urinary and faecal incontinence among female members of the Hypermobility Syndrome Association (HMSA). Obstet Gynaecol. 2009 Feb;29(2):126-8. doi: 10.1080/01443610802664747.

Asnaani A. Vonk I.J. et al - The Efficacy of Cognitive Behavioral Therapy: A Review of Meta-analyses.Hofmann SG, Cognit Ther Res. 2012 Oct 1; 36(5):427-440.

Åström E. 2011 - The Astrid Lindgren Children's Hospital. The Swedish Information Centre for Rare Diseaseswww.socialstyrelsen.se

Atzinger C.L. et al 2011 - In a cross sectional and longitudinal assessment of aortic root dilation and valvular anomalies in hypermobile and classic Ehlers-Danlos syndrome. J Pediatr. 2011 May;158(5):826-830.e1. Epub 2010 Dec 28.

Autonomic Disorders Consortium - www.rarediseasesnetwork.org/ardcrc/professional/disorders/POTS/index.htm

Ayres O., Pope J G, Reidy F M, Clark J F, Thorax T J H. - Abnormalities of the lungs and thoracic cage in Ehlers–Danlos syndrome.1985. 40300–305.305.

Baeza-Velasco C. et al 2011 - oint hypermobility syndrome: problems that require psychological intervention. Rheumatology International. 2011;31(9):1131–1136. [PubMed]

Baker V. Bennell K. Stillman B. Cowan S. Crossley K. 2002 - Abnormal knee joint position sense in individuals with patellofemoral pain syndrome. J Orthop Res. Mar;20(2):208-14

Barabas G.M. et al - The Ehlers-Danlos syndrome. A report of the oral and haematological findings in nine cases. Br Dent J. 1967;123(10): 473-9. [PubMed]

Barber J. 2012 - Hypermobility Syndrome - First published in STATNews, January 2012. www.atfriends.org/Hypermobility.htm

Barns C. 2015 - Nutritionist at the NutriCentre (www.nutricentre.com) - writing for Woman's Own magazine article on probiotics - July 2015

Barrett D. S et al 1991- Joint proprioception in normal, osteoarthritic and replaced knees. www.boneandjoint.org.uk/highwire/filestream/14461/field_highwire_article_pdf/0/53.full-text.pdf

Basbaum A.I. et al 2009 - Cellular and Molecular Mechanisms of Pain - Published in final edited form as: Cell. 2009 Oct 16; 139(2): 267–284. doi: 10.1016/j.cell.2009.09.028 PMCID: PMC2852643
NIHMSID: NIHMS155644 Cell. Author manuscript; available in PMC 2010 Oct 16.

Baum J. Larsson L-G. 2000 - Hypermobility syndrome - new diagnostic criteria. J Rheumatol 2000;27:1585-6.

Beighton P. H. et al -1969 - Gastrointestinal complications of the Ehlers-Danlos syndrome Gut 1969 10: 1004-1008

Beighton P. 1969 - Surgical aspects of the Ehlers-Danlos syndrome: a survey of 100 cases. Br J Surg. 1969;56:255-259 [PubMed]

Beighton P. et al 1989 (2nd Edition) Hypermobility of Joints - Biochemistry of Joint Hypermobility (Pages 25 - 39) - 11 DOI 10.1007/978-1-84882-085-2_2, © Springer-Verlag London Limited 2 (Updated 1999 - 3rd edition)

Beighton P. et al 1998 - Ehlers-Danlos syndromes: revised nosology, villefranche, 1997. Ehlers-Danlos National Foundation (USA) and Ehlers-Danlos Support Group (UK) American Journal of Medical Genetics. 1998;77:31–37.

Beighton P. Grahame R. Bird H. 2012 (Fourth Edition) - Hypermobility of Joints, 11 DOI 10.1007/978-1-84882-085-2_2, © Springer-Verlag London Limited 2012

Bell K.M. 1991 - Recurrent common peroneal palsy in association with the Ehlers-Danlos syndrome. A case report. Poss Refs: Pubmed.gov Acta Orthop Scand. 1991 Dec;62(6):612-3.

Benarroch E.E. 2012 - Postural tachycardia syndrome: a heterogeneous and multifactorial disorder. Mayo Clin. Proc. 87, 1214–1225. doi: 10.1016/j.mayocp.2012.08.013

Bendick E.M and Tinkle B.T. Joint hypermobility syndrome: a common clinical disorder associated with migraine in women, Cephalalgia, vol. 31, no. 5, pp. 603–613, 2011.

Benrud-Larson L.M. et al 2002 - Quality of life in patients with postural tachycardia syndrome. www.ncbi.nlm.nih.gov/pubmed/12059122

Berglund B. et al 2000 - Living a restricted life with Ehlers-Danlos syndrome. International Journals of Nursing studies 37:111-118

Berglund B. et al 2010 - Dignity not fully upheld when seeking health care experiences expressed by those suffering from ehlers-danlos 2010 32: 1-7

Bhasin S. et al 1996 - The Effects of Supraphysiologic Doses of Testosterone on Muscle Size and Strength in Normal Men. N Engl J Med 1996; 335:1-7July 4, 1996 DOI: 10.1056/NEJM199607043350101

Bird E. 2016 - Team Inspire forum June 3 - www.inspire.com

Bird H. 2007 - Joint hypermobility Musculoskeletal Care. 2007 PubMed Mar;5(1):4-19.

Bird H. (posted 2013) - University of Leeds, UK - Hormonal Aspects of Hypermobility: Living with Hypermobility Syndrome - www.hmsa.org/ - Viewed 1/1/15

Birrel F.N. et al 1994 - High prevalence of joint laxity in West Africans. Br J Rheumatol. 1994 Jan;33(1):56-9.

Bishcoff S.C. 1996 - Mucosal allergy: role of mast cells and eosinophil granulocytes in the gut. Baillieres Clin Gastroenterol. 1996 Sep;10(3): 443-59.

Blackburn J.T. et al 2009 - Comparison of hamstring neuromechanical properties between healthy males and females and the influence of musculotendinous stiffness. J Electromyogr Kinesiol. 2009 Oct; 19(5):e362-9. doi: 10.1016/j.jelekin.2008.08.005. Epub 2008 Sep 30.

Blasier R. B et al 2014 - Shoulder proprioception. Effect of joint laxity, joint position, and direction of motion. Orthop Rev. 1994 Jan;23(1): 45-50.

Blitshteyn S. et al 2012 - Pregnancy in Postural Tachycardia Syndrome: clinical course and maternal and fetal outcomes. J Matern Fetal Neonatal Med. 2012; 25: 1631-1634.

Bohora S. 2010 - Joint hypermobility syndrome and dysautonomia: expanding spectrum of disease presentation and manifestation. Indian Pacing Electrophysiol. J. 10, 158–161.

Bonafe L. et al 2015. Nosology and classification of genetic skeletal disorders: 2015 revision.

Bonfil A. - Relaxation - CBT. -cogbtherapy.com/relaxation-training-los-angeles/

Bonica J. 1990 - The Management of Pain - N Engl J Med 1990; 323:1713December 13, 1990DOI: 10.1056/NEJM199012133232426

Bønnelykke K. 2013 - Copenhagen Studies of Asthma in Childhood (COPSAC) news.ku.dk/all_news/2013/2013.11/researchers-identify-main-genes-responsible-for-asthma-attacks-in-children/

Booshanam D.S.et al. 2011 - Evaluation of posture and pain in persons with benign joint hypermobility syndrome. Rheumatol Int 2011, 31:1561–1565. 10.1007/s00296-010-1514-2

© Understanding hEDS and HSD by C. Smith

Bouhnik Y. 1996 - Effects of fructo-oligosaccharides ingestion on fecal bifidobacteria and selected metabolic indexes of colon carcinogenesis in healthy humans. Nutr Cancer 1996;26:21–9.

Boundless.com 2015 - "Muscle Tone." - Boundless Anatomy and Physiology. Boundless, 22 Jan. 2015. from https://www.boundless.com/physiology/textbooks/boundless-anatomy-and-physiology-textbook/muscle-tissue-9/control-of-muscle-tension-97/muscle-tone-545-5975/. Retrieved 22 Feb. 2015

Bowel and Cancer Research - Connective Tissue and Functional Disorders www.bowelcancerresearch.org/changing-lives/connective-tissue-and-functional-disorders/

Boyan B. et al 2013 - Hormonal modulation of connective tissue homeostasis and sex differ- ences in risk for osteoarthritis of the knee. Biol Sex Diff 4:3.

Bravo J.F. & Wolff C. 2006 - Clinical study of hereditary disorders of connective tissues in a Chilean population: joint hypermobility syndrome and vascular Ehlers-Danlos syndrome. 2006 Feb;54(2):515-23.

Bravo J. 2010 - When to Suspect" document for patients - oreds.org/uploads/3/1/5/0/3150381/drbravowhentosuspect.pdf. First 2007 - revised 2010

Bravo J. 2011 - Diagnostic criteria for Joint Hypermobility syndrome - Retrieved 14 January 2012. www.reumatologia-dr-bravo.cl/para%20medicos/crit%20y%20diag/DIAGCRITJHS.htm

Bravo J. 2013 - When to suspect Joint Hypermobility syndrome. www.reumatologia-dr-bravo.cl/index5b31.html?lang=en&p=529

Bridges A.J. et al 1992 - Joint hypermobility in adults referred to rheumatology clinics. Ann Rheum Dis. 1992;51:793-796.

Briggs J. et al 2009 - Injury and joint hypermobility syndrome in ballet dancers - a 5-year follow-up Oxford Journals Medicine & Health Rheumatology Volume 48, Issue 12 Pp. 1613-1614.

British Society for immunology - www.immunology.org

Brockway L. 2016 - Gastrointestinal manifestations of Ehlers-Danlos syndrome (hypermobility type). Wingate Institute of Neurogastroenterology. Written for For EDS Support UK and reviewd by Prof Q. Aziz - www.ehlers-danlos.org/about-eds/medical-information/gastrointestinal/gastro-and-eds/#sthash.jtPycc6D.dpuf

BSPR 2013 - British Society for Paediatric and Adolescent Rheumatology. Guidelines for Management of Joint Hypermobility Syndrome in Children and Young People. www.bspar.org.uk/DocStore/FileLibrary/PDFs/Guidelines%20for%20Management%20of%20Joint%20Hypermobility%20Syndrome%20v1.1%20June%202013.pdf

Bulbena A. 1993 - Anxiety disorder in the joint hypermobility syndrome. Psychiatry Res 1993;43:59-68.

Bulbena A. et al 2011a - Joint hypermobility syndrome is a risk factor trait for anxiety disorders: a 15-year follow-up cohort study.. Gen Hosp Psychiatry. 2011;33(4):363-70.

Bulbena A. 2011b - Joint hypermobility syndrome - Easily Missed? BMJ 2011; 342 doi: dx.doi.org/10.1136/bmj.c7167 (Published 20 January 2011) Cite this as: BMJ 2011;342:c7167

Bulbena A. et al 2017 - Psychiatric and psychological aspects in the Ehlers–Danlos syndromes. Psychiatric and psychological aspects in the Ehlers–Danlos syndromes. Am J Med Genet Part C Semin Med Genet 9999C:1–9.

Bunzli S. 2015 - What Do People Who Score Highly on the Tampa Scale of Kinesiophobia Really Believe?: A Mixed Methods Investigation in People With Chronic Nonspecific Low Back Pain. Clin J Pain. 2015 Jul;31(7):621-32. doi: 10.1097/AJP.0000000000000143.

Bupa.co.uk - Joint joint dysfunction - www.bupa.co.uk/health-information/directory/j/jaw-joint-problems

Burcharth J. 2012 - Gastrointestinal surgery and related complications in patietns with ehlers-Danlos syndrome: A systematic review. Dig Surg 29:349-357

Cabone L. et.al - Bone density in Ehlers-Danlos Syndrome. Osteoporos Int. 2000, 11 (5): 388-92)

Callaghan M.J. S et al: 2002 - The effects of patellar taping on knee joint proprioception, Journal of Athletic Training 37(1):19–24, 2002.

Callaghan M.J. et al: 2008 - Effects of patellar taping on knee joint proprioception in patients with patellofemoral pain syndrome, Man Ther 13(3):192–199, 2008.

Camerota F. et al 2010 - Ehlers-Danlos syndrome hypermobility type and the excess of affected females: possible mechanisms and perspectives. American Journal of Medical Genetics A. 2010;152(9):2406–2408. [PubMed]

Carbone L. et al 2000 - Bone density in Ehlers-Danlos syndrome.

Carley M.E. Schaffer J. 2000 - Urinary incontinence and pelvic organ prolapse in women with Marfan or Ehlers Danlos syndrome.

Cassisi G. 2014 - Pain in fibromyalgia and related conditions - Reumatismo, 2014;66(1): 72-86

Castellanos J. 1990 - Effect of habitual knuckle cracking on hand function. Ann Rheum Dis 1990;49:308-309 doi:10.1136/ard.49.5.308 Research Article

Castells M. 2006 - Mast cell mediators in allergic inflammation and mastocytosis. Immunol Allergy Clin North Am. 2006 Aug;26(3):465-85.

Castori M. et al 2010 - Ehlers-Danlos syndrome hypermobility type and the excess of affected females: possible mechanisms and perspectives. American Journal of Medical Genetics A. 2010;152(9):2406–2408. [] PubMed

Castori M. 2010a - Natural History and Manifestations of the Hypermobility Type Ehlers-Danlos Syndrome: A Pilot Study on 21 Patients - www.researchgate.net/publication/41415410_Natural_History_and_Manifestations_of_the_Hypermobility_Type_Ehlers-Danlos_Syndrome_A_Pilot_Study_on_21_Patients

Castori M. et al 2011- Symptom and joint mobility progression in the joint hypermobility syndrome (Ehlers-Danlos syndrome, hypermobility type) Clinical and Experimental Rheumatology. 2011;29:998–1005. [PubMed]

Castori M. 2011a - Unifying concept for various functional somatic syndromes edsiii- somatic-symptoms - edsinfo.wordpress.com/2014/03/06/eds-iii-unifying-concept-for-various-functional-somatic-syndromes/edsiii-somatic-symptoms-p2/

Castori M. 2011b - Chronic fatigue syndrome is commonly diagnosed in patients with Ehlers-Danlos syndrome hypermobility type / Joint hypermobility syndrome. Clin Exp Rheum (in press). www.researchgate.net/publication 51460861_Chronic_fatigue_syndrome_is_commonly_diagnosed_in_patients_with_Ehlers-Danlos_syndrome_hypermobility_typejoint_hypermobility_syndrome

Castori M. 2012 - Ehlers-Danlos Syndrome, Hypermobility Type: An Underdiagnosed Hereditary Connective Tissue Disorder with Mucocutaneous, Articular, and Systemic Manifestations' by Marco Castori, Medical Genetics Dept. of Molecular Medicine www.hindawi.com/isrn/dermatology/2012/751768/ www.ncbi.nlm.nih.gov/pmc/articles/PMC3512326/ (This is an open access article distributed under the Creative Commons Attribution License, which permits unrestricted use, distribution, and reproduction in any medium, provided the original work is properly cited).

Castori M. 2012a - Management of Pain and Fatigue in The Joint Hypermobility Syndrome (a.k.a. Ehlers–Danlos Syndrome, Hypermobility Type): Principles and Proposal for a Multidisciplinary Approach. Americal Journal of Genetics Research Review PDF and American Journal of Medical Genetics A. 2012;158:2055–2070.

Castori M. 2012b - Gynecologic and Obstetric Implications of the Joint Hypermobility Syndrome (a.k.a. Ehlers–Danlos Syndrome Hypermobility Type) in 82 Italian Patients - Wiley Periodicals, Inc. www.afadoc.it/wp/wp-content/uploads/2012/06/35506_fta.pdf

Castori M. 2013 - Joint hypermobility syndrome (a.k.a. Ehlers-Danlos Syndrome, Hypermobility Type): an updated critique. PubMed G Ital Dermatol Venereol. Feb;148(1):13-36.

Castori M. et al 2017 - A framework for the classification of joint hypermobility and related conditions. Am J Med Genet Part C Semin Med Genet 9999C:1–10.

Celletti C. et al 2013a - The multifaceted and complex hypermobility syndrome (a.k.a. Ehlers-Danlos Syndrome Hypermobility Type): Evaluation and management through a rehabilitative approach Clin Ter 2013; 164 (4):e325-335. doi: 10.7417/CT.2013.1597

Celletti. C 2013a - Evaluation of Kinesiophobia and its correlation with pain and fatigue n JHS/EDS_H. Biomed Research Int Volume 2013, Article ID 580460

Centre for FGI and Motility Disorders 2015 -www.med.unc.edu/ibs/files/educational-gi-handouts/What%20Is%20Functional%20GI.pdf

Chakraborty T.K. 1989 - Abnormal cardiovascular reflexes in patients with gastro-oesophageal reflux. Gut 30:46–49.

Chartered Society of Physiotherapy (CSP) - Physiotherapy works: Urinary incontinence - Physiotherapy for women with urinary incontinence is highly clinically effective and cost effective.www.csp.org.uk/professional-union/practice/evidence-base/physiotherapy-works/urinary-incontinence

Charvet P.Y. et al 1991 - Ehlers-Danlos syndrome and pregnancy. Apropos of a case - Service de Gynécologie-Obstétrique, Faculté de Médecine, Lyon Nord, Hôpital Claude-Bernard, Oullins. Journal de Gynecologie, Obstetrique et Biologie de la Reproduction [1991, 20(1): 75-78]

Chello M. et al 1994 - Analysis of collagen and elastin content in primary varicose veins. [J Vasc Surg. 1994

Cheung I. et al 2015 - A New Disease Cluster: Mast Cell Activation Syndrome, Postural Orthostatic Tachycardia Syndrome, and Ehlers-Danlos Syndrome - The Journal of Allergy and Clinical Immunolgy www.jacionline.org/article/S0091-6749(14)02927-3/

Cheung J.P. 2010 - Multiple triggering in a girl with Ehlers-Danlos syndrome www.mendeley.com/research/multiple-triggering-girl-ehlersdanlos-syndrome-case-report

Child A.H. (Ear nose an throat aspects of Marfan Syndrome.pdf www.marfantrust.org/assets/uploads/

Chopra P. 2013a - Complex Regional Pain syndrome updates on treatment. CRPS Partnership in Pain. crpspartnersinpain.com/wp-content/uploads/2013/12/CRPS-update-on-treatment-2013-Philly-06-Compatibility-Mode.pdf

Chopra P. 2013b - Pain management in Ehlers Danlos Syndrome ehlers-danlos.com/2013-annual-conference-files/Chopra_Chronic_pain_and_EDS_Final_1slideS.pdf

Chopra P. 2015 - Pain management in Ehlers Danlos Syndrome – 2015 https://ehlers-danlos.com/2015-annual-conference-files/Chopra.pdf

Chopra P. et al 2017 - Pain management in the Ehlers–Danlos syndromes. Am J Med Genet Part C Semin Med Genet 175C:212–219.

Chronic Pain AU - chronicpainaustralia.org.au/index.php/2013-09-04-07-54-38/pain-physiology

Clayton H.A. 2013 - Proprioceptive sensitivity in Ehlers–Danlos syndrome patients - Exp Brain Res (2013) 230:311–321 DOI 10.1007/s00221-013-3656-4 - deniseh.lab.yorku.ca/files/2013/11/Clayton-Cressman-Henriques-2013.pdf Accessed Nov 201

Cleveland Clinic - Posture for a Healthy Back - my.clevelandclinic.org/health/diseases_conditions/hic_Posture_for_a_Healthy_Back

Clinical Key - Thoracic Outlet syndrome - Anesthesiology www.clinicalkey.com/topics/anesthesiology/thoracic-outlet-syndrome.html

Coelho P.C. Santos 1994 - Osteoporosis and Ehlers Danlos syndrome. Ann Rheum Dis 1994;53:212– 13.

Colì G. 2013 - To prevent the osteoporosis playing in advance. Clin Cases Miner Bone Metab. 2013;10:83–85

College of Medicine - www.collegeofmedicine.org.uk/healthcare-professionals/specialist-groups/neuromusculoskeletal-group/).

Collier D. 2002 - FISH, flexible joints and panic: are anxiety disorders really expressions of instability in the human genome? DOI: 10.1192/bjp.181.6.457 Published 1 December 2002 bjp.rcpsych.org/content/181/6/457

Collins H. 2013 - Title: How Ehlers-Danlos Syndrome Affects Digestion, Nutrition, Bowel Function, and Gut-Related Immune Function. TCAPP Think Tank Published on Sep 15, 2013 www.youtube.com/watch?v=ivtpVu6-rNY

Conner R. 2012 - Postural Orthostatic Tachycardia Syndrome (POTS): Evaluation and Management start node.tpl.php BJMP 2012;5(4):a540

Cuckow P. - The Urinary Tract www.ehlers-danlos.org/the-urinary-tract/#sthash.yzcz53cC.dpuf (The Urinary Tract Peter Cuckow FRCS Registrar in Paediatric Surgery and Urology. St James's University Hospital, Leeds.

Czaprowski D. 2011 - Joint hypermobility in children with idiopathic scoliosis: SOSORT award 2011 winner - scoliosisjournal.biomedcentral.com/articles/10.1186/1748-7161-6-22

Davenport M. 2014 (updated 2016)- Joint Reduction, Hip Dislocation, Posterior. www.emedicine.medscape.com/article/109225-overview

Davis L.M.G. 2010 - A dose dependent impact of prebiotic galactooligosaccharides on the intestinal microbiota of healthy adults. Int J Food Microbiol 2010;144:285–92..

Day M. A. Thorn B.E & Burns J.W. - The continuing evolution of biopsychosocial interventions for chronic pain. J Cogn Psychother. 2012;26(2):114–129)

De S. 2015 - Instant Notes on Immunology Chapter 7 page 17 - ISBN 978-1516829804

De Coster P. J. 2005a - Generalized joint hypermobility and temporomandibular disorders: inherited connective tissue disease as a model with maximum expression. 2005 Winter;19(1):47-57.

De Coster P. J. et al 2005b- Oral health in prevalent types of Ehlers-Danlos syndromes. J Oral Pathol Med. 2005;34:298-307).

Deodhar A. A. et al 1994 - Ehlers Danlos syndrome & osteoporosis (letter). Ann Rheum Dis 1994;53:841–2.

De Kort L.M et al 2003 - Lower urinary tract dysfunction in children with generalised joint hypermobility of joints. Journal of Urology 170:1971-1974

De Paepe A. et al 1996 - Revised criteria for the Marfan syndrome. Am J Med Genet 62:417–426. [CrossRef][Medline][Web of Science]Google Scholar

© Understanding hEDS and HSD by C. Smith

De Paepe A. 2004 - Bleeding and bruising in patients with Ehlers–Danlos syndrome and other collagen vascular disorders. Blackwell Publishing Ltd, British Journal of Haematology, 127, 491–500. www.williams.medicine.wisc.edu/eds.pdf

Desbordes G. et al 2012. - Effects of mindful-attention and compassion medication training on amygdala response to emotional stimuli in an ordinary, non meditative state. Frontiers in human neuroscience, 6.

De Vos M. et al - Preterm premature rupture of membranes in a patient with the hypermobility type of the Ehlers-Danlos syndrome. A case report. 1999

De Wandele I. 2014 - Dysautonomia and its underlying mechanisms in the hypermobility type of Ehlers-Danlos syndrome. Semin. Arthritis Rheum. 44, 93–100. doi: 10.1016/j.semarthrit.2013.12.006

De Wandele I. et al 2014b. Autonomic symptom burden in the hypermobility type of Ehlers- Danlos syndrome: A comparative study with two other EDS types, fibromyalgia, and healthy controls. Semin Arthritis Rheum 44:353–361.

Deweber K. et al 2011 - Knuckle cracking and hand osteoarthritis. Am Board Fam Med. 2011 Mar-Apr;24(2):169-74. doi: 10.3122/jabfm.2011.02.100156.

Dickson M.J & Davis S. 2011 - www.bmj.com/rapid-response/2011/11/03/urinary-incontinence-presenting-feature-joint-hypermobility-syndrome. Writing In response to letter from Ross J & Grahame R. 2011 Hypermobility - easily missed - The British Medical Journal - BMJ 2011; 342 doi: dx.doi.org/10.1136/bmj.c7167 (Published 20 January 2011) Cite this as: BMJ 2011;342:c7167)

Dieli-Conwright CM. Spektor TM, Rice JC, et al. 2009 - Influence of hormone replace.ment therapy on eccentric exercise induced myogenic gene expression in postmenopausal women. J Appl Physiol. 2009;107:1381–8.

Dietz H.C. & Pyeritz R.E. 1995 - Mutations in the human gene for fibrillin-1 (FBN1) in the Marfan syndrome and related disorders. Hum Mol Genet. 1995;4 Spec No:1799-809.

Dinet.org - Dysautonomia Information Network - www.dinet.org

Dolan A.L. 1997. Clinical and echocardiographic survey of the Ehlers-Danlos syndrome. Br J Rheumatol 36:459–462.

Dolan A.L. et al 1998 - Assessment of bone in Ehlers Danlos syndrome by ultrasound and densitometry Ann Rheum Dis 57:630- 3 [Medline]

Dommerhault J. 2016 - Overcome Kinesiophobia www.bethesdaphysiocare.com/overcome-kinesiophobia/ accessed Dec 2016

Donkervoort S. et al 2015 - The neuromuscular differential diagnosis of joint hypermobility. Am J Med Genet C Semin Med Genet. 2015 Mar; 169C(1):23-42. doi: 10.1002/ajmg.c.31433.

Driscoll D. - The Role of External Communicating Hydrocephalus, Mast Cell Disease and CCSVI as the cause of POTS (Postural Orthostatic Tachycardia Syndrome) in Ehlers-Danlos Syndrome - https://slingsandarrowsofoutrageousfortune.wordpress.com/the-driscoll-theory/

Duke Centre for Human Genetics - Chiari Type I Malformation Research - Chiari Whole Genome Linkage Screen Completed (Chiari Malformation and Ehlers Danlos Syndrome) 2012 dmpi.duke.edu/files/inline/chiari_newsletter_2012.pdf

Dysautonomia International - Postural Orthostatic Tachycardia syndrome www.dysautonomiainternational.org/page.php?ID=30

Earley C J. (2003). "Restless Legs Syndrome". New England Journal of Medicine 348 (21): 2103–9. doi:10.1056/NEJMcp021288. PMID 12761367.

Eccles J. A. 2012 - Brain structure and joint hypermobility: relevance to the expression of psychiatric symptoms. Br. J. Psychiatry 200, 508–509. doi: 10.1192/bjp.bp.111.09246

Eccles J. A. 2014a - Joint hypermobility and autonomic hyperactivity: relevance to neurodevelopmental disorders. J. Neurol. Neurosurg. Psychiatry 85, e3–e3. doi: 10.1136/jnnp-2014-308883.9

Eccles J. A 2014b - Joint hypermobility and autonomic hyperactivity: relevance to the expression of psychiatric symptoms. Psychosom. Med. 76, A80.

Eccles J. A. 2015 - Neurovisceral phenotypes in the expression of psychiatric symptoms - REVIEW ARTICLE Front. Neurosci., 10 February 2015 | dx.doi.org/10.3389/fnins.2015.00004 - www.journal.frontiersin.org/article/10.3389/fnins.2015.00004/full

EDSInfo.org 2013 - Understanding Your Fascia - edsinfo.wordpress.com/2013/12/07/understanding-your-fascia/

1) EDS Support UK - Ehlers-Danlos Syndrome - 'Misguided' Child Protection Concerns www.ehlers-danlos.org/useful-info/ehlers-danlos-syndrome-child-protection-concerns#sthash.QT18vqMA.dpufy1

2) EDS Support UK - Fibromyalgia - www.ehlers-danlos.org/fibromyalgia-and-cf

3) EDS Support UK - Autonomic Dysfunction - Alan Hakim and Rodney Grahame writing for www.ehlers-danlos.org/about-edsautonomic-dysfunction/autonomic-dysfunction-sheet#sthash.T2s3x1uk.dpuf

4) EDS Support UK - FODMAP diet - by Marianne Williams, NHS & Private Specialist IBS & Allergy Dietitian, - See more at: www.ehlers-danlos.org/about-eds/diet-and-eds/fodmap-diet/#sthash.4pqtP8Iu.dpufmany

5) EDS Support UK - Dr Brad Tinkle writing for Fragile Links Magazine Spring 2015 page 38

6) EDS Support UK - The Urinary Tract. By Peter Cuckow FRCS Registrar in Paediatric Surgery and Urology. St James's University Hospital, Leeds. www.ehlers-danlos.org/about-eds/medical-information/the-urinary-tract/#sthash.kIEGTw5I.dpuf

7) EDS Support UK - Dr Atul A Deodhar MD MRCP - EDS and Osteoporosis - writing for EDS UK www.ehlers-danlos.org/about-eds/medical-information/osteoporosis/#sthash.5bHcVERg.dpuf

8) EDS Support UK - Hormonal Aspects of Ehlers-Danlos. plus.google.com/+Ehlers-danlosOrg/posts/Xs88rYW1jrA

9) EDS Support UK - Splinting and bracing in EDS - Redmond A and Dr Siddle writing for EDS Support UK - www.ehlers-danlos.org/patient-support/management-advice/physio-and-management/rnoh-rehabilitation/splinting-and-bracing-in-eds/#sthash.4pGKv3yF.dpuf

10) EDS Support UK - How is Ehlers-Danlos syndrome inherited? www.ehlers-danlos.org/about-eds/types-of-eds/hypermobility-ehlers-danlos-syndrome/

11) EDS Support UK - Footcare in hEDS - www.ehlers-danlos.org/about-eds/medical-information/footcare/#sthash.KZ1WG5QU.dpuf.

1) EDNF.org - Ehlers-Danlos National Foundation – What are the types of EDS - www.ednf.org/index.php?option=com_content&task=view&id=1348&Itemid=88888969 and www.ednf.org/index.php?option=com_content&task=view&id=1360&Itemid=88889296

2) EDNF.org - Pain Management Medical Resource Guide - ednf.org/sites/default/files/MRGPainManagementS.pdf

3) EDNF.org - Physiotherapy management of the hypermobile patient. ednf.org/medical-professionals/physical-therapy-management-hypermobile-patient Accessed Nov 2014
4)
5) EDNF.org - Chronic Pain and EDS. ednf.org/sites/default/files/Chopra_Chronic_pain_and_EDS_Final_1slideS.pdf

5) EDNF.org - Dysautonomia associated with hypermobility www.ednf.org/faq/dysautonomia-associated-hypermobility

6) EDNF.org - www.ednf.org/sites/default/files/loose-connections/winter2010.pdf

7) EDNF.org - Dental Manifestations And Considerations In Treating Patients With Ehlers-Danlos Syndrome/#content-header. School of Dental Medicine - University of Connecticut - Originally published in Loose Connections Vol VIII, No.4 1993

8) EDNF.org - Gastrointestinal Manifestations of Ehlers-Danlos syndrome - www.ednf.org/images/stories/pdfs_medical/2012/1996_GI_Manifestations_of_Ehlers-Danlos_Syndrome.pdf

9) EDNF.org - There are six major types of EDS - www.ednf.org/eds-types

10) EDNF.org EDS Medical Resource Guide. www.ednf.org/medical-resource-guides) - Olson T. 2010

11) EDNF.org - The Skin. www.ednf.org/medical-professionals/skin-ehlers-danlos-syndrome - 2014

12) EDNF.org - Some Obstetric and gynaecological issues www.ednf.org/faq/what-are-some-obgyn-issues-ehlers-danlos-syndrome - 2015

1) Ehlers-Danlos Society 2017 - What is Ehlers-Danlos syndrome? ehlers-danlos.com/what-is-eds/

2/Ehlers-Danlos Society 2017 - Criteria for hypermobile Ehlers-Danlos syndrome - General Comment. ehlers-danlos.com/wp-content/uploads/hEDSvHSD.pdf

3/ Ehlers-Danlos Society 2017 - International Classification: Your Questions Answered PDF

4/Ehlers-Danlos Society 2017 - EDS Diagnostics 2017 - ehlers-danlos.com/eds-diagnostics/

5/ Ehlers-Danlos Society 2017 - What is HSD? ehlers-danlos.com/what-is-hsd/

6/ Ehlers-Danlos Society 2017 - hEDS v HSD https://ehlers-danlos.com/wp-content/uploads/hEDSvHSD.pdf

Eldridge J. 2014 - Fat pad impingement and hyperextension - explained in person

el-Shahaly H.A. & el-Sherif A.K. 1991 - Is the benign joint hypermobility syndrome benign? Clin Rheumatol 10:302–307.

Em S. 2013 - Serum prolidase activity in benign joint hypermobility syndrome BMC Musculoskeletal Disorders201415:75 DOI: 10.1186/1471-2474-15-75© Em et al.; licensee BioMed Central Ltd. 2014 Received: 27 April 2013Accepted: 4 March 2014

Encyclopedia Britannica - Mast Cell - www.britannica.com/science/mast-cell

Engelbert R.H. et al 2003. Pediatric generalized joint hypermobility with and without musculoskeletal complaints: A localized or systemic disorder? Pediatrics 111: e248–e254.

Ensor H. - Stickman Communications. www.stickmancommunications.co.uk. Also, Patron and HSD Ambassador for the Hypermobility Syndromes Association.

ENTnet.org - American Academy of Otolaryngology – Head & Neck Surgery www.entnet.org/HealthInformation/deviatedSeptum.cfm

Eorthopod.com - Complex Regional Pain syndrome www.eorthopod.com/complex-regional-pain-syndrome/topic/204 emedicinehealth.com - www.emedicinehealth.com/costochondritis/article_em.htm accessed April 2015

Evans A.M. & Rome K. 2011. A Cochrane review of the evidence for non-surgical interventions for flexible pediatric flat feet. Eur J Phys Rehabil Med 47:69–89.

Faber W.J. - Fybromyalgia and Hypermobility Syndrome milwaukeepainclinic.com/alternativeTherapy/fibromyalgiaHypermobilitySyndrome

Farmer A.D. & Aziz Q. - writing for Ehlers-Danlos Support UK Gastrointestinal Manifestations of Ehlers-Danlos syndrome. nebula.wsimg.com/ea54d776ae34853f0d97622a25fa174d?AccessKeyId=F84C79052E9E63499433&disposition=0&alloworigin=1

Farmer A.D & Aziz Q. 2014 - It's a gut feeling: how the gut microbiota affects the state of mind. J Physiol. 2014 Jul 15;592(Pt 14):2981-8. doi: 10.1113/jphysiol.2013.270389. Epub 2014 Mar 24.

Farmer A.D. et al 2009 - Unexplained Gastrointestinal Symptoms in Joint Hypermobility: Is connective tissue the missing link? British Journal of Reumatology 2009

Feinberg Joseph H. -Thoracic Outlet Syndrome (TOS): An Overview www.hss.edu/conditions_thoracic-outlet-syndrome-overview.asp

Felson D.T. 2009 - The effects of impaired joint position sense on the development and progression of pain and structural damage in knee osteoarthritis Arthritis Rheum. Aug 15, 2009; 61(8): 1070–1076.doi: 10.1002/art.24606 PMCID: PMC2758271NIHMSID: NIHMS137677

Ferrar M. Sheridan P. and West J. 2012 - Postural Tachycardia Syndrome www.potsuk.org/classification Produced 30/3/12

Ferrell W. & Ferrell P. 2010 - Hypermobility, Fibromyalgia and Chronic Pain. Author/Edited by: Hakim A. & Keer R. ISBN : 9780702030055 Publication Date : 15-09-2010 Published by Elsevier

Fikree A. et al 2013 - Joint hypermobility syndrome. Rheum Dis Clin North Am. 2013 May;39(2):419-30. doi: 10.1016/j.rdc.2013.03.003.

Fikree A. et al 2014 - A Prospective Evaluation of Undiagnosed Joint Hypermobility Syndrome in Patients With Gastrointestinal Symptoms. Clin Gastroenterol Hepatol. 2014 Jan 16. pii: S1542-3565(14)00049-4. doi: 10.1016/j.cgh.2014.01.014.

Fikree A. et al 2017. Gastrointestinal involvement in the Ehlers–Danlos syndromes. Am J Med Genet Part C Semin Med Genet 9999C:1–7.

Fillingim R. B. 2009 - Sex, gender, and pain: a review of recent clinical and experimental findings. J Pain. 2009 May;10(5):447-85. doi: 10.1016/j.jpain.2008.12.001.

Finkbohner R. et al 1995 - Mafan syndrome. Long term survival and complications after aortic aneurysm repair

Foot.com - Over pronation. www.foot.com/site/foot-conditions/over-pronation Accessed 2015.

Footjax.com - Proprioception - footjax.com/technical-expertise/proprioception-kinesthetic-awareness/injuries-cause-a-proprioceptive-deficit/

Fragile Links, spring 2015, page 38 - Dr Brad Tinkle writing for EDS Support UK

Francomano C.A. 2006 - The Spine and the Craniocervical Junction in Ehlers-Danlos Syndrome. Program Nr: 285 for the 2006 ASHG Annual Meeting

Francomano C. 2011 - EDS Update - What We Know and What We Don't Know. www.ednf.org/images/2011conference/Handouts/Francomano_EDS2011_What_ We_Know.pptx

Francomano C. & Bloom L. 2017 - The 2017 EDS International Classification Webinar: Your Questions Answered 1. Transcript of March 15, 2017 https://ehlers-danlos.com/wp-content/uploads/QandA_Webinar_Transcript.pdf

Freeman M.D. 2010 - A case-control study of cerebellar tonsillar ectopia (Chiari) and head/neck trauma (whiplash). Brain Inj. 2010; 24(7-8):988-94.

Freeman R. et al., 2011 - Consensus statement on the definition of orthostatic hypotension, neurally mediated syncope and the postural tachycardia syndrome. Autonomic Neuroscience: Basic and Clinical 161 (2011) 46-48.

Freidberg F. 2016 - Cognitive-behavior therapy: why is it so vilified in the chronic fatigue syndrome community? | Fatigue: Biomedicine, Health & Behavior | 7 July 2016

Frieri M. 2013 - Mast cell activation syndrome: a review. www.ncbi.nlm.nih.gov/pubmed/23179866 - Curr Allergy Asthma Rep. 2013 Feb;13(1):27-32. doi: 10.1007/s11882-012-0322-z.

Frizzierob A. 2014 - Muscles Ligaments Tendons J. 2014 Jul-Sep; Impact of oestrogen deficiency and aging on tendon: concise review - 4(3): 324–328. Published online 2014 Nov 17.PMCID: PMC4241423

Fu, Q. 2010 - Menstrual cycle affects renal-adrenal and hemodynamic responses during prolonged standing in the postural orthostatic tachycardia syndrome. Hypertension 56, 82–90. doi: 10.1161/HYPERTENSIONAHA.110.151787

Fu Q. & Levine B. 2014 Exercise in the postural orthostatic tachycardia syndrome. Institute for Exercise and Environmental Medicine, Texas Health Presbyterian Hospital Dallas, The University of Texas Southwestern Medical Center, Dallas, TX, USA
DOI: dx.doi.org/10.1016/j.autneu.2014.11.008 |

Fuerst M.L 2014 - Mast Cell Activation Disorders On the Rise www.medpagetoday.com/resource-center/anaphylaxis-advances/mast-cells/a/46719

Gaisl T. et al 2017 - Thorax Jan 2017- The full article can be accessed at: www.ncbi.nlm.nih.gov/pubmed/28073822, and the abstract is shown below:

Gangemi. S 2012 - sock-doc.com/2013/04/case-for-orthotics/ - Accessed Dec 2014

García Campayo J. 2010 - Association between joint hypermobility syndrome and panic disorder: a case-control study. Psychosomatics. 2010 Jan-Feb; 51(1):55-61. [PubMed]

Gazit J. et al 2003 - Dystautonomia in the hypermobility syndrome. American Journal of Medicine 115:33-40

Gedalia A. et al 1993a - Joint hypermobility in pediatric practice–a review. J Rheumatol. 1993;20:371 –374.

Gedalia A. et al 1993b Joint hypermobility and fibromyalgia in schoolchildren. Ann Rheum Dis 1993 52: 494-496 doi: 10.1136/ard.52.7.494

Gerhard J. 2011 - Mast cell activation disease: a concise practical guide for diagnostic workup and therapeutic options. J Hematol Oncol. 2011; 4: 10. Published online 2011 Mar 22. doi: 10.1186/1756-8722-4-10PMCID: PMC3069946

Germain D. 2012 - Ehlers-Danlos syndrome, hypermobility September 2012 www.orpha.net/consor/cgi-bin/OC_Exp.php?Lng=EN&Expert=285

Germain D. - Ehlers-Danlos syndrome, hypermobility type www.orpha.net/consor/cgi-bin/OC_Exp.php?Lng=EN&Expert=285

Gharbiya M. et al 2009 - Ocular features in joint hypermobility syndrome/ehlers-danlos syndrome hypermobility type: a clinical and in vivo confocal microscopy study. 2009;111(1-3):84-8.

1) ghr.nlm.nih.gov - What is Ehlers-Danlos syndrome - Your guide to understanding genetic conditions - viewed Jan 2015 ghr.nlm.nih.gov/condition/ehlers-danlos-syndrome

2)ghr.nlm.nih.gov - Penetrance expressivity. viewed Feb 2015. ghr.nlm.nih.gov/handbook/inheritance/penetranceexpressivity

3)ghr.nlm.nih.gov - What is DNA? ghr.nlm.nih.gov/handbook/basics/dna
Glenny J. 2013 - Hypermobility on the mat: some pointers for teaching yoga to people with Ehlers Danlos / Hypermobility Syndrome movingprayer.wordpress.com/2013/06/05/teaching-yoga-to-people-with-hypermobility/

Glesby M. J. 1989 - Association of mitral valve prolapse and systemic abnormalities of connective tissue. A phenotypic continuum. JAMA. 1989 Jul 28;262(4):523-8. PubMed

Goldschneider K. 2013 - What Pain Feels Like For Someone With Ehlers-Danlos Syndrome

Goldstein E. 2013 - The Now Effect. Publisher: Atria Books; Reprint edition (25 April 2013) ISBN-10: 1451623895 ISBN-13: 978-1451623895

Gosney MB. Unusual presentation of a case of Ehlers-Danlos syndrome. Br Dent J. 1987;163(2):54-6. [PubMed]

Grahame R. 1981 - A clinical and echocardiographic study of patients with teh hypermobility syndrome. Annals of the Rheumatic Diseases 40:541 - 546

Grahame R. & Pyeritz 1995 - Marfan syndrome: joint and skin manifestations are prevalent and correlated. Br J Rheumatol 34:126–131.

Grahame R. 1999 - Joint hypermobility and genetic collagen disorders: are they related? Arch Dis Child 1999;80:188-191 doi:10.1136/adc.80.2.188 Archive of Diseases in Childhood

Grahame R. et al 2000 - The revised (Brighton 1998) criteria for the diagnosis of benign joint hypermobility syndrome (BJHS). Rheumatol 2000. 271777–1779.1779.

Grahame R. 2007 - The Need to Take a Fresh Look at Criteria for Hypermobility - The Journal of Rheumatology jrheum.com

Grahame R. 2012a - Pain and Joint Hypermobility syndromes - hypermobility.org/help-advice/pain-management-2/pain-and-jhs/ Accessed Nov 2014

Grahame R. 2012b - British consultant rheumatologists' perceptions about the hypermobility syndrome: a national survey - rheumatology.oxfordjournals.org/content/40/5/559.short
Grahame R. 2012c - Speech given at HMSA Residential Patient Conference.

Grahame R. & Kazkaz H. 2014 - The rheumatological heritable disorders of connective tissue May 2014 Volume 42, Issue 5, Pages 275–278 Rheumatol. 2004;31:173 –178.

Grant M. 2012 - Ten Tips For Communicating With A Person Suffering From Chronic Pain. overcomingpain.com/self-help/pain-10-tips-for-communicating-with-a-pain-sufferer/

Gratacos M. et al 2001 - A polymorphic genomic duplication on human chromosome 15 is a major susceptibility genetic factor for panic and phobic disorders. Cell. 2001;106:367-379.

Greising S.M. et al. 2009 - Hormone therapy and skeletal muscle strength: a meta-analysis. J Gerontol A Biol Sci Med Sci. 2009;64(10): 1071–81.

Grelsamer R. 2008 - Conditions interfering with patellofemoral mechanics (part 4a of a course on Patellofemoral Pain). www.kneeguru.co.uk/KNEEnotes/courses/patellofemoral-pain-course-ronald-grelsamer-md/conditions-interfering-patellofemoral

Grubb B.P. - The potential of serotonin pathogenesis of neurocardiogenic syncope and related autonomic disturbances. Journal of Interventional Cardiac Electrophysiology, 2, 325-332.

Grubb B. P. & Kanjwal K. et al 2006 - The Postural Tachycardia Syndrome - A Concise Guide to Diagnosis and Management. J. Cardiovasc Electrophysiol. 2006;17(1):108-112.

Grubb B.P. 2008 - Postural Orthostatic Tachycardia syndrome - 2008; 117: 2814-2817 doi: 10.1161/CIRCULATIONAHA.107.761643

Guinane C.M. 2013 - Role of the gut microbiota in health and chronic gastrointestinal disease: understanding a hidden metabolic organ Therap Adv Gastroenterol. 2013 Jul; 6(4): 295–308. doi: 10.1177/1756283X13482996 PMCID: PMC3667473

Gulbahar S. et al 2006 - Hypermobility Syndrome Increases the risk for low bone mass.2006 Jul;25(4):511-4. Epub 2005 Nov 26.

Gunter K.B. 2012 - Physical activity in childhood may be the key to optimizing lifespan skeletal health. Exerc Sport Sci Rev. 2012;40:13–21. doi: 10.1097/JES.0b013e318236e5ee.

Gurley-Green S. 2001 - Living with the hypermobility syndrome. Oxford Journals, Medicine & Health, Rheumatology, Volume 40, Issue 5, Pp. 487-489

Hakala R.V. 2005 - Prolotherapy (proliferation therapy) in the treatment of TMD. Cranio 23:283–288.

Hakim A. J. & Grahame R.- 2003 - A simple questionnaire to detect hypermobility: an adjunct to the assessment of patients with diffuse musculoskeletal pain. Int J Clin Practice 2003;57:163–

Hakim A. J. and Grahame R 2004. Non-musculoskeletal symptoms in joint hypermobility syndrome. Indirect evidence for autonomic dysfunction? For The Oxford Journals 04

Hakim A. J. et al 2005 - Local anaesthetic failure in joint hypermobility syndrome. J R Soc Med. 2005 Feb; 98(2): 84-5.

Hakim A. J. 2006 - Joint hypermobility and skin elasticity: the hereditary disorders of connective tissue. Clinics in Dermatology, vol. 24, no. 6, pp. 521–533, 2006.

Hakim A. J. Keer R. Grahame G. 2010 - Pain Management and Cognitive Therapy. Chapter 8 in Hypermobility, Fibromyalgia, and Chronic Pain. Eds, Churchill Livingston, London

Hakim A.J. 2011 - 3rd Edition - Oxford Handbook of Rheumatology

Hakim A.J. 2012 (HMSA) - The Brighton Criteria for JHS Oct 2012 www.hypermobility.org

Hakim A. J. 2013a (HMSA) - Genes and Inheritance www.hypermobility.org Viewed Jan 2015

Hakim A.J. 2013b (HMSA) - Is there a difference between Joint Hypermobility Syndrome (JHS) and Ehlers Danlos www.hypermobility.org

Hakim A.J. 2013c (HMSA) - Clinician's Guide to JHS www.hypermobility.org Viewed 2014

Hakim A. J. 2013d (HMSA) - Bowel in JHS & EDS www.hypermobility.org Viewed 2014

Hakim A.J. 2013e (HMSA) - Pain and Hypermobility Syndromes - www.hypermobility.org

Hakim A.J 2013f (HMSA) - Bladder and the pelvic floor - www.hypermobility.org

Hakim A.J. 2013g (HMSA) - The Skin in JHS and EDS. hypermobility.org/help-advice/the-skin/

Hakim A.J & Keer R. 2013h (HMSA) - Pregnancy - hypermobility.org/help-advice/pregnancy/

Hakim A.J. 2013i - Pain Medication and HMSs - hypermobility.org/help-advice/pain-management-2/pain-medication-information/

Hakim A.J. 2014a - Hypermobility and HDCTs - an overview - HMSA Journal Autumn 2014

Hakim A.J. 2014b - (HMSA) Trifold - Have you, or someone you know, recently been diagnosed with an HDCT v1.6

Hakim A.J 2014c (HMSA) - Chiari Malformation and EDS/JHS - www.hypermobility.org Viewed 2015

Hakim A. J. 2016a - Postural Orthostatic Tachycardia syndrome - Private email correspondence

Hakim A.J. 2016b (HMSA) - HMSA Journal Article Volume 6 - The bowel

Hakim A. J. et al 2017a - Cardiovascular autonomic dysfunction in Ehlers–Danlos syndrome—Hypermobile type. Am J Med Genet Part C Semin Med Genet 9999C:1–7.

Hakim A.J. et al 2017b - Chronic fatigue in Ehlers–Danlos syndrome—Hypermobile type. Am J Med Genet Part C Semin Med Genet 175C: 175–180.

Hakim A.J 2017c (HMSA) - Hypermobility Disorders; an update for clinicians. hypermobility.org/update-for-clinicians/ March 16th 2017

Hall M.G et al 1995 - The effect of the hypermobility syndrome on knee joint proprioception. Br J Rheumatol 34:121_5

Halmos E.P. 2014 - A diet low in FODMAPs reduces symptoms of irritable bowel syndrome. Gastroenterol 2014;146:67–75.

Hamilton M.J. 2011 - Mast cell activation syndrome: a newly recognized disorder with systemic clinical manifestations. J Allergy Clin Immunol. 2011; 128: 147–152 (e142)

Hamonet C. 2017 - Ehlers-Danlos Syndrome (EDS), an Hereditary, Frequent and Disabling Disease, Victim of Iatrogenia due to Widespread Ignorance. International Journal of Emergency Mental Health and Human Resilience, Vol. 17, No.3, pp. 661-663

Handa S. et al 2001 - Ehlers-Danlos syndrome with bladder diverticula. Br J Dermatol. 2001 - May;144(5):1084-5.

Handler C.E. et al 1985 - Mitral Valve Prolapse, aortic compliance, and skin collagen in joint hypermobility syndrome. British Heart Journal 54:501 - 508

Hargrave T. 2008 - Proprioception - the 3D Map of the Body. www.bettermovement.org/2008/proprioception-the-3-d-map-of-the-body/

Harris J.G. - Respiratory symptoms in children with Ehlers- Danlos syndrome PDF Clinical Communication

Haviland M.G. et al 2012 - Fibromyalgia: prevalence, course, and co-morbidities in hospitalized patients in the United States, 1999-2007. Clin Exp Rheumatol. 2011 Nov-Dec;29(6 Suppl 69):S79-87. Epub 2012 Jan 3.

Hawkins R. J. et al 1983 - Recurrent posterior instability (subluxation) of the shoulder. J Bone Joint Surg Am. 1984 Feb; 66(2):169-74. [PubMed]

Healthline.com Arthritis Knee Noise: Crepitus and Popping Explained - healthline.com/health/osteoarthritis/crepitus#Overview1

Hefti F. 2007 - Pediatric Orthopedics in Practice - Published by Springer-Verlag Berlin Heidelberg

Helliwell P. et al 2011, Senior Lecturer in Rhematology at the Leeds University, writing for the Arthritis Research UK - / www.arthritisresearchuk.org/health-professionals-and-students/reports/topical-reviews/topical-reviews-spring-2011.aspx

Henkel G - Function Despite Pain -Strides in recognition and management of joint hypermobility syndrome www.the-rheumatologist.org/details/article/865565/Function_Despite_Pain.html

Henderson Sr. F.C. et al 2017 - Neurological and spinal manifestations of the Ehlers–Danlos syndromes. Am J Med Genet Part C Semin Med Genet 175C:195–211.

Hermanns-Le T. et al 2007 - Ultrastructural alterations of elastic fibers and other dermal components in ehlers-danlos syndrome of the hypermobile type. Am J Dermatopathol. 2007; 29:370-3. l Article l PubMed
Hermanns-Lê T. et al 2012a - (We support the concept that BJHS represents a mild variant of EDSH) Dermal Ultrastructure in Low Beighton Score Members of 17 Families with Hypermobile-Type Ehlers-Danlos Syndrome 3 October 2012

Hermanns-Le T. et al 2012b - Fibromyalgia: an unrecognized Ehlers-Danlos syndrome hypermobile type? www.researchgate.net/publication/235748437_Fibromyalgia_an_unrecognized_Ehlers-Danlos_syndrome_hypermobile_type [accessed Jul 29, 2015]. ().

Hermanns-Lê T. et al 2014 - Gynecologic and obstetric impact of the ehlers-danlos syndrome : clues from scrutinizing dermal ultrastructural alterations. Research Journal of Women's Health - Gynecology ISSN 2052-6210. www.hoajonline.com/gynecology/2052-6210/2/1

Hertel J. 2002 - Functional Anatomy, Pathomechanics, and Pathophysiology of Lateral Ankle Instability. J Athl Train. 2002 Oct-Dec; 37(4): 364–375. PMCID: PMC164367

Hickmott R. 1987 - BAppSc (Physio); PGDip (Sports Physio); GCert Clinical Physiotherapy (Women's Health & Continence) Sports and pelvic floor physiotherapist, Riseley Physio - Joint hypermobility syndrome 1987 Dec;30(12):1426-30.

Hickmott R. 2013 - Active Wear - Joint hypermobility syndrome bodyplus.net.au/active-wear-joint-hypermobility-syndrome/ Accessed 2013

Hildebrand K. A. et al 2008 - Cellular, matrix, and growth factor components of the joint capsule are modified early in the process of posttraumatic contracture formation in a rabbit model. Published in final edited form as: Acta Orthop. Feb 2008; 79(1): 116–125. doi: 10.1080/17453670710014860 PMCID: PMC2950862 CAMSID: CAMS854 Acta Orthop. Author manuscript; available in PMC Oct 6, 2010.

1/ HMSA 2014 - Have you, or someone you know, been diagnosed with one of the hypermobility syndromes? Trifold Leaflet - Copy written by Alan Hakim, Donna Wicks and Claire Smith

2/ HMSA 2015 - Living well with a heritable disorder of connective tissue - V3.4 Heading: Relief of severe pain and using pain killers effectively. Copy written by Claire Smith, Donna Wicks and Alan Hakim

3/ HMSA 2014 - An educator's guide to the hypermobile child - V3.9 - Copy written by Claire Smith, Donna Wicks and Alan Hakim

4/ HMSA 2014 - Hormones and hypermobility - HMSA website - by Dr Howard Bird and later updated by Hakim A. hypermobility.org/help-advice/hormones-hypermobility/

5/HMSA 2014 - Hypermobility in Heritable Disorders of Connective Tissue - An Overview. Basic Essentials for medical professionals and members wanting to learn about these conditions. HMSA Journal Volume 2 Autumn/Winter 2014 v.1.2, page 31

6/HMSA 2017 - Statement of Position on 2017 International Criteria for Ehlers-Danlos syndromes - re: hypermobility.org/sop2017eds/

7/HMSA 2013 - Pain and Hypermobility Syndrome - www.hmsa.org

8/HMSA 2014 - 'Help and Advice' introduction on website. Hakim A.J. , Smith C.E. , Wicks D.

Holman A. 2008 - Positional cervical spinal cord compression and fibromyalgia: a novel comorbidity with important diagnostic and treatment implications. J Pain. 2008 Jul;9(7):613-22. doi: 10.1016/j.jpain. 2008.01.339. Epub 2008 May 22.

Hongliang L. et al 2014 - Autoimmune Basis for Postural Tachycardia Syndrome. J Am Heart Assoc. 2014; 3: e000755 originally published February 26, 2014 doi: 10.1161/JAHA.113.000755

Houben R.M.A..et al 2005 - Fear of movement/injury in the general population: factor structure and psychometric properties of an adapted version of the Tampa Scale for Kinesiophobia. Journal of Behavioral Medicine. 2005;28(5):415–424. [PubMed]

Houglum P.A. 2001 - Therapeutic Exercise for Athletic Injuries by (2001). Peggy A. Houglum I ISBN-10: 0880118431 I ISBN-13: 9780880118439.

Hows J. 2000 - Dance Technique and Injury Prevention Page 97

Hueber A.J. et al 2010 - Mast cells express IL-17A in rheumatoid arthritis synovium J. Immunol., 184 (2010), pp. 3336–3340
Hughes C.L. 2015 - Odontectomy in treatment of Ehlers-Danlos syndrome: report of case. J Oral Surg. 1970;28(8):612-4. [PubMed]

Hughston J.C.1968 - Subluxation of the patella. J Bone Joint Surg (Am) 50:1003-1026,1968

Hughston J.C. 1979 - Proximal and distal reconstruction of the extensor mechanism for patella subluxation. Clin Orthop 144:36-42,1979

Hugon-Rodin J. et al 2016 - Gynecologic symptoms and the influence on reproductive life in 386 women with hypermobility type ehlers-danlos syndrome: a cohort study. Orphanet J Rare Dis. 2016 Sep 13;11(1):124. doi: 10.1186/s13023-016-0511-2.

Hunt, B. E. 2001 - Estrogen replacement therapy improves baroreflex regulation of vascular sympathetic outflow in postmenopausal women. Circulation 103, 2909–2914. doi: 10.1161/01.CIR.103.24.2909

Hunt K. - Hip and Knee Pain www.spinalphysio.co.uk/hip-and-knee-pain

Huygen F.J. 2004 - Mast cells are involved in inflammatory reactions during Complex Regional Pain Syndrome type 1.Immunol Lett. 2004 Feb 15;91(2-3):147-154. Pain Treatment Center, Department of Anesthesiology, P.O. Box 2040, 3000 CA Rotterdam, The Netherlands.

Ireland P.D. et al 1996 - Evaluation of the autonomic cardiovascular response in Ar- nold-Chiari deformities and cough syncope syndrome. Arch Neurol 53:526–531.

In^es M. 2008 - Prevalence of temporomandibular dysfunction in patients with cervical pain under physiotherapy treatment. Fisioter Mov 21:63–70.

Inspire.com/groups/ehlers-danlos-national-foundation/ Accessed November 2014

Ions G. - What is EDS - Medical Information. www.ehlers-danlos.org/what-is-eds/medical-information/9-medical-information/151-chiari-1-malformation

Jacob G. 2000 - The neuropathic postural tachycardia syndrome. N Engl J Med2000;343:1008–1014.

Jacome D.E. 1999 - Headache in Ehlers-Danlos syndrome. Cephalalgia. 1999;19(9):791–796. [PubMed]

Janz K.F. 2010 - Early physical activity provides sustained bone health benefits later in childhood. Med Sci Sports Exerc. 2010;42:1072–1078.

Järvinen M. et al 1997 - Histopathological findings in chronic tendon disorders. Scand J Med Sci Sports. 1997 Apr;7(2):86-95.

Jarvis S. 2013 - How to calm restless legs - www.goodhousekeeping.co.uk/health/health-advice/calming-restless-legs

Jha S. et al 2007 - Prevalence of incontinence in women with benign joint hypermobility syndrome. Int Urogynecol J Pelvic Floor Dysfunct. 2007 Jan;18(1):61-4. Epub 2006 Mar 31. PubMed PMID: 16575484.

Johnson S.M. 2010 - Shoulder instability in patients with joint hyperlaxity. J Bone Joint Surg Am. 2010 Jun; 92(6):1545-57.

Johnston B.A. 2006 Ehlers-Danlos syndrome: complications and solutions concerning anesthetic management. Middle East J Anesthesiol. 2006;18:1171-1184 [PubMed])

Jones T.L,. 2008 - Anaesthesia for caesarean section in a patient with Ehlers-Danlos syndrome associated with postural orthostatic tachycardia syndrome. Int J Obstet Anesth. 2008 Oct; 17(4):365-9.

Jordan J. 2002 - Increased sympathetic activation in idiopathic orthostatic intolerance: Role of systemic adrenoreceptor sensitivity. Hypertension 2002;39:173–178.

Judge D.P 2005 - Marfan's syndrome. Lancet. Author manuscript; available in PMC 2006 Jul 19. Published in final edited form as: Lancet. 2005 Dec 3; 366(9501): 1965–1976. doi: 10.1016/ S0140-6736(05)67789-6 PMCID: PMC1513064 NIHMSID: NIHMS10620

© Understanding hEDS and HSD by C. Smith

Jung M. 2013). (J Biol Chem. 2013 Feb 1;288(5):3289-304. doi: 10.1074/jbc.M112.387811. Epub 2012 Dec 12. Mast cells produce novel shorter forms of perlecan that contain functional endorepellin: a role in angiogenesis and wound healing.

Juul-Kristensen B, et al 2007. Inter-examiner reproducibility of tests and criteria for generalized joint hyper- mobility and benign joint hypermobility syndrome. Rheumatology 46:1835–1841.

Juul-Kristensen B. et al 2017 - Measurement properties of clinical assessment methods for classifying generalized joint hypermobility—A systematic review. Am J Med Genet Part C Semin Med Genet 175C:116–147.

Kakadia N. et al 2011 - Ehlers-Danlos syndrome and overview JCPR-2011-3-3-98-107.pdf - jocpr.com/vol3-iss3-2011/JCPR-2011-3-3-98-107.pdf and J. Chem. Pharm. Res., 2011, 3(3):98-107

Kanjwal K. et al 2009 - Outcomes of pregnancy in patients with Postural Orthostatic Tachycardia Syndrome. PACE 2009; 32:1000-1003.

Kanjwal K. et al. 2010 - Retrospective study - Comparative Clinical profile of postural orthostatic tachycardia patients with and without joint hypermobility syndrome. Indian Pacing Electrophysiol J. 2010;10:173.

Kaplan R.E. et al 2001- Recurrent Nursemaid's Elbow (Annular Ligament Displacement)

Kavi L. 2015 - Personal correspondence and review of cardiovascular autonomic dysfunction section of this book.

Keer R. & Grahame R. 2003 - Recognition and Management for Physiotherapists - Butterworth Heinemann, London, 2003, ISBN 0750653906

Keer R. & Butler K. 2010 - Physiotherapy and occupational therapy in the hypermobile adult Elsevier Ltd. DOI: 10.1016/B978-0-7020-3005-5.00013-6

Keer R. & Simmonds, J. 2011 - Joint protection and physical rehabilitation of the adult with hypermobility syndrome, Current Opinion in Rheumatology. 2011; 23, 2: 131–136.

Kerr A. J. 2000 - Physiotherapy for children with hypermobility syndrome. Physiotherapy 2000;86(6):313-7.

Kimpinski K. 2010 - Effect of pregnancy on Postural Tachycardia Syndrome. Mayo Clin Proc 2010; 85: 639-644.

Kirby A. 2007 - Developmental coordination disorder and joint Hypermobility syndrome—overlapping disorders? Implications for research and clinical practice, Child: Care, Health and Development, vol. 33, no. 5, pp. 513–519, 2007.

Kirk J A. et al. - The hypermobility syndrome: musculoskeletal complaints associated with generalized joint hypermobility. Ann Rheum Dis 1967. 26419–425.425.

Kjaer, M. 2004 - Role of Extracellular Matrix in Adaptation of Tendon and Skeletal Muscle to Mechanical Loading. Physiol Rev 84: 649–698, 2004; 10.1152/physrev.00031.2003.)

Kjaer M. 2005 Metabolic activity and collagen turnover in human tendon in response to physical activity. J Musculoskelet Neuronal Interact. 2005 Mar;5(1):41-52.

Kjaer M. et al 2006 - Extracellular matrix adaptation of tendon and skeletal muscle to exercise. J Anat. 2006 Apr; 208(4): 445–450. doi: 10.1111/j.1469-7580.2006.00549.x

Klekamp J. 2012. Neurological deterioration after foramen magnum decompression for Chiari malformation Type I: Old or new pathol- ogy? J Neurosurg Pediatr 10:538–547.

Knight I. 2011 - A Guide to living with Hypermobility Syndrome: bending without breaking. Singing Dragon ed. London

Knight I. 2013 - Managing EDS (Type III) - Hypermobility Syndrome

Kochharn P.K. 2011 - Consultant Anaesthetist, St Marys Hospital, Central Manchester - Anaesthesia and positioning - LABOUR - Joint hypermobility disorder - challenges in an Obstetric and perioperative setting BMJ 2011; 342 doi: dx.doi.org/10.1136/bmj.c7167 (Published 20 January 2011) Cite this as: BMJ 2011;342:c7167

Kok B.E. et al 2013 - How positive emotions build physical health perceived positive social connections account for the upward spiral between positive emotions and vagal tone. Psychological science 24(7): 1123-1132

Koralewicz L.M. 2000 - Comparison of proprioception in arthritic and age-matched normal knees. J Bone Joint Surg Am. 2000 Nov;82-A(11): 1582-8.

Kramer P.G. 1986 - Patella Malalignment Syndrome: Rationale to Reduce Excessive Lateral Pressure. The Journal of Orthopaedic and Sports Physical Therapy 0196-6011/86/0806-0301

Kubo K. et al 2003 - Gender differences in the viscoelastic properties of tendon structures (find rest) / Kubo K, Kanehisa H, Fukunaga T. 2003. Gender differences in the viscoelastic properties of tendon structures. Eur J Appl Physiol 88: (find rest)

Kumar A. 2012 - Joint Proprioception in Normal and Osteoarthritic Knees. J Yoga Phys Ther 2012, 2:4 dx.doi.org/10.4172/2157-7595.1000119

Lane J.M. Spine Osteoporosis. Medical prevention and treatment 1997 Dec 15;22(24 Suppl): 32S-37S).

Langevin H M. 2013 - The Science of Stretch - The study of connective tissue is shedding light on pain and providing new explanations for alternative medicine.Scientist »May 2013 Issue

Larson R.L. 1978 - The patellar compression syndrome: surgical treat-ment by lateral retinacular release. Clin Orthop 134:158-167, 1978

Larsson L.G. 1987- Hypermobility: features and differential incidence between the sexes. Arthritis Rheum. 1987 Dec;30(12):1426-30.

Laserspineinstitute.com/back_problems/spondylosis/spondylolisthesis/ - Accessed November 2014

Lazar S. W. et al 2005 - Meditation experience is associated with increased cortical thickness. Neuroreport, 16(17), 1893

Lee, J. K. 2008 - Whittaker, SJ; Enns, RA; Zetler, P (Dec 7, 2008). "Gastrointestinal manifestations of systemic mastocytosis". World journal of gastroenterology : WJG 14 (45): 7005–8. doi:10.3748/wjg.14.7005. PMID 19058339.

Létourneau Y. 2001 - Oral manifestations of Ehler-Danlos syndrome. J Can Dent Assoc. 2001;67:330-334.

Levard G et al 1989 - Urinary bladder diverticula and the Ehlers- Danlos syndrome in children. J Pediatr Surg 1989:24:1184–1186. www.ehlers-danlos.org/about-eds/medical-information/the-urinary-tract/#sthash.aoyG7T2l.dpuf)

Levy H. P. et al 1999 - Gastroesophageal reflux and irritable bowel syndrome in classical and hypermobile Ehlers Danlos syndrome (EDS). Program Nr: 362 from the 1999 ASHG Annual Meeting . H.P. 1) NHGRI, NIH, Bethesda, MD; 2) Georgetown University Medical Center, Washington, DC. www.ashg.org/genetics/abstracts/abs99/f362.htm

Levy H.P. 2004 (updated 2007) - Ehlers-Danlos Syndrome, Hypermobility Type - , PhD GeneReviews - www.ncbi.nlm.nih.gov/books/NBK1279/ (www.ncbi.nlm.nih.gov/books/NBK1116/) and copyright (University of Washington, Seattle)

Levy H.P. 2010 - Ehlers-Danlos Syndrome, Hypermobility Type. www.ncbi.nlm.nih.gov/books/NBK1279/

Levy H.P. 2012 (posted update) - Ehlers-Danlos Syndrome, Hypermobility Type - , PhD GeneReviews - www.ncbi.nlm.nih.gov/books/NBK1279/ (www.ncbi.nlm.nih.gov/books/NBK1116/) and copyright (University of Washington, Seattle)

Lind J. and Wallenburg H.C. 2002 - Pregnancy and the Ehlers-Danlos syndrome: a retrospective study in a Dutch population. 2002 Apr;81(4): 293-300.

Louisias M. et al 2013 - Prevalence of allergic disorders and mast cell activation syndrome in patients with Ehlers Danlos syndrome. Ann Allergy Asthma Immunol 111:A12

Low P.A. 2000 - Orthostatic Intolerance - National Dysautonomia Research Foundation patient Conference - Patient notes July 2010.

Low P.A. 2009 - Postural Tachycardia Syndrome (POTS) www.ncbi.nlm.nih.gov › NCBI › Literature › PubMed Central (PMC)

Macgregor K., Gerlach S., Mellor R., et al: 2005 - Cutaneous stimulation from patellar tape causes a differential increase in vasti muscle activity in people with patellofemoral pain, Journal of Orthopaedic Research 23(2): 351–358, 2005.

Magee D.J. 2008 - Orthopedic Physical Assessment - Sunders Elsevier ISBN 13:978-0-7216-0571-5

Maillard, S. et al 2010 - Review of an Out-Patient Self Management Exercise Programme. [abstract]; Physiotherapy Management of Children with Hypermobility: Arthritis Rheum 2010;62 Suppl 10 :1342 DOI: 10.1002/art.29108

Maillard S. 2012 'Flexible Kids' - hypermobility.org/help-advice/physio-and-occupational-therapy/flexible-kids/)

Malfait F. et al 2017 - The 2017 international classification of the Ehlers–Danlos syndromes - American Journal of Medical Genetics Volume 175, Issue 1, March 2017, Pages 8–26

Mallik A.K. et al., 1994 - Impared proprioreceptive acuity at the PIP joint in patients with hypermobility syndrome. BR J Rheumatol 33:631-7

Mantle D. A. 2005 - novel therapeutic strategy for Ehlers-Danlos syndrome based on nutritional supplements. Med Hypotheses. 2005; 64(2):279-83.

Mao J. 2001 - The Ehlers-Danlos syndrome: on beyond collagens. www.jci.org/articles/view/12881

Mar P.L. 2014 - Neuronal and hormonal perturbations in postural tachycardia syndrome. Front Physiol 5: 220. doi:10.3389/fphys. 2014.00220. PMC 4059278. PMID 24982638.

Marini I. 2010 - Effects of superpulsed low-level laser therapy on temporomandibular joint pain. Clin J Pain 26:611–616.

Marks I.M. 1986 - Genetics of fear and anxiety disorders. Br J Psychiatry. 1986 Oct;149:406-18.

Martin S.D. - What is the difference between open-chain and closed-chain exercises? https://www.sharecare.com/health/types-exercise/what-open-closed-chain-exercises, Orthopedic Surgery

Martin-Santos R. et al., 1998 - Association between joint hypermobility syndrome and panic disorder. Am J Psychiatry. 1998 Nov;155(11): 1578-83.

Mastocytosis Society Canada www.mastocytosis.ca - Mastocytosis /Mast Cell Activation Syndrome

Mastoroudes H. et al 2013 - Lower urinary tract symptoms in women with benign joint hypermobility syndrome: a case–control study - full text article: link.springer.com/article/10.1007/s00192-013-2065-3/

Masuki S et al 2007 - Excessive heart rate response to orthostatic stress in postural tachycardia syndrome is not caused by anxiety. J Appl Physiol 2007;102:896–903.

Mathias C.J. 2010 - Other Autonomic Disorders - National Dysautonomia Rsearch Foundation Patient Conference - conference notes July 2010.

Mathias C.J. 2011 - Postural tachycardia syndrome--current experience and concepts. 2011 Dec 6;8(1):22-34. doi: 10.1038/nrneurol.2011.187. Autonomic and Neurovascular Medicine Unit, Imperial College London and Nature Reviews Neurology. 2011;8:22–34.

Mayer K. 2013 ˙ Clinical utility gene card for: Ehlers–Danlos syndrome types I–VII and variants - update 2012˙ European Journal of Human Genetics 21, doi:10.1038/ejhg.2012.162; published online 15 August 2012

Mayfield Clinic - Posture for a Heathly Back www.mayfieldclinic.com/PE-POSTURE.htm#.Vo6xsElmaJU

1/Mayo Clinic - Complex Regional Pain syndrome. www.mayoclinic.org/diseases-conditions/complex-regional-pain-syndrome/basics/definition/con-20022844

2/Mayo Clinic 2015 - First aid for dislocations www.mayoclinic.org/first-aid/first-aid-dislocation/basics/art-20056693

3/Mayo Clinic - Thoracic Outlet syndrome. www.mayoclinic.org/diseases-conditions/thoracic-outlet-syndrome/basics/causes/con-20040509

McCormack M. et al 2004 - Joint laxity and the benign joint hypermobility syndrome in student and professional ballet dancers. J.Rheumatol, 31, 173-8.

McDonnell N.B. 2006 - Echocardiographic findings in classical and hypermobile Ehlers-Danlos syndromes. Am J Med Genet Part A 140A: 129–136.

McGhee J.R. 2012 - Inside the mucosal immune system. journals.plos.org/plosbiology/article?id=10.1371/journal.pbio.1001397

McIntosh L.J. 1995 - J Soc Gynecol Investig. 1995 May-Jun;2(3):559-64. Gynecologic disorders in women with Ehlers-Danlos syndrome.

McIntosh L.J. 1996 et al - Ehlers-Danlos Syndrome: relationship between joint hypermobility, urinary incontinence, and pelvic floor prolapse. Gynecol Obstet Invest. 1996;41:135-139.

McLuckie F. 2015 HMSA - commenting on behalf of the HMSA during HMSAware week 2016

McIver H. 2014 Writing for EDS Support UK - Hormonal Aspects of EDS www.facebook.com/EhlersDanlosUK/photos/a.230651766986895.80779.153693304682742/776626052389461/?type=1&theater

Medical News Today - Why being double-jointed can be a pain in the gut. www.medicalnewstoday.com/releases/275642.php

Medicine.org - Neuromusculoskeletal Group. medicine.org.ukhealthcare-professionals/specialist-groups/neuromusculoskeletal-group/

Mehta N.R. 2013 - Temporomandibular Disorders - www.merckmanuals.com/home/mouth_and_dental_disorders/temporomandibular_disorders/temporomandibular_disorders.html Accessed Nov 2014

Melson P. & Riddle O. 2010 - Physical Therapy Section - Writing for Dr Brad Tinkle's book, entitled The Hypermobility Handbook 2010 (Chapter 22).

Metlaine A. et al 2012 - Prevalence of sleep disorders in Ehlers-Danlos syndrome: a questionnaire study - Wednesday, September 05, 2012 - 21st Congress of the European Sleep Research Society - Paris, France - 04.09.2012 - 08.09.2012 Neurosurgery. 1999 May;44(5):1005-17.

Mielenz T.J. et al - 2010 - First item response theory analysis on Tampa Scale for Kinesiophobia in arthritis. The Journal of Clinical Epidemiology. 2010,63(3):315-20)

Milhorat T.H. et al 1999 - Chiari I malformation redefined: clinical and radiographic findings for 364 symptomatic patients.

Milhorat T.H. et al 2007 - Syndrome of occipitoatlantoaxial hypermobility, cranial settling, and chiari malformation type I in patients with hereditary disorders of connective tissue. J Neurosurg Spine. 2007 Dec;7(6):601-9.

Milhorat T.H et al 2009 - Association of Chiari Malformation type 1 and tethered cord syndrome: preliminary results of sectioning filum terminale. Surgical Neurology 72: 20-25, 2009).

Milhorat T.H. et al 2010. Mechanisms of cerebellar tonsil herniation in patients with Chiari malformations as guide to clinical management. Acta Neurochir. 152:1117–1127.

Mishra B.P. et al 1996 - "Extra-articular features of benign joint hypermobility syndrome," British Journal of Rheumatology, vol. 35, no. 9, pp. 861–866, 1996.

Mitakides J. et al 2017. Oral and mandibular manifestations in the Ehlers–Danlos syndromes. Am J Med Genet Part C Semin Med Genet 175C:220–225.

Mohammed et al 2010 - Joint hypermobility and rectal evacuatory dysfunction: an etiological link in abnormal connective tissue? Neurogastroenterol Motil. 2010 Oct;22(10):1085-e283. doi: 10.1111/j. 1365-2982.2010.01562.x. Epub 2010 Jul 5

Molloholli M. 2011 - Implications for obstetric care. BMJ 2011; 342: d1003. And article by Molloholli M., Specialty Registrar in Obstetrics and Gynaecology,Horton General Hospital, Oxford Radcliffe Hospitals NHS Trust

Moolenaar J. - www.mindfulpilates.co.uk contributing to a chapter on Pilates and EDS to Isobel Knight's newest book, Managing EDS (Type III)-Hypermobility Syndrome (2013)

Moore J.R. 1985 - Painful subluxation of the carpometacarpal joint of the thumb in Ehlers-Danlos syndrome, J Hand Surg Am 10(5):661–663, 1985.

Morgan A. W. and Bird H. 2007 - Asthma and airways collapse in two heritable disorders of connective tissue Ann Rheum Dis. 2007 Oct; 66(10): 1369–1373. Published online 2007 Apr 5. doi: 10.1136/ard. 2006.062224 PMCID: PMC1994284

Morhart M. 2015 - Wrist Fractures and Dislocations - emedicine.medscape.com/article/1285825-overview

Morris S.L. et al 2016. Hypermobility and musculoskeletal pain in adolecents. J Pediatr 16:31044–31047.

Morrison J. Health Advisor and volunteer for EDS UK - Splinting and bracing in EDS www.ehlers-danlos.org/patient-support/management-advice/physio-and-management/rnoh-rehabilitation/splinting-and-bracing-in-eds/#sthash.4pGKv3yF.dpuf

Morrison J. Health Advisor and volunteer for EDS UK - Managing Fatigue, Sleeping Problems and Brain Fog. www.ehlers-danlos.org/patient-support/management-advice/living-with-ehlers-danlos-syndrome/managing-fatigue-sleeping-problems-and-brain-fog/

Morrison S.C. et al 2013. Assessment of gait characteristics and orthotic management in children with Developmen- tal Coordination Disorder: Preliminary findings to inform multidisciplinary care. Res Dev Disabil 34:3197–3201.

Morris-Rosendahl D.J. 2002 - Are there anxious genes? Dialogues Clin Neurosci. 2002 Sep; 4(3): 251–260. PMCID: PMC3181683

Moulderings G.J. 2011 - Mast cell activation disease: a concise practical guide for diagnostic workup and therapeutic options J Hematol Oncol. 2011; 4: 10. Published online 2011 Mar 22. doi: 10.1186/1756-8722-4-10 PMCID: PMC3069946

Mrugacz M et al - Myopia in systemic disorders. English translation - https://www.ncbi.nlm.nih.gov/pubmed/19517854

Muaidi Q.I. 2009 - Do elite athletes exhibit enhanced proprioceptive acuity, range and strength of knee rotation compared with non-athletes? Scand J Med Sci Sports. 2009;19:103–112. doi: 10.1111/j. 1600-0838.2008.00783.x. [PubMed] [Cross Ref]

Mulvey M.R. et al 2013. Modest association of joint hypermobility with disabling and limiting musculoskeletal pain: Results from a large- scale general population-based survey. Ar- thritis Care Res (Hoboken) 65:1325–1333.

Murray K.J.and Woo P. 2001 Benign joint hypermobility in childhood rheumatology.oxfordjournals.org/content/40/5/489.long NHS/conditions/ehlers-danlos-syndrome/Pages/Introduction.aspx - Accessed January 2014

Murray K.J. 2006 - Hypermobility disorders in children and adolescents. Best Practice and Research, Clin Rheumatol 20(2):329–351, 2006.

Myers W. 2012 - The Best and Worst Ways to Cope With Pain. www.everydayhealth.com/pain-management/the-best-and-worst-ways-to-cope-with-pain.aspx

Napolitano C. et al 2000 - Risk factors that may adversely modify the natural history of the pediatric pronated foot. Clinics in Podiatric Medicine and Surgery 17:397-414

National Institute of Allergy and Infectious Disease 2013 - Mastocytosis. - www.niaid.nih.gov/topics/mastocytosis/pages/default.aspx

Neubauer H. 2011 - Popliteal Cysts in Paediatric Patients: Clinical Characteristics and Imaging Features on Ultrasound and MRI Arthritis Volume 2011 (2011), Article ID 751593, 7 pages dx.doi.org/ 10.1155/2011/751593 Clinical Study

NHS Direct Wales - Hypotonia - nhsdirect.wales.nhs.uk/encyclopaedia/h/ article/hypotonia/

1/ NHS.uk - Dry eye syndrome - www.nhs.uk/conditions/dry-eye-syndrome/Pages/Introduction.aspx

2/ NHS.uk - Fibromyalgia - www.nhs.uk/Conditions/Fibromyalgia/Pages/ Introduction.aspx

3/ NHS.uk - Fibromyalgia Help - www.nhs.uk/Conditions/Fibromyalgia/ Pages/SelfHelp.aspx

4/ NHS.uk - GP appointments - nhs.uk/choiceintheNHS/Yourchoices/ GPchoice/Pages/GPappointments.aspx

5/ NHS.uk - Joint hypermobility symptoms - www.nhs.uk/Conditions/ Joint-hypermobility/Pages/Symptoms.aspx

6/ NHS.uk - Varicose Veins - www.nhs.uk/conditions/Varicose-veins/ Pages/Whatarevaricoseveins.aspx

7/ NHS.uk - What is Fibromyalgia PDF for South Devon Healthcare NHS Trust - www.sdhct.nhs.uk/uploads/what-is-fibromyalgia.pdf

8/ NHS.uk - Postural tachycardia syndrome www.nhs.uk/Conditions/ postural-tachycardia-syndrome/Pages/Introduction.aspx

9/ NHS.uk - Pelvic Organ Prolapse - www.nhs.uk/conditions/Prolapse-of-the-uterus/Pages/Introduction.aspx

10/ NHS.uk - Pelvic Pain in pregnancy - www.nhs.uk/conditions/ pregnancy-and-baby/pages/pelvic-pain-pregnant-spd.aspx? tabname=Getting%20pregnant

11/ NHS.uk - Mindfulness www.nhs.uk/conditions/stress-anxiety-depression/pages/mindfulness.aspx

12/ NHS.uk - EMDR Therapy - www.nhs.uk/Conditions/Counselling/ Pages/Talking-therapies.aspx

13/ NHS.uk - Bursitis - www.nhs.uk/Conditions/Bursitis/Pages/ Introduction.aspx

14/ NHS.uk - Complex Regional Pain Syndrome www.nhs.uk/Conditions/ Complex-Regional-Pain-Syndrome/Pages/Treatment.aspx.

15/ NHS.uk - Costochondritis - www.nhs.uk/conditions/Tietzes-syndrome/pages/introduction.aspx

© Understanding hEDS and HSD by C. Smith

16/NHS.uk - Heavy periods (menorrhagia). www.bupa.co.uk/health-information/directory/m/menorrhagia

17/NHS.uk - Cognitive behavioural therapy - How it works. www.nhs.uk/Conditions/Cognitive-behavioural-therapy/Pages/How-does-it-work.aspx

18/ NHS.uk - Chiari Malformations www.nhs.uk/conditions/chiari-malformation/Pages/Introduction.aspx

NIH - What are proteins and what do they do? ghr.nlm.nih.gov/primer/howgeneswork/protein

1/ NIH - What are proteins and what do they do? ghr.nlm.nih.gov/primer/howgeneswork/protein

2/ NIH - National of Health - Institute of Allergy and Infectious Diseases - niaid.nih.gov

Nijs J. A. Aerts, and K. De Meirleir 2006 - Generalized joint hypermobility is more common in chronic fatigue syndrome than in healthy control subjects 2006

Nochi T. 2006 - immunity in the mucosal immune system. Curr Pharm Des. 2006;12(32):4203-13.

Norton L.A. for EDS Support UK - Orthodontics and EDS viewed 2017

Noyes Knee Institute - The Unstable Patella (Kneecap): Everything You Need to Know to Make the Right Treatment Decision." eBooks, see: noyeskneebookseries.com/.

Ofluoglu D 2006 - . Hypermobility in women with fibromyalgia syndrome. Clin Rheumatol. 2006 May;25(3):291-3. Epub 2005 Oct 16. Department of Physical Medicine and Rehabilitation, School of Medicine, Marmara University, Istanbul, Turkey. dofluoglu@hotmail.com

Ogilive A.L. 1985 - Impairment of vagal function in reflux oesophagitis. Q J Med 54:61–74.

Oguntona S. and Adelowo O. 2014 - Frequency of benign hypermobility syndrome in females with knee pain - Global Advanced Research Journal of Medicine and Medical Science (ISSN: 2315-5159) Vol. 3(4) pp. 076-079, April 2014 Available online garj.org/garjmms/index.htm

Oliver J. 2005 - Hypermobility - Reports on the Rheumatic Diseases Series 5, Hands On - www.arthritisresearchuk.org/~/media/Files/.../Hands.../HO07-Oct-2005.ashx

Olson T.S. 2005 - Physical Therapy Management of the Hypermobile Patient. www.ednf.org/medical-professionals/physical-therapy-management-hypermobile-patient

Olson T.S. 2012 (updated) - Physical Therapy Management of the Hypermobile Patient. orpha.net/consor/cgi-bin/OC_Exp.php?Lng=EN&Expert=285. - 2012 accessed 1/1/15

Oro J. 2010 - Treatment of Chiari Malformation - csfinfo.org/research/csf-funded-research/csf-ehlers-danlos-syndrome-colloquium/treatment-chiari-malformation/

Pacak D.K. 2009 - The Journal of Professional Excellence - Dimensions of dental hygine Ehlers-Danlos syndrome April 2009; 7(4): 42-45. www.dimensionsofdentalhygiene.com/ddhright.aspx?id=4356

Pacey V. et al 2013 . - Exercise in children with joint hypermobility syndrome and knee pain: a randomised controlled trial comparing exercise into hypermobile versus neutral knee extension - Pediatric Rheumatology 2013, 11:30 www.ped-rheum.com/content/11/1/30 Oreds.org (Oregon Area Ehlers-Danlos Syndrome Support - Mast Cell Activation Disorder. www.oreds.org/uploads/3/1/5/0/3150381/mcadsymptomslist.pdf

Pacey V. 2014 - Proprioceptive acuity into knee hypermobile range in children with Joint Hypermobility Syndrome - Pediatric Rheumatology 2014, 12:40 doi:10.1186/1546-0096-12-40 or www.ped-rheum.com/content/12/1/40

Palm S. Pelvic Organ Prolapse Support - www.pelvicorganprolapsesupport.org/enterocele-rectocele-or-both/

Palmer S. 2004 - Quoted in - Stretching a point by Jane Wright 2004 - Hypermobility, joints and physiotherapy research www.csp.org.uk/frontline/article/stretching-point-hypermobility-joints-physiotherapy-research Volume 10, issue 20

Palmer S. 2014 - The effectiveness of therapeutic exercise for joint hypermobility syndrome: a systematic review. Physiotherapy Journal Volume 100, Issue 3, Pages 220–227. eprints.uwe.ac.uk/23637/7/1-s2.0-S0031940613000849-main.pdf

Palmer S. et al. 2015 - Physiotherapy management of joint hypermobility syndrome - a focus group study of patient and health professional perspectives. Physiotherapy.

Palmer S. et al 2016 - The feasibility of a randomised controlled trial of physiotherapy for adults with joint hypermobility syndrome Health Technology Assessment, No. 20.47

Palmer S. 2017 - Personal discussion

Park Clinic Orthopaedics - FemoroAcetabular Impingement. www.parkclinic.com.au/home/conditions-treatment/hip/femoroacetabular-impingement-fai/

Partners Against Pain - www.partnersagainstpain.com/pain-management/communicating.aspx

1) Patient.co.uk - Postural Orthostatic Tachycardia www.patient.co.uk/health/postural-orthostatic-tachycardia-syndrome Accessed 2014.

2) Patient.co.uk - Chronic Fatigue Syndrome (ME) - www.patient.co.uk/health/chronic-fatigue-syndromeme - Accessed 2015

3) Patient.co.uk - Wrist fractures and dislocations www.patient.co.uk/doctor/carpal-fractures-and-dislocations#ref-1

4) Patient.co.uk - Halux Valgus (Bunions). www.patient.co.uk/doctor/hallux-valgus

5) Patient.co.uk - Ehlers Danlos syndrome - Hypermobile EDS (formerly known as type III) - www.patient.co.uk/doctor/ehlers-danlos-syndrome-pro

6) Patient.co.uk - Fibromyalgia - patient.info/health/fibromyalgia-leaflet

7) Patient.co.uk - Mast Cell Activation Disorder - patient.info/doctor/mastocytosis-and-mast-cell-disorders

8) Patient.co.uk - Raynaud's Phenomenon - patient.info/health/raynauds-phenomenon

9) Patient.co.uk - Dry eye syndrome patient.info/health/dry-eyes-leaflet

10)Patient.co.uk - Restless Legs syndrome. www.patient.co.uk/health/restless-legs-syndrome-leaflet

11) Patient.co.uk - Tendinopathy - patient.info/health/tendinopathy-and-tenosynovitis

Pauker S.P. et al 2014 - Clinical manifestations and diagnosis of Ehlers-Danlos syndromes - www.uptodate.com/contents/clinical-manifestations-and-diagnosis-of-ehlers-danlos-syndromes - Accessed Nov 2014 and May 2015

Paulson P.E. et al 1998 - Gender differences in pain perception and patterns of cerebral activation during noxious heat stimulation in humans. Author manuscript; available in PMC 2007 Mar 15. Published in final edited form as: Pain 1998 May; 76(1-2): 223–229. PMCID: MC1828033 NIHMSID: NIHMS16320

PCDS.org 2014 - Clinical Guidance re: Piezongenic Papules. www.pcds.org.uk/clinical-guidance/piezogenic-pedal-papules Accessed 2 Dec 2014

Peggs K. J. et al 2012 - Gynecologic disorders and menstrual cycle lightheadedness in postural tachycardiasyndrome. Int. J. Gynaecol. Obstet. 118, 242–246. doi: 10.1016/j.ijgo.2012.04.014

1/ Physiopedia - Slipping rib syndrome. www.physio-pedia.com/Slipping_rib_syndrome

2/ Physiopedia - Ehlers-Danlos syndrome. www.physio-pedia.com/Ehlers-Danlos_Syndrome

Picard M. et al 2013 - Expanding spectrum of mast cell activation disorders: monoclonal and idiopathic mast cell activation syndromes. Clin Ther. 2013 May;35(5):548-62. doi: 10.1016/j.clinthera.2013.04.001. Epub 2013 May 1.

Pierard G.E. et al 1988 - Morphometric study of cauliflower collagen fibrils in Ehlers-Danlos syndrome type I. Coll Relat Res. 1988; 8:453-7. I Article I PubMed

Pilates Foundation - Pilates for hypermobility. www.pilatesfoundation.com/articles/show/pilates-for-hypermobility/

Pocinki A.G. 2010 - Joint Hypermobility and Joint Hypermobility Syndrome. www.cfids.org/pdf/joint-hypermobility-guide.pdf 2141 K Street, NW, Suite 600. Washington, DC 20037.

1) PoTS UK - A guide for medical professionals PDF - www.potsuk.org/UserFiles/File/MPIL2_Medical_professionals_guide_to_POTSJW.pdf

2)PoTS UK 2017 Exercise - www.potsuk.org/exercise

Pocinki A.G. 2011- Understanding CFS. George Washington University Hospital - General Awareness, Managing CFS, Understanding CFS I 31. Oct, 2011 - solvecfs.org

Pollock J. 2006 - The Regenerative Medicine Partnership in Education - Duquense University - sepa.duq.edu/regmed/immune/histamine.html

Pool-Goudzwaard A.L. 1998 - Insufficient lumbopelvic stability: a clinical, anatomical and biomechanical approach to 'a-specific' low back pain. Man Ther. 1998 Feb;3(1):12-20.

Porter S. 2016 - Dental implications for those with Ehlers-Danlos syndrome. HMSA Journal Edition 6.

Pritchard, J. A. 1965. Changes in the blood volume during pregnancy and delivery. Anesthesiology 26, 393–399. doi: 10.1097/00000542-196507000-00004

Protopapas M. et al May 2002. - Joint cracking and popping: understanding noises that accompany articular release.

Prussin C. & Metcalfe D.D. 2003 - IgE, mast cells, basophils, and eosinophils". The Journal of Allergy and Clinical Immunology 111 (2 Suppl): S486–94. doi:10.1067/mai.2003.120. PMID 12592295.)

Puckett K., National Director of Mind-body Medicine - www.cancercenter.com/midwestern/doctors-and-clinicians/katherine-puckett/

Punzi L. et al 2000 - Pro–inflammatory interleukins in the synovial fluid of rheumatoid arthritis associated with joint hypermobility - Oxford Journals Rheumatology, Medicine & Health Rheumatology, Volume 40, Issue 2, Pp. 202-204

Rahi A. et al 1977 - Br J Ophthalmol. 1977 Dec; 61(12): 761–764. PMCID: PMC1043115 Keratoconus and coexisting atopic disease.

Raj S. et al 2005 Arrhythmia/Electrophysiology Renin-Aldosterone Paradox and Perturbed Blood Volume Regulation Underlying Postural Tachycardia Syndrome. circ.ahajournals.org/content/111/13/1574.full

Rarediseases.org - Mastocytois - rarediseases.org/rare-diseases/mastocytosis/

Rawlings J. 2014 - Hypermobility versus flexibility - do you know the difference - www.jennirawlings.com/blog/2014/9/4/hypermobility-vs-flexibility-do-you-know-the-difference

Raynaud's and Scleroderma Association - Chilblains - www.raynauds.org.uk/raynauds/raynauds/133

Rees J.D. 2006 - Current concepts in the management of tendon disorders - Oxford Journals Medicine & Health - Rheumatology Volume 45, Issue 5 Pp. 508-521.

Redmond A.C. et al 2006a - Pain and health status in people with hypermobility syndrome are associated with overall joint mobility and selected local mechanical factors. Rheumatology (Oxford) 2006;45 Suppl 1:i108(254).

Redmond A.C. 2006b - The distribution and prevalence of symptoms associated with hypermobility syndrome. Ann Rheum Dis 2006;65 Suppl II:ii241(352).

Remvig L. 2007 et al - Epidemiology of general joint hypermobility and basis for the proposed criteria for benign joint hypermobility syndrome: review of the literature. J Rheumatol. 2007 Apr;34(4):804-9. Epub 2007 Jan 15.

Richards A. J. et al 1998 - A single base mutation in COL5A2 causes Ehlers-Danlos syndrome type II. J Med Genet. Oct 1998; 35(10): 846–848. PMCID: PMC1051462

Richards K. L 2009 - Pain central - Fibromyalgia and hypermobility - www.healthcentral.com/article/joint-hypermobility-and-fibromyalgia

Richeimer S. 2000 - helpforpain.com 2000 - helpforpain.com/arch2000dec.htm - Accessed March 2015

Rinne K.M. & Kirkinen PP. 1999 - What predisposes young women to genital prolapse? Eur J Obstet Gynecol Reprod Biol. 1999;84:23-25.

Robert-McComb J.J. - 2014 - The Active Female: Health Issues Throughout the Lifespan ISBN: 978-1-4614-8883-5 (Print) Page: 773

Rombaut L. et al 2010 - Musculoskeletal complaints, physical activity and health-related quality of life among patients with the Ehlers-Danlos syndrome hypermobility type. 2010;32(16):1339-45. doi: 10.3109/09638280903514739

Ronstein R. 2011 - New York City–based Pilates instructor - How to handle the hypermobile client - www.ideafit.com/fitness-library/how-to-handle-the-hypermobile-client

Rothblum K. et al 2004 - Constitutive release of a4 Type V collagen N-terminal domain by Schwann cells and binding to cell surface and extracellular matrix heparan sulfate proteoglycans. J Biol Chem 2004;279:51282–8.

Rothstein M. et al 2009 - THE GHOST IN OUR GENES: LEGAL AND ETHICAL IMPLICATIONS OF EPIGENETICS. Health Matrix Clevel. Author manuscript; available in PMC 2011 Feb 7.Published in final edited form as: Health Matrix Clevel. 2009 Winter; 19(1): 1–62.

Rowe P.C. 1999 - Orthostatic intolerance and chronic fatigue syndrome associated with Ehlers-Danlos syndrome. J Pediatr. 1999 Oct;135(4): 494-9.

Rozen T. D., Roth J. M., Denenberg N, "Cervical spine joint hypermobility: a possible predisposing factor for new daily persistent headache," Cephalalgia, vol. 26, no. 10, pp. 1182–1185, 2006

Rozniecki J.J. 1995 - Elevated mast cell tryptase in cerebrospinal fluid of multiple sclerosis patients Ann. Neurol., 37 (1995), pp. 63–66

Rozzi S. et al. 1999 - Knee Joint Laxity and Neuromuscula Characterisitcs of Male and Female Soccer and Basketball Players - The Americal Journal of Sports Medicine Vol. 27 No 3

RSD.org - Reflex Sympathetic Dystrophy Syndrome Association (www.rsds.org/OLD/web/content/newsletter/Mast_Cell_Activation_Syndrome_and_CRPS.html)

© Understanding hEDS and HSD by C. Smith

Russek L. N. 1999 - Joint Hypermobility. Physical Therapy 1999;79(6): 591-9.

Russek L. N. 2000 - Examination and treatment of a patient with hypermobility syndrome Physical Therapy 2000;80:386-98. Available at: www.ptjournal.org/cgi/content/full/80/4/386. Accessed August 29, 2006.

Sacheti A. et al - Chronic pain is a manifestation of the Ehlers-Danlos syndrome. Journal of Pain and Symptom Management. 1997;14(2):88–93. [PubMed]

Santa Maria School of Medicine 2013- POTs and Periods. santamariamedicine.com/2013/04/p-o-t-s-periods-postural-orthostatic-tachycardia-patients-menstrual-cycles/

Sayed B.A. 2008 - The master switch: the role of mast cells in autoimmunity and tolerance Annu. Rev. Immunol., 26 (2008), pp. 705–739

Schmidt-Wilcke T. et al 2007 - Striatal grey matter increase in patients suffering from fibromyalgia--a voxel-based morphometry study. Pain. 2007 Nov;132 Suppl 1:S109-16. Epub 2007 Jun 22.

Schmidt-Wilcke T. et al 2014 - Pain in Fibromyalgia Patients Correlate with Changes in Brain Activation in the Cingulate Cortex in a Response Inhibition Task - www.researchgate.net/publication/263670266_2014

Schondorf R. & Lowe P.A.1993 - Idiopathic postural orthostatic tachycardia syndrome: An attenuated form of acute pandysautonomia? Neurology 1993;43:132–137.

Schondorf R. et al 1999 - Orthostatic intolerance in the chronic fatigue syndrome. J Auton Nerv Syst 75:192–201.

Schwartzman R. J. 2009 - The natural history of complex regional pain syndrome. Clin J Pain. 2009 May;25(4):273-80. doi: 10.1097/AJP. 0b013e31818ecea5.

Schwartzman R.J. 2012 - Systemic Complications of Complex Regional Pain Syndrome. Department of Neurology, Drexel University College of Medicine, Philadelphia, PA, USA Received July 17, 2012. Neuroscience & Medicine 2012, and https://pdfs.semanticscholar.org/e723/ d9f58a7318c834a9ff33fb9a975261b99de3.pdf

Selfcare4rsi.com/fascia.html - Facia. Accessed Feb 2015

Self Management UK - selfmanagementuk.org/what-self-management

Sendur O.F. et al 2007 - The frequency of hypermobility and its relationship with clinical findings of fibromyalgia patients. Clin Rheumatol. 2007 Apr;26(4):485-7. Epub 2006 Apr 25.

Seneviratne S. 2016 - By email correspondence

Seneviratne S.L. et al 2017. Mast cell disorders in Ehlers–Danlos syndrome. Am J Med Genet Part C Semin Med Genet 9999C:1–11.

Sheehan F.T. et al 2008 - Understanding patellofemoral pain with maltracking in the presence of joint laxity: complete 3D in vivo patellofemoral and tibiofemoral kinematics. Journal of Orthopaedic Research 27:561-570

Sheldon R.S. et al 2015 - 2015 heart rhythm society expert consensus statement on the diagnosis and treatment of postural tachycardia syndrome, inappropriate sinus tachycardia, and vasovagal syncope. Heart Rhythm. 2015 Jun;12(6):e41-63. doi: 10.1016/j.hrthm.2015.03.029. Epub 2015 May 14.

Shibao C. et al 2005 - Hyperadrenergic postural tachycardia syndrome in mast cell activation disorders. Hypertension. 2005 Mar;45(3):385-90. Epub 2005 Feb 14.

Shirley E.D. et al 2012 - Ehlers-Danlos Syndrome in Orthopaedics - Etiology, Diagnosis, and Treatment Implications www.ncbi.nlm.nih.gov/ pmc/articles/PMC3435946/ports Health. 2012 Sep; 4(5): 394–403. doi: 10.1177/1941738112452385 PMCID: PMC3435946

Shoen R et al 1982). The hyypermobility syndrome, Postgraduate Medicine, 71, 199-208

Shultz S.J. et al 2012. Changes in serum collagen markers, IGF-I, and knee joint laxity across the menstrual cycle. J Orthop Res 30:1405–1412.

Siqueira C.M et al 2011 - Misalignment of the knees: Does it affect human stance stability. Journal of Bodywork and Movement Therapies, v. 15, n. 2, p. 235-241, 2011.

Silliman J.F. 1993 - Classification and physical diagnosis of instability of the shoulder. Clin Orthop Relat Res. 1993 Jun; (291):7-19. [PubMed]

Silva J.A. - Retropulsion and vertigo in the Chiari malformation: case report. Arq Neuropsiquiatr. 2005 Sep; 63(3B):870-3.

Simmonds J.V. & Keer R. 2007 - Hypermobility and the Hypermobility Syndrome (Patient Masterclass) using content from Manual Therapy. 2007; 13: 492-495.

Simmonds J.V. 2013 - Posture, Supports, Orthotics. hypermobility.org/ help-advice/physio-and-occupational-therapy/supports-orthotics/) Published by the Hypermobility Syndromes Association

Simmonds J.V. 2014 - (Updated version) - Posture, Supports, Orthotics hypermobility.org/help-advice/physio-and-occupational-therapy/ supports-orthotics/) Published by the Hypermobility Syndromes Association

Simmonds J.V. 2014 - PE and Sport - The hypermobile child - a guide for schools - HMSA guide 2014

Simmonds J.V. 2015 - Speaking on 'Physiotherapy and children with EDS' at the EDS UK conference.

Simmonds J.V. 2016 - Splints, Braces and Taping - HMSA Journal Volume 5

Simpson M.R. 2006 - Benign Joint Hypermobility Syndrome: Evaluation, Diagnosis, and Management DO, MC, USA www.jaoa.osteopathic.org/ content/106/9/531.full#ref-20

Shultz S.J. et al 2012 - Changes in serum collagen markers, IGF-I, and knee joint laxity across the menstrual cycle. J Orthop Res 30:1405–1412.

Slosar P.J. 2000 - Spine (Phila Pa 1976). 2000 Mar 15;25(6):722-6. Patient satisfaction after circumferential lumbar fusion.

Smith D.B. - 2012 Female Pelvic Floor Health: A Developmental Review www.nursingcenter.com/journalarticle?Article_ID=507289

Smith T.O. et al 2013 - Do people with benign joint hypermobility syndrome (BJHS) have reduced joint proprioception? A systematic review and meta-analysis. link.springer.com/article/10.1007/ s00296-013-2790-4#page-2

Smith M.D. et al 2012 - Stress urinary incontinence as the presenting complaint of benign joint hypermobility syndrome - Short Rep. 2012 Sep; 3(9): 66.Published online 2012 Sep 26. doi: 10.1258/shorts. 2012.012005 PMCID: PMC3545343.

Soliman K. et al 2010 - Postural orthostatic tachycardia syndrome (POTS): a diagnostic dilemma February 2010 Volume 17, Issue 1 Br J Cardiol 2010;17:36-9

Solomon J.A. 1999 - "Gastrointestinal Manifestations of EDS." Am J Gastroenterol 1996 Nov; 91 (11): 2282–8. Available from bit.ly/UzmCCX.

Sorokin Y. et al. 1994 - Obstetric and gynecologic dysfunction in the Ehlers-Danlos syndrome.

Soyucen E. & Esen F.-2010 - Benign joint hypermobility syndrome: a cause of childhood asthma? www.ncbi.nlm.nih.gov/books/NBK1279/ 2010 May;74(5):823-4. doi: 10.1016/j.mehy.2009.12.004. Epub 2010

Spaziani R.M. et al 1996 - A low resting vagal tone predicts response to acid perfusion in patients with esophageal symptoms. Gastroenterology 110:A762.

1/ Spine-Health.com. Types of Back Pain - Spine-health.com/conditions/chronic-pain/types-back-pain-acute-pain-chronic-pain-and-neuropathic-pain - Accessed March 2015

2/ Spine-health.com. Why Does it Hurt" - Spine-health.com/conditions/chronic-pain/chronic-pain-a-disease-why-does-it-still-hurt - Accessed Jan 2015

3/ Spine-Health.com. Pars Interarticularis - www.spine-health.com/glossary/pars-interarticularis

4/ Spine-Health.com - Using your brain to combat pain - www.spine-health.com/blog/how-stop-your-pain-your-mind
Stachenfeld N. S. and Taylor H. S. 2005 - Progesterone increases plasma volume independent of estradiol. J. Appl. Physiol. (1985) 98, 1991–1997. doi: 10.1152/japplphysiol.00031.2005

Staheli L.T. 2008 - Fundamentals of Paediatric Orthopaedics 4th Edition Wolters kluwer, Lippincott, Williams and Wilkins.

Stanitski D.F. et al - 2000 - Orthopaedic manifestations of Ehlers-Danlos syndrome. Clin Orthop Relat Res. 2000;376:213-221 [PubMed]

STARS (Syncope trust and Reflex Anoxic Seizures) - www.stars.org.uk/patient-info/conditions/pots

Stauffer R. et al 1977 - Force and motion analysis of the normal, diseased, and prosthetic ankle joint. Clinical Orthopaedics and Related Research, Vol.127, pp. 189-196.

Steenbergen L. et al 2015 - A randomized controlled trial to test the effect of multispecies probiotics on cognitive reactivity to sad mood. Brain Behav Immun. 2015 Aug;48:258-64. doi: 10.1016/j.bbi.2015.04.003. Epub 2015 Apr 7.

Steering Committee for the Workshop on Work-Related Musculoskeletal Injuries - Work- Related Musculoskeletal disorders, page 82)

Steinmann B. et al. 2002. The Ehlers-Danlos syndrome. In: Royce PM, Steinmann B, editors. Connective tissue and its heritable disorders, 2nd edition. New York (US): Wiley-Liss. pp 431–524.

Stiles L. 2015 (co-founder of Dysautonomia International) - writing for: Crowd Med. blog.crowdmed.com/pots-the-most-common-medical-condition-you-never-heard-of/

Stodolna-Tukendorf J. 2011 - Spinal pain syndromes and constitutional hypermobility. Chir Narzadow Ruchu Ortop Pol. 2011 May-Jun;76(3):138-44.

Stoler J.M. & Oaklander A.L. 2006 - Patients with Ehlers Danlos syndrome and CRPS: a possible association? Genetics and Teratology Unit, Department of Pediatrics, Massachusetts General Hospital, Harvard Medical School, Boston www.rsds.org/pdfsall/Stoler_Pain_2010.pdf and also at: Pain. 2006 Jul;123(1-2):204-9. Epub 2006 Apr 4 www.ncbi.nlm.nih.gov/pubmed/16600507

Streepey J.W. et al 2010 - Effects of quadriceps and hamstrings proprioceptive neuromuscular facilitation stretching on knee movement sensation. J Strength Cond Res. 2010 Apr;24(4):1037-42. doi: 10.1519/JSC.0b013e3181d09e87.

Sugimoto J. et al 2000. A patient with mitochondrial myopathy associated with isolated succinate dehydro- genase deficiency. Brain Dev 22:158–162.

Sundelin H.E. et al 2016 - Pregnancy outcome in Joint Hypermobility Syndrome and Ehlers-Danlos Syndrome. Acta Obstet Gynecol Scand. 2016 Oct 14. doi: 10.1111/aogs.13043. [Epub ahead of print]

Syx D. et al 2015 - Ehlers-Danlos Syndrome, Hypermobility Type, Is Linked to Chromosome 8p22-8p21.1 in an Extended Belgian Family. Disease Markers Volume 2015 (2015), Article ID 828970, 9 pages dx.doi.org/10.1155/2015/828970

Tarrant M.L. 2003 - How to Improve Proprioception. www.ideafit.com/fitness-library/focus-on-the-lower-body-to-train-balancehow-to-improveproprioception

Taylor D. et al 1981 - Ehlers-Danlos syndrome during pregnancy - a casre report and review of the literature. Obstretical and gynecological Survey 36:277-281

Temporomandibular Disorders, Dental Care and You 2016. The TMJ Association. www.tmj.org/site/page?pageId=332

The Chartered Society of Physiotherapy Stretching a point - Hypermobility, joints and physiotherapy research - www.csp.org.uk/frontline/article/stretching-point-hypermobility-joints-physiotherapy-research)

The Mastocytosis Society Inc - Mast Cell Activation Disorders - tmsforacure.org/patients/mastocytosis_explained_6.php#sthash.g57QuGZ5.dpuf

Theodorou S. et al 2012 - Low bone mass in Ehlers-Danlos syndrome. Intern Med. 2012;51(22):3225-6. Epub 2012 Nov 15.

Thieben M. et al 2007 - Postural orthostatic tachycardia syndrome – Mayo Clinic experience. Mayo Clin Proc 2007;82:308–313.

Ting T.V. et al 2012 - The role of benign joint hypermobility in the pain experience in Juvenile Fibromyalgia: an observational study Pediatric Rheumatology201210:16 DOI: 10.1186/1546-0096-10-16

Tinkle B.T. et al 2009 - The lack of clinical distinction between the hypermobility type of Ehlers–Danlos syndrome and the joint hypermobility syndrome (a.k.a. hypermobility syndrome) Part A 149A:2368–2370

Tinkle B.T. 2010 - Joint Hypermobility Handbook - A Guide for the Issues & Management of Ehlers-Danlos syndrome hypermobility type and the hypermobility syndrome

Tinkle B. Writing for Fragile Links Magazine Spring 2015 page 38 - EDS Support UK - Dr Brad

Tinkle B.T et al 2017 - Hypermobile Ehlers-Danlos syndrome (a.k.a. Ehlers-Danlos syndrome Type III and Ehlers-Danlos syndrome hypermobility type): Clinical description and natural history. Am J Med Genet Part C Semin Med Genet 9999C:1-22

Tougas G. 1999 - The autonomic nervous system in functional bowel disorders. Gut 2000;47:iv78-iv80 doi:10.1136/gut.47.suppl_4.iv78 Chapter 7

Tougas G. 2000 - Am J Gastroenterol. 2000 Jun;95(6):1456-62. Assessment of gastric emptying using a low fat meal: establishment of international control values.

Trost Z. et al 2007 Exposure To Movement in Chronic Back Pain: Evidence of Successful Generalization Across a Reaching Task. In Pain. ugly construction to get trailing dot after citation, or after journals slug if citation is not defined PubMed Journals - Pain 137 (1), 26-33. 2007 Sep 14.

Tulandi T. et al (Lit review 2016) - Spontaneous abortion: Risk factors, etiology, clinical manifestations, and diagnostic evaluation. www.uptodate.com/contents/spontaneous-abortion-risk-factors-etiology-clinical-manifestations-and-diagnostic-evaluation

Turk D.C. et al 1983. - Pain and behavioral medicine: A cognitive behavioral perspective. New York: Guilford Press.

Udermann B.E. 2005 - Slipping Rib Syndrome in a Collegiate Swimmer: A Case Report J Athl Train. 2005 Apr-Jun; 40(2): 120–122.

Unsworth A. et al 1971 - 'Cracking joints.' A bioengineering study of cavitation in the metacarpophalangeal joint. Ann Rheum Dis 1971;30:348–58.

Valent P. et al 2007 - Standards and standardization in mastocytosis: consensus statements on diagnostics, treatment recommendations and response criteria. Eur J Clin Invest. 2007; 37: 435–453

Verbraecken J. et al 2001 - "Evaluation for sleep apnea in patients with EDS and Marfan: a questionnaire study." Clin Genet. 2001 Nov; 60 (5): 360–5.]

Vernino S. et al 2000 - Autoantibodies to ganglionic acetylcholine receptors in autoimmune autonomic neuropathies. N Engl J Med. 2000; 343: 847–855

Virginia Spine Institute - Sacroiliac joint dysfunction - www.spinemd.com/symptoms-conditions/sacroiliac-joint-pain

Vlaeyen, J.W. and S.J. Linton 2000 - Fear-avoidance and its consequences in chronic musculoskeletal pain: a state of the art. Pain, 2000. 85(3): p. 317-32.

Voermans N.C. et al 2009 - Joint hypermobility as a distinctive feature in the differential diagnosis of myopathies - Journal of Neurology 256(1): 13-27 March 2009 DOI: 10.1007/s00415-009-0105-1 - PubMed

Voermans N.C. et al 2010. - Pain in Ehlers-Danlos syndrome is common, severe, and associated with functional impairment. J Pain Symptom Manage. 2010;40:370-378 [PubMed]

Voermans N.C. et al 2011 - Fatigue is associated with muscle weakness in Ehlers-Danlos syndrome: an explorative study. Physiotherapy. 2011;97(2):170–174. [PubMed]

Walker M.E. et al 2012 - New insights into the role of mast cells in autoimmunity: Evidence for a common mechanism of action? Biochimica et Biophysica Acta (BBA) - Molecular Basis of Disease Volume 1822, Issue 1, January 2012, Pages 57–65 Mast Cells in inflammation

Wallman D. et al 2014. Ehlers- Danlos syndrome and postural tachycardia syndrome: A relationship study. J Neurol Sci 340:99–102.

Watson P. et al 1989. A study of the cracking sounds from the metacarpophalangeal joint. Proc Inst Mech Eng 1989;203:109–18.

Webmd.com 2013 - Plantar Fasciitis - Symptoms, Treatments, Causes of Plantar ... www.webmd.com/a-to-z-guides/plantar-fasciitis-topic-overview

Webmd.com 2014 - Urinary Incontinence and repair of the bladder or urethra - www.webmd.com/urinary-incontinence-oab/repair-of-the-bladder-or-urethra Last Updated: March 12, 2014

Wedemeyer J. & Galli S.J. 2000 - Mast cells and basophils in acquired immunity British Med Bull (2000) 56 (4): 936-955.

Weinberg J. et al 1999 - Joint surgery in Ehlers-Danlos patients: results of a survey. Am J Orthop (Belle Mead NJ). 1999 Jul; 28(7):406-9. PubMed

Weinberger A. 1997 (For EDNF.org) - The role of rheumatologist in Ehlers-Danlos syndrome Loose Connections - EDNF May 1997 (213) 651-3038 www.ednf.org/images/stories/Loose_Connections_Archived/lc_1997-05.pdf

White A. 2015 - A tale of two syndromes Dysautonomia Dispatch Feb 2015 - Dysautonomia International www.dysautonomiainternational.org/blog/wordpress/a-tale-of-two-syndromes-pots-and-mcas/)

Wicks D. 2015 - Persistent Fatigue and Heritable Disorders of Connective Tissue - HMSA Journal Spring 2005

Wicks D. and Hakim A.J. 2017 - Spectrum of JH/HSD/hEDS - Explained in person.

Wikilectures - The threshold model - www.wikilectures.eu/index.php/Genetic_Liability,_Threshold_Model. Accessed 2015.

Williams J.M.G. (Prof.) - Former director of the Oxford Mindfulness Centre, contributing to NHS.uk - Mindfulness. www.nhs.uk/conditions/stress-anxiety-depression/pages/mindfulness.aspx?tabname=what%20you%20can%20do%20now. His book: Mindfulness - Diverse Perspectives on its Meaning, Origins and Applications. SBN-13: 978-0415636476

Winterowd C. 2003 - Cognitive therapy with chronic pain patients - ISBN 0-8261-4595-7

Wolf J.M. 2009 - Influence of ligamentous laxity and gender: Implications for hand surgeon. J Hand Surg 34A:161–163.

Wolfe F. et al 1990 - Criteria for the Classification of Fibromyalgia. Report of the Multicenter Criteria Committee. Arthritis Rheum. 1990 Feb;33(2): 160-72. The American College of Rheumatology 1990

Yen J.L. et al 2006 - Clinical features of Ehlers-Danlos syndrome. J Formos Med Assoc 2006, 105:475-480.

You J.S. et al 2007 - The usefulness of CT for patients with carpal bone fractures in the emergency department. Emerg Med J. 2007 Apr;24(4): 248-50.

Zarate N. et al 2010 - Unexplained gastrointestinal symptoms and joint hypermobility: is connective tissue the missing link? Neurogastroenterology & Motility - Volume 22, Issue 3, pages 252–e78, March 2010

Zhang H. and Francomano C.A. 2010 - High prevalence of Food Allergies in Patients with Ehlers-Danlos Syndromes. LCI, NIA/NIH, Baltimore, MD; 2) GBMC, Baltimore, MD; 3) IUSM, South Bend, IN. The American Society of Human Genetics. Translation: Alejandra Guasp, Ehlers-Danlos Network Argentina, December 2010 - www.ashg.org/genetics/ashg07s/f21352.htm

Image Attribution

The author of this book has done their utmost to establish and provide attribution in the format required (where required) for the images used.

Cover image - author's own archive - all rights reserved

Page 4 licence purchased from Istock

Page 18 (dancer stretching) by irulandotnet 04. ShareAlike 2.0 Generic

Page 20 (hand) author's own archive, all rights reserved

Page 23 (inheritance patterns) author's own archive - all rights reserved

Page 24 (variable expressivity diagram - author's own archive - all rights reserved

Page 24: (family) licence purchased from istock

Page 27: (conference) author's own archive, all rights reserved

Page 29 - Pixabay.com - no author attribution required

Page 32 - (diagram image) based on image by the HMSA (with permission)

Page 33 - (girl dancing) by orthomed - Creative Commons Licence

Page 33 (girl in wheelchair) created by Freepik

Page 36 (down arrow) by Stuart Miles - Freedigitaldownloads.net

Page 36 (man with question mark) by: Freedom Wiki

Page 37 (conference) copyright HMSA 2014 - used with permission

Page 45 - (musculoskeletal) by Pixabay.com - no author attribution required

Page 47 - (elbow, knees, w-sitting) - author's own archive, all rights reserved.

Page 48 (pain) by Bandita - Creative Commons Licence

Page 53 (CRPS) image by: Timsong311 2013

Page 55 (girl with fatigue) by Jcomp -Freepik

© Understanding hEDS and HSD by C. Smith

Page 57 - (girl tripping) by Jamie Campbell - Creative Commons Licence

Page 59 (muscle stiffness) - Pexels.com - no author attribution required

Page 60 (joint cracking) by jweski - freedigitalimages.net

Page 61 (shoulder) by Hellerhoff - Creative Commons Licence

Page 61 (knee) - Pexels.com - no author attribution required

Page 62 (bone) by Wardel - Creative Commons Licence

Page 63 (scars and bruising) all authors own - all rights reserved

Page 64 (skin hyperextensibility x 3) author's own archive, all rights reserved

Page 64 (stretch marks, underarm) by Micheal Astor - Creative Commons Licience

Page 64 (stretch marks, back) by Josephrockz4 - Creative Commons Licence

Page 64 (varicose vein / piezogenic papules) - author's own archive - all rights reserved

Page 65 by: David Castillo Dominici -FreeDigitalPhotos.net

Page 65 by: Conor Lawless - Creative Commons Licence

Page 69 (autonomic dysfuntions) - author's own archive - all rights reserved

Page 73 (POTs) - author's own archive - all rights reserved

Page 77 (mast cells) by fillim - Creative Commons Licence

Page 79 (mast cell rash, sore eyes) - author's own archive - all rights reserved

Page 79 (hives) - James Heilman, MD - Creative Commons Licence

Page 79 (dermatographia) - fillim - Creative Commons Licence

Page 81 (Raynauds) - author's own archive - all rights reserved

Page 82 by: Arocamora - Creative Commons Licence

Page 83 by www.jointessentials.com - Creative commons licence

Page 85 (girl holding head) by marcolm - FreeDigitalPhotos.net

Page 85 (blue sclerea) by National Eye Institute

Page 86 (devited setum) - autor's own archive - all rights reserved

Page 86 by: (inhailer) photo by marin, FreeDigitalPhotos.net

Page 86 (teeth) - Istock licence

Page 87 (neck) by marcolm - FreeDigitalPhotos.net

Page 88 by: (shoulder) sixninepixels - FreeDigitalPhotos.net

Page 89 (ribs) by yodiyim - FreeDigitalPhotos.net

Page 90 (heart) by yodiyim - FreeDigitalPhotos.net

Page 90 (elbow) author's own archive - all rights reserved

Page 91 (wirst) Pixabay - no author attribution required

Page 91 (hand) author's own archive - all rights reserved

Page 91 (gangolion) by Cieslaw '06

Page 91 (arachnodactyly) BQmUB2010144

Page 91 (Spine) by yodiyim - FreeDigitalPhotos.net

Page 93 (scoliosis) author's own archive - all rights reserved

Page 93 (chiari) - Wikipedia - Creative Commons Licence

Page 94 (cord) - Wikipedia - Creative Commons Licence

Page 95 (pelvis) by: Henry Gray - Anatomy of the Human Body 1918

Page 96 (hip) by: cnx.org/contents/FPtK1zmh@8.25:fEl3C8Ot@10/ Prefacecreativecommons.org/licences/by-sa/3.0/

Page 97 (bowel) by: yodiyim - FreeDigitalPhotos.net

Page 101 (prolapse) - Wikipedia - Creative Commons Licence

Page 101 (pregnancy) by: nenetus FreeDigitalPhotos.net

Page 105 (gyneacology) - Shutterstock Licence

Page 105 (diagram) by: National Cancer Institute
Page 110 (urology) - Shutterstock Licience

Page 110 (diagram) by: National Cancer Institute

Page 111 (leg massage) by: imagerymajesticv - under Creative Commons Licence

Page 111 (feet image) by Pixabay - no attributation required

Page 112 (knee) by: jk1991 - under Creative Commons Licence

Page 114 (flat foot) Esther Max - under Creative Commons Licence

Page 114 (hallux valgus) - Lamiot - under Creative Commons

Page 114 (Plantar fasciitis) - Daniel Max - under Creative Commons Licence

Page 119 © Hypermobility Syndromes Association 2014 - All rights reserved. Design Redcliff-House Publications 2014

Page 122 - Bieghton score images all author's own archive

Page 123 - (goniometer - various) - youtube, Creative Commons Licience

Page 125 (doctor and baby) Jim Gathany, CDC - under Creative Commons Licence

Page 130 (physical exam) Image by: Flare- Freedigitalphotos.net

Page 133 - healthcare - author's own archive - all rights reserved

Page 134 by: © Claire Smith, Redcliff-House Publications - All rights reserved

Page 135 (physio) Flare- Freedigitalphotos.net

Page 138 (hydro) - Istock Licience

Page 140 - (posture) based on image by Freepik

Page 145 by: (OT) Istock licence

Page 145 (Joints) by: Esther Max under Creative Commons Licence

Page 146 (orthotics / tape) by: Pixabay - no author attribution required

Page 148 (consultation) NCI under Creative Commons Licence

Page 149 (tablets) - Istock Licence

Page 156 (cogs) by: David Castillo Dominici - Freedigitalphotos.net

Page 157 (massage) by: Nenelus - Creative Commons Licence

Page 159 (patient) by: Selmaemiliano - Creative Commons Licence

Page 162 (dentist) by: Stockimages - Freedigitalphotos.net

Page 163 (retainer) Pixabay.com - no author attribution required

Page 164 (jaw) by: Stockimages - Freedigitalphotos.net

Page 165 (surgery) Pexels.com - no author attribution required

All other images are either attribution free, from Pixabay.com, Pexels.com or Freepik.com, or are the property of the author of this book (all rights reserved).

Resources

Please note: The likelihood is that this list is not exhaustive and will be updated in future editions. Listings are displayed alphabetically. Inclusion in this section does not constitute recommendation. Individual readers must make their own assessment with regard to suitability. The author of this publication accepts no liability for any claims made in the text or websites featured.

Charities, non profit, & support organisations

Supporting those with EDS / HSD

Asociación Síndromes De Ehlers-Danlos E Hiperlaxitud (Spain)
asedh.org

Bindweefsel.be (Belgium)
www.bindweefsel.be

Canadian Ehlers-Danlos Foundation
www.caneds.org.

EDS Canada
www.ehlers-danlossyndromecanada.org

EDS Riksförbund (Sweden & Norway)
www.ehlers-danlos.se

EDS Wellness (USA)
edswellness.org

Ehlers-Danlos Foreningen (Denmark)
ehlersdanlos.dk

Ehlers-Danlos Initiative (Germany)
www.ehlers-danlos-initiative.de

Ehlers-Danlos Italy
www.ehlersdanlos.it

Ehlers-Danlos Selbsthilfe e.V. (Germany)
eds-selbsthilfe-ev.de

Ehlers-Danlos Society (USA)
www.ehlers-danlos.com
(previously known as: Ehlers-Danlos National Foundation - www.ednf.org)

Ehlers-Danlos Support UK
www.ehlers-danlos.org

Hypermobility Syndromes Association (UK)
hypermobility.org

Inspire Support Community (USA)
www.inspire.com/groups/ehlers-danlos-syndromes/

Irish EDS & HMS (Ireland)
irishedsandhms.ie

Israel Ehlers Danlos Support Group
edsisrael.wordpress.com

Les Amis de l'ASED (France)
Les syndromes Ehlers-Danlos
www.ased.fr

Swiss EDS (Switzerland)
www.swiss-eds.ch

Union Nationale des Syndromes d'Ehlers-Danlos (France)
www.unsed.org

Verneniging van Ehlers-Danlos patienten (Netherlands)
www.ehlers-danlos.nl

Also of interest:

Action on Disability and Work UK
www.adwuk.org
Brings employees and businesses together with advice and support to facilitate a successful pathway that works perfectly for everyone.

Burning Knights (complex regional pain syndrome)
www.burningnightscrps.org

Carer's Allowance Unit
Tel: 0845 608 4321
www.gov.uk/carers-allowance-unit

Carers Trust
www.carers.org

Chronic Pain Partners / EDS Awareness (USA)
www.chronicpainpartners.com

Contact a family (UK)
www.cafamily.org.uk
Provides support to families, whatever their child's disability or health condition, with a wide range of life-changing help and class-leading services.

CRPS UK (Complex regional pain syndrome)
support@CRPS-UK.org

© Understanding hEDS and HSD by C. Smith

Dysautonomia International (USA)
www.dysautonomiainternational.org

Enquire
The Scottish advice service for additional support for learning.
www.enquire.org.uk

Fibromyalgia Action UK
www.fmauk.org

Fibromyalgia Association UK
www.fibromyalgia-associationuk.org

Financial Advice if you are disabled
www.gov.uk/financial-help-disabled/overview

Genetic Alliance
www.geneticalliance.org.uk

Hormones and hypermobility
hypermobility.org/help-advice/hormones-hypermobility/

Inspire
Ehlers-Danlos Syndromes and Hypermobility Spectrum Disorders Support Community
inspire.com

Pain UK
www.painuk.org

PALS (Patient Advice and Liaison Services)
www.nhs.uk/Service-Search/Patient-advice-and-liaison-services-(PALS)/LocationSearch/363

POTs UK (Postural Orthostatic Tachycardia)
www.potsuk.org
(Accredited under NHS England's Information Standard)

Occupational Therapy, Life Experience & Creative Thinking
jboccupationaltherapy.co.uk/sleep-hygiene/

Rare Disease Connection Site (Worldwide)
www.rareconnect.org

Scoliosis Association UK
www.sauk.org.uk

SCOPE (UK)
www.scope.org.uk

Scleroderma & Raynaud's UK
www.sruk.co.uk

SOS!SEN
A national charity aiming to empower parents and carers of children with special educational needs (SEN) to tackle successfully, themselves, the difficulties they face when battling for their children's rights.
www.sossen.org.uk

Special Needs Jungle
A not-for-profit organisation, offering parent-led information, resources and informed opinion about children and young people with SEN, special needs, disability, health conditions and rare diseases.
www.specialneedsjungle.com

Understanding EDS-H & JHS (Website)
www.edhs.info

Useful items:

Annica Wheat Bags
www.annicawheatbags.co.uk

Complete Care Shop - disability aids
www.completecareshop.co.uk

HMSA Shop - Ergonomic scissors, kitchen implements and gardening tools
www.hypermobilityshop.org (Useful products section)

Medic Alert
ID jewellery enabling emergency professionals to gain vital information from members' secure emergency personal records, 24/7, 365 days a year.
www.medicalert.org.uk

Ring Splints by Zomile
Affordable, contemporary silver and gold ring splints for the customer in need of stabilising fingers and thumbs
ringsplintsbyzomile.co.uk

Silver Ring Splint Company
Providing a beautiful and comfortable solution to long-term splint therapy.
www.silverringsplint.com

Stickman Communications
A refreshing, stylish, light-hearted yet true-to-life approach to disability. Using stickmen and simple phrases, an array of products have been created to break down barriers, challenge preconceptions, promote understanding and acceptance, and enable communication.
www.stickmancommunications.co.uk

Literature and printable material

Ehlers-Danlos Society
A wide range of printable materials including educational leaflets and posters
Visit: www.ehlers-danlos.com

Ehlers-Danlos Support UK offer a wide range of printable information covering Ehlers-Danlos syndrome
Visit: www.ehlers-danlos.org

Publications include the following:
• Pregnancy & Childbirth in Ehlers-Danlos syndrome
• Learning to be Different (written for 4-7 year olds)

The Hypermobility Syndromes Association offer a wide range of printable information covering Ehlers-Danlos syndrome, joint hypermobility syndrome, Marfan syndrome, Osteogenesis imperfecta and Stickler syndrome is available from the Hypermobility Syndromes Association website. A range of purchasable publications are available from their online shop
(visit: www.hypermobilityshop.org)

Their range of publications includes:

• Living well with a heritable disorder of connective tissue
• An Educator's Guide to the hypermobile student
• Have you, or someone you know, been diagnosed with one of the hypermobility syndromes
• Persistent fatigue and heritable disorders of connective tissue.

NHS Choices
A health A-Z of symptoms, conditions, medications and treatments
www.NHS.uk

Patient
A wide range of information on all medical conditions for lay people and professionals.
www.patient.info

Books

Hypermobility, Fibromyalgia and Chronic Pain, 1e
by Hakim, Keer and Grahame, 2010
Published by Churchill Livingstone
ISBN-13: 978-0702030055

Hypermobility Syndrome: Diagnosis and Management for Physiotherapists
by Rosemary J. Keer & Rodney Grahame.
Published by Butterworth Heinemann
ISBN-10: 0750653906
ISBN-13: 978-0750653909

Guide to Living with Ehlers-Danlos Syndrome – Hypermobility Type – Bending without Breaking
by Isobel Knight, (2nd Edition) Revised 2015
ISBN-10: 1848192312
ISBN-13: 978-1848192317

Joint Hypermobility Handbook
by Dr. Brad Tinkle
ISBN: 10: 098257715X
ISBN: 13: 978-0982577158

Multi-Disciplinary Approach to Managing Ehlers-Danlos (Type III) – Hypermobility Syndrome
by Isobel Knight 2013
ISBN: B00XWQXT2K

Never Bet Against Occam: Mast Cell Activation Disease and the Modern Epidemics of Chronic Illness and Medical Complexity
by Afrin, L. MD 2016
ISBN-10: 0997319615
ISBN-13: 978-0997319613

Our Stories of Strength: Living With Ehlers-Danlos Syndrome
by Reutlinger, Myles, Francomano et al,
ISBN-10: 0996302905
ISBN-13: 978-0996302906

Redcliff-House Publications
Books that raise awareness of EDS/HSD and associated conditions
Visit: www.redcliffhousepublications.co.uk

Centres for patient referral

Please note:
All referrals must be made via a GP; self-referral is not accepted. Great Ormond Street's Clinic for children requires a consultant's referral. Clinic availability can vary; patient lists may be closed at short notice, so please check the clinic status before asking for a referral. This list is not exhaustive. Inclusion in this section does not constitute recommendation. Individual readers must make their own assessment with regard to suitability.

Ehlers-Danlos syndrome / Hypermobility Spectrum Disorder

EDS Centre for Research & Clinical Care (USA)
Harvey Institute for Human Genetics
Greater Baltimore Medical Centre
Dr Clair Francomano

EDS Diagnostic Services for complex cases (UK)
The Mount, Glossop Rd, Sheffield S10 3FL
A specialist service for individuals and families who are suspected to have complex Ehlers-Danlos syndrome (EDS).

Gastroenterology and EDS Clinic (Private) (UK)
Princess Grace Hospital, Nottingham
Professor Qasim Aziz

Glasgow Royal Infirmary (UK)
Centre for Rheumatic Diseases
Glasgow (Adult Clinic).

Great Ormond Street (UK)
Rheumatology Clinic, Great Ormond Street
London
Susan Maillard
(Children's Clinic)

Hospital of St John and St Elizabeth (Private) (UK)
The Hypermobility Unit
London
A large multidisciplinary team comprising many of the world's leading experts on hypermobility.
Dr. Alan J Hakim, Consultant Rheumatologist.
(Child, adolescent and adult clinics)

Manchester Royal Infirmary (UK)
Manchester
Dr Pauline Ho, Consultant Rheumatologist

Royal National Hospital for Rheumatic Diseases (UK)
Hypermobility Clinic
Bath
Dr Tim Jenkinson, Consultant Rheumatologist

Royal National Orthopaedic Hospital (UK)
Rheumatology and Hypermobility Unit
Stanmore
Dr. R. L. Wolman, Consultant in Rheumatology and Sport and Exercise Medicine

Royal National Orthopaedic Hospital (Private) (UK)
45 Bolsover Street
London
Dr. R Wolman, Consultant in Rheumatology and Sport and Exercise Medicine

University College Hospital (Adult Clinic) (UK)
The Hypermobility Clinic
Department of Rheumatology,
London

Postural Orthostatic Tachycardia syndrome

The Royal London Hospital (UK)
London
(Abdominal symptoms associated with EDS/HSD and PoTS)
Professor Qasim Aziz (From age 16)

Derriford Hospital (UK)
Plymouth
(PoTS, syncope, dysautonomia, EDS)
Dr Jamie Fulton
Consultant General Medicine
From age 16

The University of Toledo Medical Centre (USA)
Dr Blair Grubb
Distinguished University Professor of Medicine and Pediatrics
(PoTS, hypermobility)

Royal Devon and Exeter Foundation Trust (UK)
Dr Mike Jeffreys (UK) (From age 18)
Consultant Physician/Geriatrician
(POTS, EDS, CFS & Autonomic Failure)

Bradford Teaching Hospital Foundation Trust (UK)
Bradford (From aged 16)
Dr Chris Morley
Consultant Cardiologist
(Syncope, PoTS including patients with HSD)